DEFORMABLE AVATARS

IFIP - The International Federation for Information Processing

IFIP was founded in 1960 under the auspices of UNESCO, following the First World Computer Congress held in Paris the previous year. An umbrella organization for societies working in information processing, IFIP's aim is two-fold: to support information processing within its member countries and to encourage technology transfer to developing nations. As its mission statement clearly states,

IFIP's mission is to be the leading, truly international, apolitical organization which encourages and assists in the development, exploitation and application of information technology for the benefit of all people.

IFIP is a non-profitmaking organization, run almost solely by 2500 volunteers. It operates through a number of technical committees, which organize events and publications. IFIP's events range from an international congress to local seminars, but the most important are:

- The IFIP World Computer Congress, held every second year;
- open conferences;
- working conferences.

The flagship event is the IFIP World Computer Congress, at which both invited and contributed papers are presented. Contributed papers are rigorously refereed and the rejection rate is high.

As with the Congress, participation in the open conferences is open to all and papers may be invited or submitted. Again, submitted papers are stringently refereed.

The working conferences are structured differently. They are usually run by a working group and attendance is small and by invitation only. Their purpose is to create an atmosphere conducive to innovation and development. Refereeing is less rigorous and papers are subjected to extensive group discussion.

Publications arising from IFIP events vary. The papers presented at the IFIP World Computer Congress and at open conferences are published as conference proceedings, while the results of the working conferences are often published as collections of selected and edited papers.

Any national society whose primary activity is in information may apply to become a full member of IFIP, although full membership is restricted to one society per country. Full members are entitled to vote at the annual General Assembly, National societies preferring a less committed involvement may apply for associate or corresponding membership. Associate members enjoy the same benefits as full members, but without voting rights. Corresponding members are not represented in IFIP bodies. Affiliated membership is open to non-national societies, and individual and honorary membership schemes are also offered.

DEFORMABLE AVATARS

IFIP TC5/WG5.10
DEFORM'2000 Workshop
November 29-30, 2000
Geneva, Switzerland
and
AVATARS'2000 Workshop
November 30–December 1, 2000
Lausanne, Switzerland

Edited by

Nadia Magnenat-Thalmann
University of Geneva
MIRALab
Switzerland

Daniel Thalmann
Swiss Federal Institute of Technology (EPFL)
Computer Graphics Lab
Switzerland

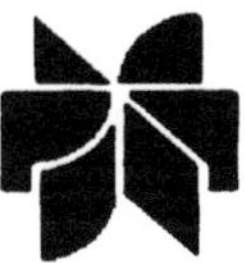

SPRINGER SCIENCE+BUSINESS MEDIA, LLC

Library of Congress Cataloging-in-Publication Data

DEFORM'2000 (2000 : University of Geneva)
Deformable avatars : IFIP TC5/WG5.10 DEFORM'2000 Workshop, November 29-30, 2000, Geneva, Switzerland and AVATARS'2000 Workshop, November 30-December 1, 2000, Lausanne, Switzerland / edited Nadia Magnenat-Thalmann, Daniel Thalmann.
p. cm. — (International Federation for Information Processing; 68)
"Most of the papers were presented during the IFIP workshop 'DEFORM'2000' that was held at the University of Geneva in December 2000, followed by 'AVATARS'2000' held at EPFL, Lausanne" —Pref.
Includes bibliographical references.

DOI 10.1007/978-0-306-47002-8
1. Computer animation—Congresses. 2. Virtual reality—Congresses. I. Magnenat-Thalmann, Nadia, 1946– II. Thalmann, Daniel. III. AVATARS'2000 (2000 : Ecole polytechnique fédérale de Lausanne). IV. Title. V. International Federation for Information Processing (Series); 68.

TR897.7 .D38 2000
006.6'96—dc21 2001038126

Printed on acid-free paper.
www.springer.com/mycopy

Contents

Preface ix

1. Animated Heads: From 3D Motion Fields to Action Descriptions 1
   Jan Neumann, Cornelia Fermüller and Yiannis Aloimonos

2. A Muscle-based 3D Parametric Lip Model for Speech-Synchronized Facial Animation 12
   Scott A.King, Richard E. Parent and Barbara L. Olsafsky

3. Feature Point Based Mesh Deformation Applied to MPEG-4 Facial Animation 24
   Sumedha Kshirsagar, Stephane Garchery, Nadia Magnenat-Thalmann

4. A Feature-based Deformable Model for Photo-Realistic Head Modelling 35
   Yong-Jin Liu, Matthew Ming-Fai Yuen, Shan Xiong

5. Multiresolution Modeling and Interactive Deformation of Large 3D Meshes 46
   Jens Vorsatz and Hans-Peter Seidel

6. Locally Interpolating Subdivision Surfaces Supporting Free-Form 2D Deformations 59
   Johan Claes, Franck van Reeth and Marc Ramaekers

7. Object-Oriented Reformulation and Extension of Implicit Free-Form Deformations 72
Olivier Parisy and Christophe Schlick

8. Soft Tissue Modeling from 3D Scanned Data 85
Jean-Christophe Nebel

9. Contextually Embodied Agents 98
Catherine Pelachaud

10. On Implicit Modelling for Fitting Purposes 109
Ralf Plänkers and Pascal Fua

11. Interactive Modelling of MPEG-4 Deformable Human Body Models 120
Hyewon Seo, Frederic Cordier, Laurent Philippon and Nadia Magnenat-Thalmann

12. Efficient Muscle Shape Deformation 132
Amaury Aubel and Daniel Thalmann

13. Towards the Ultimate Motion Capture Technology 143
Bradley Stuart, Patrick Baker and Yiannis Aloimonos

14. Delaunay Triangles Model for Image-Based Motion Retargeting 158
Dong Hoon Lee and Soon Ki Jung

15. A Vector-Space Representation of Motion Data for Example-based Motion Synthesis 169
Ik Soo Lim and Daniel Thalmann

16. Parametrization and Range of Motion of the Ball-and-Socket Joint 180
Paolo Baerlocher and Ronan Boulic

17. Towards Behavioral Consistency in Animated Agents 191
Jan M. Allbeck and Norman I. Badler

18. PECS
A Reference Model for Human-Like Agents 206
Christophe Urban

19. Communicative Autonomous Agents 217
Angela Caicedo, Jean-Sébastien Monzani and Daniel Thalmann

20. Design Issues for Conversational User Interfaces: Animating and Controlling 3D Faces 228
Wolfgang Müller, Ulrike Spierling, Marc Alexa, Ido Iurgel

21. Constructing Virtual Human Life Simulations 240
Marcelo Kallmann, Etienne de Sevin and Daniel Thalmann

Preface

Deformable avatars are virtual humans that deform themselves during motion. This implies facial deformations, body deformations at joints, and global deformations. Simulating deformable avatars ensures a more realistic simulation of virtual humans.

The research requires models for capturing of geometric and kinematic data, the synthesis of the realistic human shape and motion, the parametrisation and motion retargeting, and several appropriate deformation models. Once a deformable avatar has been created and animated, the researcher must model high-level behavior and introduce agent technology.

The book can be divided into 5 subtopics:

1. Motion capture and 3D reconstruction
2. Parametric motion and retargeting
3. Muscles and deformation models
4. Facial animation and communication
5. High-level behaviors and autonomous agents

Most of the papers were presented during the IFIP workshop "DEFORM '2000" that was held at the University of Geneva in December 2000, followed by "AVATARS 2000" held at EPFL, Lausanne. The two workshops were sponsored by the "Troisième Cycle Romand d'Informatique" and allowed participants to discuss the state of research in these important areas.

We would like to thank IFIP for its support and Yana Lambert from Kluwer Academic Publishers for her advice. Finally, we are very grateful to Zerrin Celebi, who has prepared the edited version of this book and Dr. Laurent Moccozet for his collaboration.

ANIMATED HEADS: FROM 3D MOTION FIELDS TO ACTION DESCRIPTIONS

Jan Neumann, Cornelia Fermüller and Yiannis Aloimonos
Center for Automation Research
University of Maryland
College Park, MD 20742-3275, USA
(jneumann, fer, yiannis)@cfar.umd.edu

Abstract We demonstrate a method to compute three-dimensional (3D) motion fields on a face. Twelve synchronized and calibrated cameras are positioned around a talking person, and observe its head in motion. We represent the head as a deformable mesh, which is fitted in a global optimization step to silhouette-contour and multi-camera stereo data derived from all images. The non-rigid displacement of the mesh from frame to frame, the 3D motion field, is determined from the spatio-temporal derivatives in all the images. We integrate these cues over time, thus producing an animated representation of the talking head. Our ability to estimate 3D motion fields points to a new framework for the study of action. The 3D motion fields can serve as an intermediate representation, which can be analyzed using geometrical and statistical tools for the purpose of extracting representations of generic human actions.

1. INTRODUCTION

What does it mean to understand an action? *One understands an action if one is able to imagine performing an action with images that are sufficient for serving as a guide in actual performance.* To be able to visualize or virtualize an action in our mental theater, we have to develop a spatio-temporal action description of the object in space that is performing the action. What are the key points in figuring out the nature of action representations?

1 Action representations are view independent. We are able to recognize and visualize actions regardless of viewpoint.

2 Action representations capture dynamic information which is manifested in a long image sequence. Put simply, it is not possible to understand an action on the basis of a small sequence of frames (viewpoints).

3 Action representations are made up of a combination of shape and movement.

To gain insights on action representations we consider them in a hierarchy. First there is the image data, that is, videos of humans in action. Considering the cue of motion, then our image data amounts to a sequence of normal flow fields computed from the videos. The second kind of representations are intermediate descriptions encoding information about 3D space and 3D motion, estimated from the input (video). These representations consist of a whole range of descriptions of different sophistication encoding partially the space-time geometry, and they are view and scene dependent. Finally, we have representations encoding the characteristics of actions, and these representations are view and scene independent. The most sophisticated intermediate representation for the specific action in view that could be obtained is then a sequence of evolving 3D motion fields (also known as *range flow* (Spies et al., 2000) or *scene flow* (Vedula et al., 1999)). Acquiring this representation is no simple matter, but it can be achieved by employing a very large number of viewpoints (e.g., for a general overview about human motion modeling see (Aggarwal and Cai, 1999) and (Gavrila, 1999)).

As an example for an interesting action, we will examine facial expressions. Several image sequences of a talking and moving head were simultaneously recorded by a large number of cameras. From these image sequences a three-dimensional mesh model of the head was constructed and the trajectories of the mesh vertices in space-time, the evolving motion fields, were determined.

Due to the large number of possible applications, for example in the field of human-computer-interaction or in entertainment (e.g., "Motion Capturing"), a lot of work has been done on the creation of 3D models of faces and the synthesized and recognition of facial expressions. Most approaches made use only of a few viewpoints at a time, thus they were not utilizing all the available constraints and information. For example, (Fua and Miccio, 1999) and (Pighin et al., 1998) fitted a predefined animation model to image data from few views and (Vetter and Blanz, 1998) used a single image in an analysis-by-synthesis loop.

Other methods need complicated prior motion and face models (e.g., (Terzopoulos and Waters, 1993) and (Essa and Pentland, 1997) use a physics-based model with anatomically correct muscles) or tracking markers on the face (.e.g, (Guenter et al., 1998)) to extract the facial expressions. The difference to our approach is that we construct a full three-dimensional model without manual intervention and without relying on any prior model. The 3D motion flow on the head surface is computed directly from image derivatives, not on the basis of optical flow. Stereo and motion estimation were combined into one framework similar as in (Zhang and Kambhamettu, 2000) and (Malassiotis and Strintzis, 1997). But in their work in contrast to our approach the scene is still parameterized in the image space of the base view, whereas we use the more natural object space parameterization. By moving the representation from image to object space, the algorithm can handle arbitrary camera arrangements and can make use of robust regularization constraints on the object surface, because physical tissue deforms in a continuous and smooth manner. The use of multi-camera setups for the computation of full 3D flow has only recently become feasible due to sinking costs of image capture and computer equipment (for an example see Vedula et. al., 2000).

In building scene-independent representations for facial expressions, it is essential to separate the 3D motion flow field into a component due changes of pose and a component due to the facial expression. Former approaches used simplified models such as planar models plus parallax for the head motion and affine motion models for the facial expressions (e.g., Bascle and Blake, 1998 and Black and Yacoob, 1997). By using the changing silhouettes and the rigid surface regions of the object to determine the rigid motion, we can compensate for the change in pose. After subtracting the rigid motion flow component from the full flow, we are left with the non-rigid residual motion describing the facial expression that can be analyzed or used for reanimation of other models.

2. PRELIMINARIES AND DEFINITIONS

We have established in our laboratory a multi-camera network consisting of sixty-four cameras, Kodak ES-310, providing images at a rate of up to eighty-five frames per second; the video is collected directly on disk –the cameras are connected by a high-speed network consisting of sixteen dual processor Pentium 450s with 1 GB of RAM each (Davis et al., 1999).

The camera configuration is parameterized by the camera positions $\mathbf{T}_k$, the rotation matrices R_k that relate the camera coordinate system to the fiducial system, and the intrinsic camera parameters K_k (bold-face letters denote vectors, small letters scalars, and large letters matrices). The calibration is done using images of a large calibration object. In

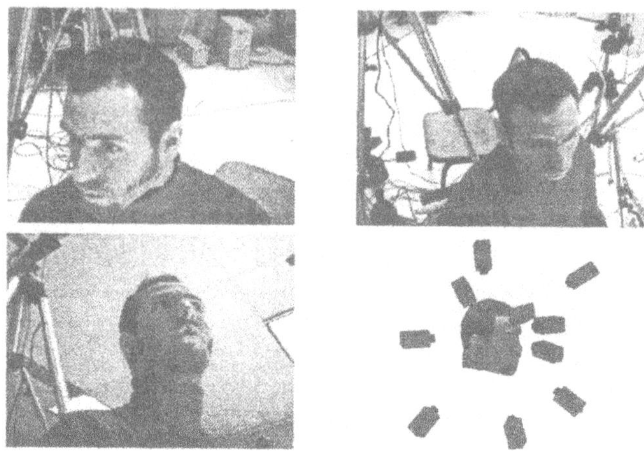

Figure 1 Calibrated Camera Setup with Example Input Views

the following we assume that the images have already been corrected for radial distortion. The image formation process is described by the conventional pinhole camera model, where the point $\mathbf{P}$ in fiducial world coordinates is related to its projection $\mathbf{p}_k$ in camera k as follows ($\hat{\mathbf{z}} = [0\,0\,1]^\mathsf{T}$):

$$\mathbf{p}_k = K_k \frac{R_k(\mathbf{P} - \mathbf{T}_k)}{\hat{\mathbf{z}} \cdot R_k(\mathbf{P} - \mathbf{T}_k)} \tag{1}$$

The head surface is approximated by a closed mesh with vertices $\mathbf{V}_i$ and triangular facets $\mathbf{F}_j$. The world coordinates of $\mathbf{V}_i(t) = [x_i(t), y_i(t), z_i(t)]$ are dependent on time t. Since we formulate the structure and motion estimation in object space, the image information needs to be sampled in regular patterns on the mesh surface instead of in regular patterns on the images. Therefore, a set of regularly spaced sampling points is associated with each triangle. The number of sampling points is dependent on the visible area of the triangle in the different cameras.

It is assumed that the head is the only moving object in all the image sequences, although this assumption is not essential and can be eliminated by applying the algorithm in turn to each independently-moving object. The following sections describe the algorithm that computes the spatio-temporal representation of the moving and talking head (from now on called the "object"):

- Section 3: Motion-based segmentation of the input images to locate the moving object, compute its silhouettes, and initialize the deformable 3D mesh.

- Section 4: Multi-camera stereo refinement of the deformable mesh where the search space is constrained by the silhouettes.
- Section 5: Computation of the 3D motion field on the mesh surface from image derivatives based on the normal flow constraint.

3. IMAGE SEGMENTATION

We incrementally construct an image of the background by modeling the temporal evolution of the changing foreground pixels and the static background pixels. The magnitude of the temporal image derivatives and image statistics such as mean and variance are computed for each pixel on ten consecutive frames in the sequence and then used to segment the image into fore- and background. We integrate information over time to make the segmentation more robust by applying order-statistic filters over small spatio-temporal volumes. After the initial segmentation , we intersect the cone-shaped spaces formed by reprojecting the convex hulls of the head silhouettes into space. The intersection is a convex approximation of the head and it defines the initial 3D surface mesh. The mesh is now back-projected into each image and the segmentation is refined by fitting the mesh to all silhouette contours simultaneously.

4. MULTI-CAMERA STEREO ESTIMATION

Using only information from silhouettes, it is not possible to compute more than the visual hull (Laurentini, 1994) of the object in view. Therefore, to refine our 3D surface estimate of the object, we adapt the vertices of the mesh to optimize the correlation between corresponding image regions in the different camera views. The search range for the vertex positions is constrained by the displacement boundaries computed in the silhouette estimation step in Section 3. To determine the visibility of each triangle, a z-buffer algorithm computes the index of the closest triangle patch for each pixel location. Next, a regular sampling point pattern is assigned to each mesh triangle as described before in Section 2, so that the sampling density of the closest image is about one projected sampling point per pixel.

We optimize orientation and position of each triangle by displacing each triangle vertex along the surface normal direction of the mesh and maximizing a similarity criterion among the triangle projections. The criterion to be optimized is the normalized cross-correlation between the projections of each triangle into all the cameras in which the triangle is visible (we denote this set of cameras as the set of "visible cameras"). For all combinations of normal displacements of the three vertices we compute the 3D coordinates of the sampling points on the triangle surface and project the sampling points into all the visible cameras. The image brightness of a projected sampling point is determined by bilinear interpolation. The cross-correlation is now computed between the corresponding image brightness samples for all pairs of cameras that mutually see the triangle. We combine the correlation scores from all the camera pairs by taking a weighted average with the weights depending on the angle between camera plane and triangle plane.

The pairwise scores between all the cameras are also used to correct the visibility information. If a bimodal distribution of high and low correlation scores can be detected, then it is possible to estimate which cameras are visible and which are not, and the occluded cameras can be excluded from the score. For each vertex we collect the normal displacements corresponding to the highest correlation score for each of the surrounding triangles and determine the final normal displacement subject to global smoothness and rigidity constraints which have been added to regularize the solution.

5. MOTION ESTIMATION

Following the description of the photometric properties of a surface in space in (Horn, 1986) and (Vedula et al., 1999), the head surface is assumed to have Lambertian reflectance properties, thus the brightness intensity of a pixel $\mathbf{p}_k$ in camera k is given by

$$I(\mathbf{p}_k;t) = -c_k \cdot \rho(\mathbf{P}) \cdot [\mathbf{n}(\mathbf{P};t) \cdot \mathbf{s}(\mathbf{P};t)] \tag{2}$$

with an albedo $\rho(\mathbf{P})$ that is constant over time ($d\rho/dt = 0$) and where c_k is the constant that describes the brightness gain for each camera, $\mathbf{n}$ is the normal to the surface at $\mathbf{P}$, and $\mathbf{s}$ the direction of incoming light. Taking the derivative with respect to time on both sides, we get the following expression for the change of the image brightness $I(\mathbf{p}_k)$ at pixel location $\mathbf{p}_k$ in camera k:

$$\frac{dI(\mathbf{p}_k)}{dt} = \nabla I(\mathbf{p}_k) \cdot \frac{d\mathbf{p}_k}{dt} + \frac{\partial I(\mathbf{p}_k)}{\partial t} = -c_k \cdot \rho(\mathbf{P}) \cdot \frac{d}{dt}[\mathbf{n}(\mathbf{P};t) \cdot \mathbf{s}(\mathbf{P};t)] \tag{3}$$

Since our sequences were recorded with a frame rate of 60 Hz and under fixed illumination, we can assume that $\frac{d}{dt}[\mathbf{n} \cdot \mathbf{s}] = 0$, and we end up with the well-known *normal flow constraint* equation.

$$-\frac{\partial I(\mathbf{p}_k)}{\partial t} = \nabla I(\mathbf{p}_k) \cdot \frac{d\mathbf{p}_k}{dt} \tag{4}$$

This equation gives us one constraint per measurement, we can only determine the component of the optic flow that is normal to the image gradient, the normal flow. The estimation of the tangential flow along the iso-brightness contour is ill-posed. Regularizing the problem by imposing image-based smoothness conditions on the solution to equation (4) introduces artifacts at depth discontinuities and biases due to inhomogeneous gradient distributions (Fermüller et al., 2000).

Each normal flow vector in an image constrains the projection of the 3D motion flow to lie along a line parallel to the iso-brightness contour in the image, the normal flow constraint line. Thus the 3D motion flow vector has to lie on the plane defined by the normal flow constraint line and the optical center of the camera. The component of the 3D motion along the iso-brightness contour on the object surface is not recoverable. This is the aperture problem revisited in 3D. Nevertheless, if we assume that neighboring patches on the surface will move in an elastic manner, we can impose smoothness constraints on the motion of neighboring points. This smoothness assumption is physically justified as long as our mesh model has the same topology as the object in view, because nearly all real materials deform elastically when strain is applied.

The mesh representation of the head defines a correspondence map between the cameras, and the full 3D motion flow at each mesh vertex is determined by combining the information from all the sampling points of the triangles neighboring the mesh vertex. To relate image derivatives and 3D motion flow using the normal flow constraint, we have to determine the Jacobian of the image formation equation (1) (R_3 is third row of matrix R and $K, R, \mathbf{T}$ refer to the calibration parameters of camera k):

$$\frac{d\mathbf{p}_k}{dt} = \frac{\partial \mathbf{p}_k}{\partial \mathbf{P}_k}\frac{\partial \mathbf{P}_k}{\partial t} = \frac{\partial P}{\partial t}K\frac{R(\mathbf{P}-\mathbf{T})}{R_3(\mathbf{P}-\mathbf{T})} = \left(\frac{KR - \mathbf{p}_k R_3}{R_3(\mathbf{P}-\mathbf{T})}\right)\frac{\partial \mathbf{P}}{\partial t} \qquad (5)$$

The derivative images are sampled at all locations where the sampling points associated with each triangle are visible. Let a given triangle of the mesh be defined by the vertices $\mathbf{V}_1, \mathbf{V}_2, \mathbf{V}_3$, then for each sampling point $P = \sum_{j=1,2,3} \lambda_j \mathbf{V}_j$ of this triangle we get the following constraint equation for each measurement:

$$-\frac{\partial I(\mathbf{p}_k)}{\partial t} = \sum_{j=1,2,3} \lambda_j \left(\nabla I(\mathbf{p}_k) \cdot \frac{KR - \mathbf{p}_k R_3}{R_3(\mathbf{P}-\mathbf{T})}\right)\frac{\partial \mathbf{P}_j}{\partial t} \qquad (6)$$

There is one equation per sampling point per visible image. To integrate these constraints, we stack these equations to form the $m \times n$ matrix L where m is the number of sampling points over all the triangles and their projections into all the visible cameras and n the number of vertices of the mesh times the three spatial dimensions. The matrices for the models presented are on the order of $100\,000 \times 3000$. To regularize the solution we add smoothness constraints as extra rows to L.

Since it is computationally infeasible to solve this large system directly, we form the normal equations of the over-constrained system and solve them with a preconditioned conjugate gradient method with either the motion field of the previous frame or the solution to a rigid motion approximation as starting vectors. The second choice worked very well to initialize the optimization, because most parts of a human head move rigidly. The magnitude of the residual non-rigid flow is used to segment the mesh into rigidly and non-rigidly moving areas. This enables us to separate the motion field into two parts, one due to the change of pose and one due to the expression on the face.

6. RESULTS

For our experiments we used eleven cameras placed in a dome-like arrangement around the head of a person that was expressing surprise (Figure 1). After the initial structure estimation stage of our algorithm, we are able to synthesize texture-mapped views of the head from arbitrary viewing directions (Figures 2a-2c). The textures, coming always from the least oblique camera with respect to a given triangle, were not blended together to demonstrate the good agreement between adjacent texture region boundaries. This demonstrates that the spatial structure of the head was recovered very well.

The 3D motion flow field for the current frame is computed and used to propagate the mesh to the next frame. The propagated mesh is refined by new stereo and silhouette data, before the next 3D motion flow field is computed, and the process is repeated. The 3D motion field shown in (Figures 2d-2fl) was computed by integrating the 3D flows of frames 40 to 45.

The rigid motion flow was computed by parameterizing the 3D motion flow vectors by the instantaneous rigid motion $\partial \mathbf{P}/\partial t = \mathbf{v} + \boldsymbol{\omega} \times \mathbf{P}$, where $\mathbf{v}$ and $\boldsymbol{\omega}$ are the instantaneous translation, and rotation (Horn, 1986). This parameterized flow field was then fitted to the image derivative information in the images. By subtracting the rigid motion flow from the full flow, we extract the non-rigid flow. It can be seen that the rigid motion part (the turning of the head to the upper left) is recovered well, as the magnitude of the residual non-rigid flow on the rigid part of the head (e.g., forehead, nose and ears) in Figure (2e) is significantly smaller than the full flow in Figure (2d).

The non-rigid motion is also computed accurately, as we can easily see in the close up of the mouth region (Figure 2f), how the mouth opens, and the skin of the jaw stretches recedes. Animations of the re-

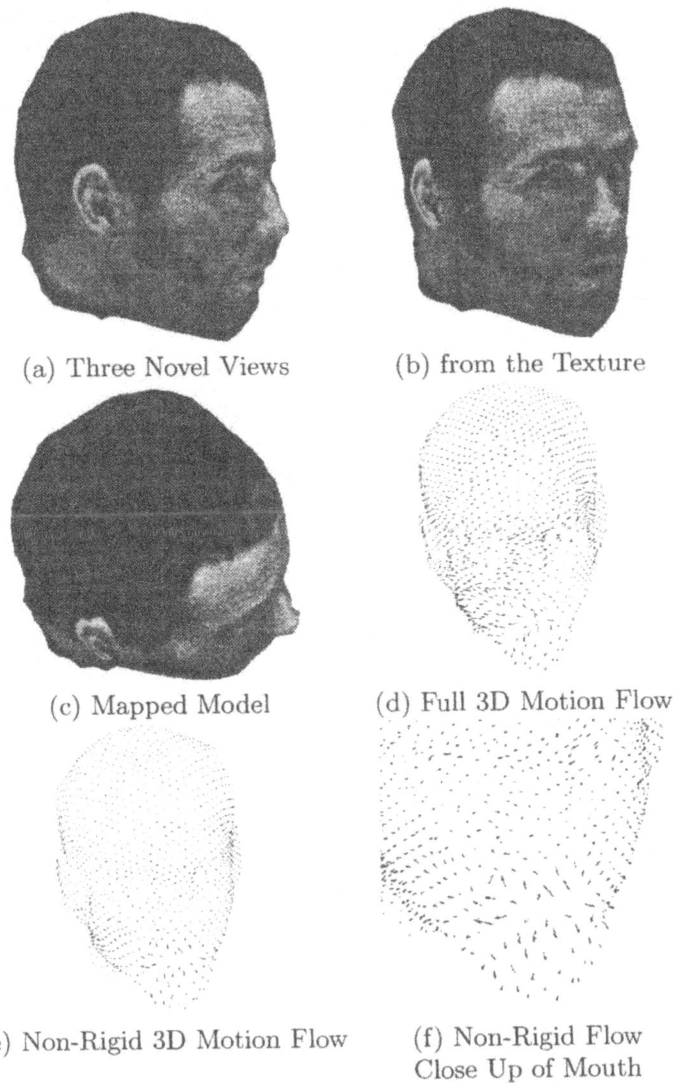

Figure 2 Results of 3D Structure and Motion Flow Estimation

covered model and flow fields can be found at the following web address: *http://www.videogeometry.com/TalkingHeads.*

7. CONCLUSION AND FUTURE WORK

We presented an algorithm that computes an accurate spatio-temporal description of a non-rigidly moving human head. The description consists of the spatio-temporal trajectories of the mesh vertices, the evolving motion fields.

To see how these motion fields can be used, let us now consider the mapping from the 3D motion fields to the scene independent action representations. This mapping should be such that it extracts from a specific action quantities of a generic character common to all actions of the same type. These quantities most probably take the form of spatio-temporal patterns in four dimensions.

One way of obtaining such patterns is to perform statistics on a large enough sample (e.g., Reynard et al., 1996). Considering, a particular action (e.g., talking or dancing), we can obtain data in the multi-camera laboratory described before for a large number of individuals. In each case we can obtain a 3D motion field and thus are able to build up a large data base of 3D motion fields. To this database a number of statistical techniques, such as principal component analysis, can be applied to reduce the dimensionality of the space and describe it with a small number of parameters. Another way of obtaining these patterns would be to study invariances related to symmetry, and geometric quantities in space-time (e.g., angles, velocities, accelerations, periodicity, etc. (Bottema and Roth, 1979)).

In our future work, we will apply the above mentioned statistical and geometrical methods to the evolving 3D motion fields and try to extract the action representations. To improve the presented algorithm we plan to incorporate explicit visibility updating into the stereo part of the algorithm and include further information such as range flow constraints (see Spies et al., 2000) between the consecutive stereo reconstructions.

References

Aggarwal, J. and Cai, Q. (1999). Human motion analysis: A review. *Computer Vision and Image Understanding*, 73(3):428–440.

Bascle, B. and Blake, A. (1998). Separability of pose and expression in facial tracing and animation. In *ICCV98*, pages 323–328.

Black, M. and Yacoob, Y. (1997). Recognizing facial expressions in image sequences using local parameterized models of image motion. *IJCV*, 25(1):23–48.

Bottema, O. and Roth, B. (1979). *Theoretical Kinematics*. North-Holland.

Davis, L., Borovikov, E., Cutler, R., Harwood, D., and Horprasert, T. (1999). Multi-perspective analysis of human action. In *Proc. of Third*

International Workshop on Cooperative Distributed Vision, Kyoto, Japan.

Essa, I. and Pentland, A. (1997). Coding, analysis, interpretation, and recognition of facial expressions. *IEEE Trans. PAMI*, 19(7):757–763.

Fermüller, C., Pless, R., and Aloimonos, Y. (2000). The Ouchi illusion as an artifact of biased flow estimation. *Vision Research*, 40:77–96.

Fua, P. and Miccio, C. (1999). Animated heads from ordinary images: A least-squares approach. *Computer Vision and Image Understanding*, 75(3):247–259.

Gavrila, D. (1999). The visual analysis of human movement: A survey. *Computer Vision and Image Understanding*, 73(1):82–98.

Guenter, B., Grimm, C., Wood, D., Malvar, H., and Pighin, F. (1998). Making faces. In *Proc. of SIGGRAPH*, pages 55–66.

Horn, B. K. P. (1986). *Robot Vision.* McGraw Hill, New York.

Laurentini, A. (1994). The visual hull concept for silhouette-based image understanding. *IEEE Trans. PAMI*, 16(2):150–162.

Malassiotis, S. and Strintzis, M. (1997). Model-based joint motion and structure estimation from stereo images. *Computer Vision and Image Understanding*, 65(1):79–94.

Pighin, F., Hecker, J., Lischinski, D., Szeliski, R., and Salesin, D. (1998). Synthesizing realistic facial expressions from photographs.

Reynard, D., Wildenberg, A., Blake, A., and Marchant, J. (1996). Learning dynamics of complex motions from image sequences. In *ECCV96*, pages I:357–368.

Spies, H., Jaehne, B., and Barron, J. (2000). Dense range flow from depth and intensity data. In *ICPR00.*

Terzopoulos, D. and Waters, K. (1993). Analysis and synthesis of facial image sequences using physical and anatomical models. *IEEE Trans. PAMI*, 15(6):569–579.

Vedula, S., Baker, S., Rander, P., Collins, R., and Kanade, T. (1999). Three-dimensional scene flow. In *ICCV99*, pages 722–729.

Vedula, S., Baker, S., Seitz, S., and Kanade, T. (2000). Shape and motion carving in 6d. In *CVPR00*, pages II:592–598.

Vetter, T. and Blanz, V. (1998). Estimating coloured 3-d face models from single images: An example-based approach. In *ECCV98*, pages 499–513.

Zhang, Y. and Kambhamettu, C. (2000). Integrated 3d scene flow and structure recovery from multiview image sequences. In *CVPR00*, pages II:674–681.

A MUSCLE-BASED 3D PARAMETRIC LIP MODEL FOR SPEECH-SYNCHRONIZED FACIAL ANIMATION

Scott A. King, Richard E. Parent and Barbara L. Olsafsky
Department of Computer and Information Science, The Ohio State University

Key words: Facial animation, facial modelling, speech synchronization, lip modelling.

Abstract: We present work on a new anatomically based 3D parametric lip model for synchronized speech that also supports the lip motion required for facial expressions. The lip model is represented with a B-spline surface and high-level parameters which define the articulation of the surface. The model parameterization is muscle-based to allow for specification of a wide range of lip motion. The B-spline surface specifies not only the external portion of the lips, but the internal surface as well. This complete geometric representation replaces the original lip geometry of any facial model.

We also describe a method to render the lip model using a procedural texturing paradigm to give color, lighting and surface texture for increased realism. We use our lip model in a text-to-audio-visual-speech system to achieve speech-synchronized facial animation.

1. INTRODUCTION

Facial animation is becoming more important as a communicative technique between man and machine. In addition, it is pivotal in the development of synthetic actors. The lips play an extremely important role in almost all facial animation. They are a significant component of expressing emotion as well as being instrumental in the intelligibility of speech. Therefore, in order to achieve realism and effective communication, a facial animation system needs extremely good lip motion with the deformation of the lips synchronized with the audial portion of the speech.

In order to animate a pair of lips a mapping between the desired motion and lip deformations is needed. For example, a mapping between speech segments and lip shapes could be used. We develop a generic lip model with such a mapping already embedded. Using a generic lip model guarantees required resolution for both deformation and rendering plus fitting the generic lip model is easier than fitting the mapping to new geometry.

Our lip model consists of a B-spline surface and high-level parameters that control the articulation of the surface. The lip model can be used with any human-like facial model and provides:

- a sufficiently controllable model to support lip synchronization as well as supporting other motions used in expressing emotions,
- a sufficiently smooth model to support quality rendering,
- internal geometry (the part of the lips in the oral cavity not visible when the mouth is closed) which is usually not provided in digitized facial models,
- support for procedural texture maps for high quality rendering.

We choose a B-spline surface for its c^2 continuity and the ease of deforming the surface by simply moving the vertices of the control mesh. The drawbacks of B-splines include difficulty in placing a part of the surface exactly in $\Re^3$, preserving volume, detecting collisions and rendering. Fortunately, by polygonalizing the model, post processing after deformations can achieve volume preservation and collision detection while rendering the polygons is straightforward. Polygonalization loses the c^2 continuity of the B-spline surface, but the quality is controllable and with Phong shading the impact is minimal. Volume preservation and collision detection are the subject of ongoing research and are not presented here.

The lip model is fit to the input geometry as a pre-processing step with a user guided process, shown in Section 4, that replaces the lip region in a given facial model and grafts the generic lip model onto the rest of the facial geometry. The lip model is parameterized based on the muscles that cause the lips to change shape. The parameterization is presented in Section 3. As the parameters change, the lips deform which drives deformation in the surrounding area. The formulas for calculating the change in the lip shapes are given in Section 4. Animation of the lip model, presented in Section 6, is achieved by interpolating between keyframes. The model is rendered with procedural textures, described in Section 5, that create realistic surface detail and lighting.

2. PREVIOUS WORK

Over the last three decades, many techniques have been used in an attempt to create convincing speech-synchronized facial animation. It has proven a difficult task due to the complexity of the system and the low tolerance for inconsistencies in the animation from a human audience. Concentration on the lips for the synchronization has been a theme, but only one research team has created a separate lip model. Generally, the speech is broken into phonetic elements, called phonemes, and the model is placed in a position that represents the phonemes, known as visemes.

Early work in speech-synchronized facial animation involved creating animation using traditional hand-drawn animation techniques [2, 16]. Meanwhile, early work in the speech and hearing community involved the use of oscilloscopes to generate lip shapes. Research by the speech community on lip reading involved drawing lip outlines on an oscilloscope [4, 7] or a CRT [5, 15]. The resulting lip shapes formed utterances that could be recognized showing the utility of using computers to teach lip reading. These techniques are concerned with speech intelligibility only, whereas, we require visual realism as well as intelligibility and are interested in a 3D solution instead of a 2D one.

Guiard-Marigny [11] measures the lip contours of French speakers articulating 22 visemes in the coronal plane. Assuming symmetry, the vermilion region of the lips is split into three sections and mathematical formulas are created to approximate the lip contours. From polynomial and sinusoidal equations, the 14 coefficients are reduced to three using regression analysis. The three parameters are internal lip width, internal lip height and lip contact protrusion. With the same technique on lip contours in the axial plane, Adjoudani [1] identifies two extra parameters to extend the lip model to 3D. The new parameters are upper and lower lip protrusion.

Guiard-Marigny et al. [12] replace the polygonal lip model with an implicit surface model using point primitives for fast collision detection and contact surfaces. Implicit surfaces give an exact contact surface [10] that allows modelling the interaction of the lips with other objects (a cigarette in their examples.) This lip model was designed for analyzing speech and is only capable of representing lip shapes produced during speech production. To create realistic facial animation we require a model capable of non-speech related facial expressions such as smiling.

3. LIP PARAMETERIZATION

Parameterizing the motion of the lips allows us to reduce the number of degrees of freedom of the system. The goal is to minimize the number of degrees of freedom while still providing flexibility and generality. Besides a minimal set, we need a parameterization for the lip motion that is intuitive to use; easily defined and modified for different mouths; and supports speech synchronization and the wide range of other lip motions needed for facial animation.

Fromkin [9] reports on a set of lip parameters that characterize lip positions for American English vowels using frontal and lateral photographs, lateral x-rays, and plaster casts of lips. The seven lip parameters identified are: width, height and area of lip opening; protrusion of the upper and lower lip; the distance between the outer-most points of the lips; and the distance between the upper and lower front teeth. This parameterization of the lips is very good for speech but it does not allow for other lip motions, such as those required to express emotion. We instead base our parameterization on muscle actions.

The lips deform due to the contraction of the connected muscles and the movement of the mandible. We use the muscles that affect the lips as the basis for our parameterization resulting in anatomy-based deformations. The parameterization must also include the movement of the mandible, which when moved affects the position of the lower lips, and thus the position of the upper lips. *Table 1* briefly describes the 21 parameters we use to deform our lip model.

Table 1. The parameters of our lip model along with a description of their actions. Muscles with a separate parameter for the left and right sides are denoted by an *.

Parameter	Action
Open Jaw	Rotates the jaw open
Jaw In	Moves the lower lip inward or outward.
Jaw Side	Lateral movements of the jaw moving the lower lip laterally.
Orbicularis Oris	Causes the lips to pucker and protrude.
Risorius*	Pulls the corner of the mouth back.
Platysma*	Pulls the corner of the mouth down and back.
Zygomaticus*	Pulls the corner of the mouth up and back.
Levitator Superior*	Raises the outer portion of the upper lip.
Left Levitator Nasi*	Raises the outer part of the upper lip as well as the wing of the nostril.
Depressor Inferious	Depresses the lower lip.
Depressor Oris	Draws the corners of the mouth downward and medial-ward.
Mentalis	Raises and protrudes the lower lip.
Buccinator*	Retracts the corner of the mouth.
Incisive Superior	Pulls the upper lip in towards the teeth.
Incisive Inferior	Pulls the lower lip in towards the teeth.

Muscles make a good choice to base a parameterization because their action is mostly along a vector allowing their effect on the lips to easily be defined. This works for all muscles except the orbicularis oris, which actually constricts and protrudes the lips. Generally, a parameter controls each muscle with a separate parameter for the left and right side. Exceptions are made for the depressor inferioris, depressor oris, mentalis, incisive inferior and incisive superior since individual control is rare. Lastly, we treat the levator labii superioris and the zygomaticus minor as a single muscle since the zygomaticus minor is usually not well developed and their actions are very similar.

An added benefit of using a muscle-based parameterization is that the muscles also affect other parts of the face and the parameters can be used to also deform these other parts. Examples are nose wrinkling, platysma affecting the neck, mentalis affecting the chin, the zygomaticus affecting the lower eyelid, and so forth. As well, when the muscles contract they bulge, which affects the surface of the face.

4. IMPLEMENTATION

We represent the lips as a B-spline surface with a 16x9 control grid. The parameters itemized above are mapped to changes in the positions of the control grid vertices. The geometry contains all of the vermilion zone (the red area of the lips) as well as the part of the mucous membrane that covers the lips internally. The geometry also contains a little extra of the mucous membrane to avoid observing an edge when looking at the lips from the outside. *Figure 1* shows the control points of the lip model along with a polygonalization of the B-spline surface.

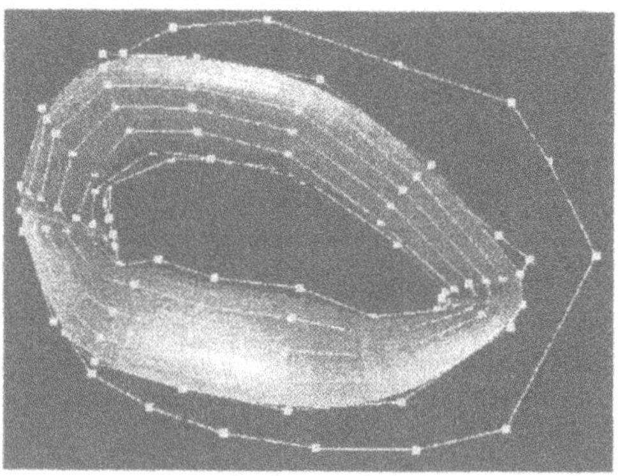

Figure 1. The B-spline control mesh and the surface used for the geometry of our lip model

All of the muscles, except the orbicularis oris, are treated as vector displacements acting upon the insertion points. The orbicularis oris constricts the shape of the lips into an oval while also extruding them. The parameters for the jaw articulate a virtual mandible and the resulting transform is used to move the lower lip.

For each control point, p_i, we calculate its position based on the parameters by the following formula

$$p_i = O_i(\hat{p}_i + L_i + J_i + A_i)$$

where $\hat{p}_i$ is the starting value for control point i, L_i is the contribution of the linear muscles, J_i is the contribution of the jaw, O_i is the contribution of the orbicularis oris and A_i is the adjustments made due to the control points being connected.

The contribution from the linear muscles involves summing the displacements from all of the individual muscles and is calculated by

$$L_i = \sum_{j=0}^{m} \rho_j M_j \delta_{ij}$$

where ρ_j is the parameter value for muscle j, M_j is the maximum displacement for muscle j, and σ_{ij} is the influence of muscle j on control point i. σ_{ij} is zero when the muscle has no influence and one when the muscle is inserted very near the control point. Intermediate values allow for creating a zone of influence on the muscle. This is used for the upper lip only, as the lower lip moves mostly as a unit. σ comes into play particularly in the middle of the upper lip and lower values tend to create a stiffer upper lip as in most males. Higher σ values will allow for more gum to be shown when the corners are raised giving a more feminine appearance.

The effect of jaw movement on the lips is calculated by

$$J_i = J_{open} + J_{in} + J_{side}$$

where J_{open} is the rotation about the axis through the condyles, J_{in} is the movement of jaw in or out and J_{side} is the lateral movement of the jaw.

The lips are made of muscle fibers that can stretch slightly but will maintain a mostly constant circumference. Adjustments to the control points to keep the lip shape more natural are done with

$$A_i = LD\alpha_i + \rho_{open}\gamma_i$$

where LD is the motion vector for the lower lip, α_i is how much the lower lip affects the upper lip, ρ_{open} is the parameter value for the jaw being open and γ_i is the effect of tightening the lips. The lower lip moves mostly in unison and individuals rarely have control over it. LD is the lower delta and represents the movement of the lower lip. As the lower lip moves it will pull on the corners of the mouth and therefore the upper lips. The α weights take care of this effect. As the mouth opens the lips stretch and tighten. As they tighten, they move medially toward the mouth center. The weights allow for this medial motion.

The orbicularis oris constricts and protrudes the lips as it contracts. This effect is handled after all the other displacements are taken into account to make combining the muscle displacements less complex. The linear displacements are additive and have constraints on the maximum displacement. However, the orbicularis oris causes complex motion and does not simply add to the other displacements. The contribution of the orbicularis oris is calculated as

$$O_i = R(\rho_{oris}\theta) + \rho_{oris}[e_i(p) + \chi_i]$$

where ρ_{oris} is the parameter value for the orbicularis oris, θ is the maximum angle of rotation from puckering the lips, $R(\theta)$ is the rotation due to contraction of the orbicularis oris, $e_i(p)$ keeps the point p on the ellipse created by the lips and χ_i is the maximum extrusion from the contraction of the orbicularis oris.

The weights and muscle displacement vectors are data to the lip model allowing the behavior of the lips to be changed by simply changing data files. Besides different geometry, characters will potentially have a separate datafile for the lip model behavior. It may also be desirable to change the lip behavior for the same character such as for slurred speech when intoxicated.

Another option is to calculate the forces of each muscle and using a Newtonian physics model, numerically solve the differential equations to find the new locations of the control points. This would have allowed us to constrain the lip shape using springs, but we would have had to numerically integrate. We instead wanted a closed-form solution that would avoid the rubbery look of spring-based systems

Grafting of the lip model geometry onto the input face geometry is done interactively. First an interactive tool is used to align the lip model with the input geometry depicted in *Figure 2a*. All vertices, and thus all triangles, inside the convex hull of the input lip geometry in a cylindrical projection are removed, thereby removing the input lips. The fitted lip model is polygonalized and triangulated along with the remaining input geometry as shown in *Figure 2b*. The new triangles and the lip model geometry are then added to the input facial geometry, effectively replacing the input lips with the lip model geometry as seen in *Figure 2c*.

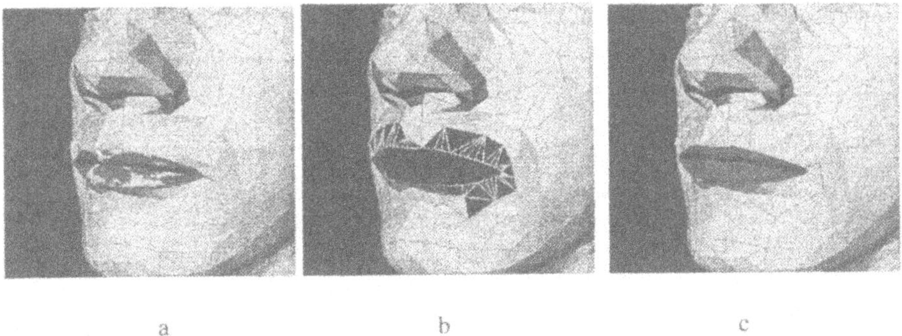

Figure 2. First, the lip model is aligned with the input geometry (a). Overlapping triangles are then removed and the boundary of the lip model and the boundary of the removed triangles are retriangulated (b). Finally the lip model geometry is added to the input geometry (c).

5. RENDERING

In order to create realism, the rendering of the lips is important. A common method to improve realism is the use of texture maps. The same problems associated with gathering the geometry of the lips also exist for gathering color information. Incomplete texture information will leave visible artifacts. We could use methods to warp what texture information is obtained, but there is no clear-cut way to do this. This would also exacerbate the problems associated with texture maps, such as limited resolution and lighting inherent in texture acquisition. We instead choose a different approach using a procedural texture shader to increase realism. Besides color information, we also add surface detail with a bump shader.

Lips are covered with very thin skin that tends to wrinkly easily. Besides the constant fine to medium wrinkles, when the lips are compressed (as in a pucker) there are large undulations of the surface. We currently ignore the finer wrinkles and instead concentrate on the larger wave-like wrinkles created during compression.

Another shader determines the color of the lips. We can simulate natural lip colors as well as lipstick and lipgloss. When the lips are licked, this results in differing depths of saliva across the lips. We model this affect by creating a second layer, using a noise function, which represents the wetness pattern. This pattern is then mixed with the current lip color to increase the specular component. Lipstick and lipgloss are implemented as a uniform color change across the lips with transparency and glossiness components controlling matte versus glossy. Flecked lipstick is modeled by adding a flecked silver pattern to the lipstick color.

Figure 3 shows examples of wrinkled lips, both dry and wet. This method only works for offline generation of animations since it is too slow for our real-time version, where we choose a single color for the lips.

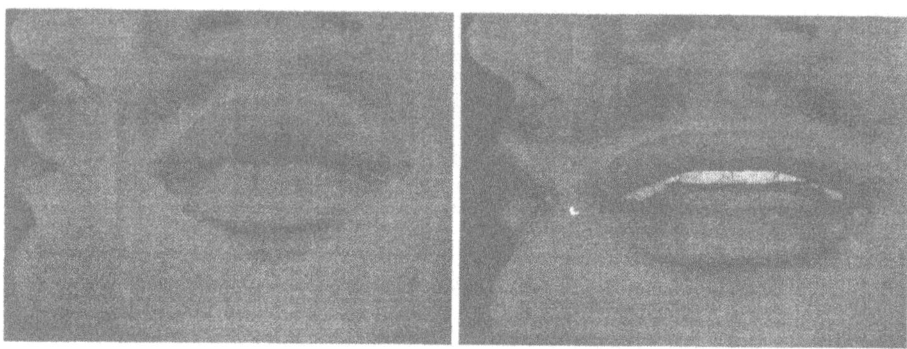

Figure 3. Rendering of the lip model using our custom shaders. The left image is of wrinkled dry lips in a pucker. The right image is of slightly wet lips being closed showing motion blur.

6. ANIMATION

In our TTAVS system [13] we use a keyframing approach. Text is input to Festival [3], which converts the text into phonemes and creates a waveform. The phonemes are then sent to MBROLA [14] to generate a waveform and to the viseme generator to produce a series of keyframes that match the audio. A viseme specifies the parameters for the lips, tongue and jaw. The facial model then takes the visemes and the waveform and generates a synchronized animation. The waveform is simply a sound track, and using t, the time from the beginning of the waveform, along with the visemes, the facial model is deformed to produce the correct shape that corresponds to the audio.

The facial model parameters associated with each phoneme are found, thus creating a viseme and the definition of the Festival voice is modified to contain this extra information. We do this by interactively setting the facial model to the keyframe position for each phoneme. When text is parsed into phonemes, it is also parsed into visemes with the same timing as the phonemes that make up the waveform. Playing the waveform and using the time t to interpolate the visemes achieves lip-synchronized animation.

7. RESULTS

We have successfully incorporated our lip model into the facial model used by our TTAVS system. Our TTAVS system creates animations from text creating a stream of visemes, or keyframes, to be interpolated between. *Figure 3* displays frames from an offline rendering using our rendering process for the lips. With our rendering technique we can achieve wrinkled and wet lips for increased realism. *Figure 3* depicts frames from an offline rendering and demonstrates motion blurring of the lips, which can move extremely fast during speech. The motion blur increases realism by giving visual cues that support fast movement of the lips.

Figure 4 shows close-ups of the mouth area of the facial model rendered with our TTAVS system in various expressions that our lip model is capable of depicting. *Figure 4a* is the viseme for /aw/, while *Figure 4b* is the viseme /aw/ while also activating the zygomaticus major muscle creating a happy /aw/. *Figure 4c* is a half smile, created by activating only the right zygomaticus major muscle.

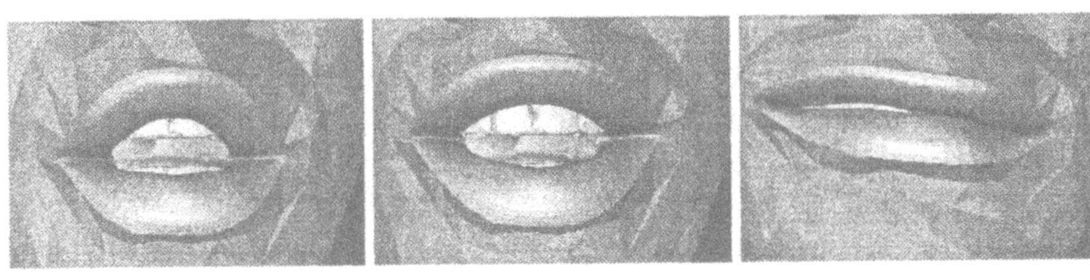

Figure 4. These are frames rendered by our TTAVS system showing various expressions that our lip model is capable of achieving. Image a depicts the viseme for /aw/ from "how", while image b is a happy /aw/. Frame c shows a half smile.

8. CONCLUSIONS AND FUTURE WORK

Our anatomically based lip model improves our ability to create realistic speech-synchronized facial animation with more realistic deformations of the lips. Because it is muscle-based, the effects of contraction of the muscles that affect the lips on other parts of the face are more easily calculated. Our lip model has both internal and external lip geometry, and by replacing the input lip geometry with the lip model's geometry we guarantee the internal geometry, which would otherwise be often missing, especially when the input geometry is acquired via a laser scan of the subject. This internal geometry is important to have when the mouth opens to avoid loss of realism. With our generic lip model that is fitted to the subject, we also do not need to redefine the insertion of the muscles for each new subject.

Our lip model is capable of highly realistic lip shapes and controlling it to produce realistic animation is an open question. Having a single keyframe for each phoneme is not adequate since a phoneme is actually a dynamic shaping of the vocal tract. As well, the same phoneme does not always visually look the same but instead depends on the phonemes before and after. This effect, called coarticulation, is a byproduct of the laws of physics and human anatomy. The vocal tract parts do not move and stop instantaneously so we must anticipate or lag behind, blurring the lines between phonemes. Coarticulation has been tackled with look ahead [17], triphones [8], nonlinear interpolation and masses [18] and using a coarticulation model such as the Lofqvist model [6]. In addition to coarticulation affects there are differences due to prosody (stress and intonation) that should be considered.

Our current focus has been on the motion of the lips due to muscle contractions, however, we also need to consider deformations due to collisions between the lips and other parts of the face. The lips must flow around the teeth and not penetrate them. Furthermore, when the tongue presses against the lips for creating sounds or when wetting them, there is a slight deformation that is needed to improve realism. Finally, when the upper and lower lips come into contact with each other there are subtle changes that need to be shown. However, these deformations can be done without collision detection between the lips. And the spatial relationship between the upper and lower lips makes interpenetration hard to notice.

The lip model does not have a concept of state, that is, it does not know what came before, therefore, certain shapes are indistinguishable without further information. For example, to rotate the lower lip outward into a pout the lower lip is pushed upward toward the upper lip, which is tensed, causing the lower lip to slide over the upper lip and outward. However, if the upper lip is not tensed it will be pushed upward by the lower lip. These two distinctly different positions can have the same parameters values. Adding state to the model would change this, however, the model would then have multiple shapes for the same parameter set. Adding new parameters would also work but requires a parameter to handle each of the special cases.

To see more results and animation from this work, please visit our web page at http://www.cis.ohio-state.edu/graphics/research/FacialAnimation/.

9. ACKNOWLEDGMENTS

This work was partially funded by a grant from Texas Instruments.

10. REFERENCES

[1] Ali Adjoudani, *Élaboration d'un modéle de lèvres 3D pour animation en temps réel*, Masters thesis, *Mémoire de D.E.A. Signal-Image-Parole*, Institut National Polytechnique, Grenoble, France, 1993.

[2] Philippe Bergeron, *3-D Character Animation on the Symbolics System, SIGGRAPH '87 course notes: 3-D Character Animation by Computer*, jul 1987.

[3] Alan W Black, Paul Taylor, Richard Caley and Rob Clark, *The Festival Speech Synthesis System*, http://www.cstr.ed.ac.uk/projects/festival/.

[4] D. W. Boston, *Synthetic Facial Communication*, British Journal of Audiology, 7 (1973), pp. 95-101.

[5] N. M. Brooke and Quentin Summerfield, *Analysis, Synthesis and Perception of Visible Articulatory Movements*, Journal of Phonetics, 11 (jan 1983), pp. 63-76.

[6] Michael Cohen and Dominic Massaro, *Modeling coarticulation in synthetic visual speech*,in N. M.-T. a. D. Thalmann, ed., *Models and Techniques in Computer Animation*, Springer-Verlag, Tokyo, 1993, pp. 139-156.

[7] Norman P. Erber, Richard L. Sachs and Carol Lee De Filippo, *Optical synthesis of articulatory images for lipreading evaluation and instruction*, in D. L. McPhearson, ed., *Advances in Prosthetic Devices for the Deaf: A Technical Workshop*, Rochester, NY: NTID, 1979, pp. 228-231.

[8] Tony Ezzat and Tomaso Poggio, *MikeTalk: A Talking Facial Display Based on Morphing Visemes*, , *Computer Animation '98*, IEEE Computer Society, Philadelphia, University of Pennsylvania, jun 1998, pp. 96-102.

[9] Victoria Fromkin, *Lip positions in American English vowels*, Language and Speech, 7 (1964), pp. 215-225.

[10] Marie-Paul Gascuel, *An implicit formulation for precise contact modeling between flexible solids*, , *SIGGRAPH '93*, 1993, pp. 313-320.

[11] Thierry Guiard-Marigny, *Animation en temps réel d'un modèle paramétrique de lèvres*, Masters thesis, *Mémoire de D.E.A Signal-Image-Parole*, Institut National Polytechnique, Grenoble, France, 1992.

[12] Thierry Guiard-Marigny, Nicolas Tsingos, Ali Adjoudani, Christian Benoit and Marie-Paule Gascuel, *3D Models of the Lips for Realistic Speech Animation*, , *Computer Graphic '96*, Geneve, 1996.

[13] Scott A. King and Richard E. Parent, *TalkingHead: A text-to-audiovisual-speech system*, OSU-CISRC-2/80-TR05, Computer and Information Science, The Ohio State University, Columbus, Ohio, 2000.

[14] MBROLA, *The MBROLA Project*, http://www.tcts.fpms.ac.be/synthesis/.

[15] A. A. Montgomery, *Development of a model for generating synthetic animated lip shapes*, Journal of the Acoustical Society of America, 68 (1980), pp. S58(A).

[16] Frederic I. Parke, *A parametric model for human faces*, Ph.D. thesis, University of Utah, Salt Lake City, Utah, dec 1974.

[17] J A Provine and L T Bruton, *Lip Synchronization in 3-D Model Based Coding for Video-conferencing, Proc. of the IEEE Int. Symposium on Circuits and Systems*, Seattle, May 1995, pp. 453-456.

[18] Keith Waters and Thomas M. Levergood, *DECface: An Automatic Lip-Synchronization Algorithm for Synthetic Faces*, Technical Report CRL 93/4, Digital Equipment Corporation Cambridge Research Lab, Sep 1993.

FEATURE POINT BASED MESH DEFORMATION APPLIED TO MPEG-4 FACIAL ANIMATION

Sumedha Kshirsagar, Stephane Garchery, Nadia Magnenat-Thalmann
MIRALab, CUI, University of Geneva

Key words: mesh deformation, real-time facial animation, performance driven animation, optical tracking

Abstract: Robustness and speed are primary considerations when developing deformation methodologies for animatable mesh objects. The goal of this paper is to present such a robust and fast geometric mesh deformation algorithm. The algorithm is feature points based *i.e.* it can be applied to enable the animation of various mesh objects defined by the placement of their feature points. As a specific application, we describe the use of the algorithm for MPEG-4 facial mesh deformation and animation. The MPEG-4 face object is characterized by the Face Definition Parameters (FDP), which are defined by the locations of the key feature points on the face. The MPEG-4 compatible facial animation system developed using this algorithm can be effectively used for real time applications. We extract MPEG-4 Facial Animation Parameters (FAP) using an optical tracking system and apply the results to several synthetic facial mesh objects to assess the results of the deformation algorithm.

1. INTRODUCTION

In this paper, we present a robust, fast, and simple geometric mesh deformation algorithm. A geometric mesh can be characterized by the locations of key feature points. Further, the animation of the mesh can be defined by the displacements of these feature points. The algorithm described here can be applied for animation of such meshes. As a specific application, we describe the use of the algorithm for MPEG-4 facial mesh, which is characterized by the Face Definition Parameters (FDP). We examine the results of the mesh deformation applied to facial animation by using the Facial Animation Parameters (FAP) obtained from an optical tracking system used for facial feature capture.

There are a variety of ways possible to represent animatable objects geometrically. The choice depends on the considerations such as precise shape, effective animation and efficient rendering. Barr introduced geometric modeling deformations using abstract data manipulation operators creating a useful sculpting metaphor [1]. Bearle applied surface patch descriptions to model smooth character form [2]. Free Form Deformation (FFD) and its variants have been used extensively for a variety of modeling and animation applications [3][4][9][13]. They involve the definition and deformation of a lattice of control points. An object embedded within the lattice is then deformed by defining a mapping from the lattice to the object.

FFDs allow volume deformation using control points while keeping the surface continuity. They provide the sculptural flexibility of deformations. FFDs have been successfully used for synthetic objects like face [6] and hand deformation [11]. FFDs have some limitations though. The locations of the control points are not very well controllable with respect to the actual mesh object. Also, the discontinuities or holes in the mesh are difficult to handle as a general case. Recently, Singh *et. al.*[15], proposed a new approach of using *wire* curves to define an object and for shaping its deformation. They illustrated the applications of animating figures with flexible articulations, modeling wrinkled surfaces and stitching geometry together.

In order to define shape and animation of a geometric mesh object, we concentrate on the use of feature points. We assume that the shape of the object is defined by the locations of the predefined feature points on the surface of the mesh. Further, the deformation of the mesh can be completely defined by the movements of these feature points (alternatively referred as control points) from their neutral positions either in absolute or in normalized units. This method of definition and animation provides a concise and efficient way of representing an object. Since the control points lie on the geometric surface, their locations are predictable, unlike in FFD.

2. GEOMETRIC MESH DEFINITION AND DEFORMATION

In this section, we describe in detail the feature point based mesh deformation algorithm. The algorithm is usable on any generic surface mesh. To begin with, the feature points or the control points with movement constraint are defined for a given mesh. A constraint in a direction indicates the behaviour of the control point in that direction. For example, if a control point is constrained along the *x* axis, but not along the *y* and *z* axes, means that it still acts as an ordinary vertex of the mesh along the *y* and *z* axes. Its movement along these axes will be controlled by the other control points in the vicinity.

Given a geometric mesh with control point locations, we need to compute the regions influenced by each of the control points. In order to get realistic looking deformation and animation, it is necessary that the mesh has a good definition of the feature points; *i.e.* the control point locations should be defined considering the animation properties and real-life topology of the object under consideration. Each vertex of the mesh should be controlled by not only the nearest feature point, but other feature points in the vicinity, in order to avoid patchy animation. The number of feature points influencing a vertex and the factor by which each feature point influences the movement of this vertex is decided by the following:

- The distances between the feature points *i.e.* if the feature points are spread densely or sparsely on the mesh
- The distances between the ordinary (non-feature point) vertices of the mesh and the nearest feature point
- The relative spread of the feature points around a given vertex

The algorithm is divided into two steps. In the *Initialization* step, the above mentioned information is extracted and the coefficients or *weights* for each of the vertices corresponding to the nearest feature points are calculated. The distance between two points is computed as the sum of the edge lengths encountered while traversing from one point to the other. We call this *surface distance*. This *surface distance* measure is useful to handle holes and discontinuities in the mesh, *e.g.* mouth and eye openings in the facial mesh models. The *Deformation* step actually takes place during the real-time animation for each frame.

2.1 Initialization

The initialization can further be divided into two substeps.

2.1.1 Computing Feature Point Distribution

In this step, the information about all the neighbouring feature points for each of the feature point is extracted. The mesh is traversed starting from each feature point, advancing only one step in all the possible directions at a time, thus growing a mesh region for each feature point, called *feature point region*. Neighbouring feature points are those feature points that have a common *feature point region* boundary. As a result, for each feature point defined on the mesh surface, we get a list of the neighbouring feature points with *surface distances* between them. This information is further used in the next step.

2.1.2 Computing Weights

The goal of this step is to extract possible overlapping influence regions for each feature point and to compute the corresponding weight for deformation for all the vertices in this influence region. Consider a general surface mesh as shown in Figure 1. During the process of mesh traversal starting from the feature points, assume that the vertex P is approached from a feature point FP_1. FP_1 is added to the list of the influencing feature points of P.

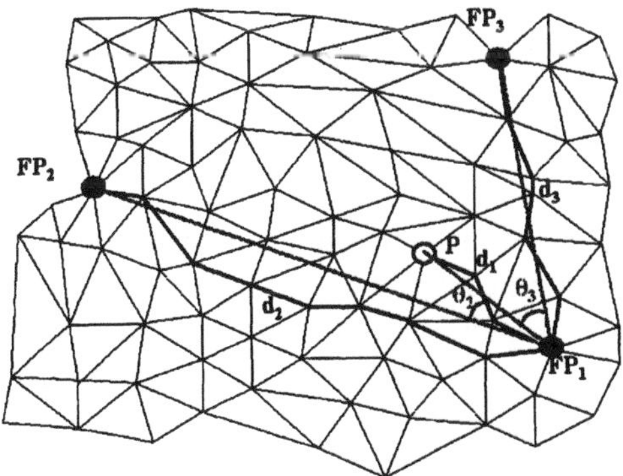

Figure 1. Computing weights for animation

From the information extracted in the previous step of mesh traversal, FP_2, and FP_3 are the neighbouring feature points of FP_1. FP_2 and FP_3 are chosen such that the angles θ_2 and θ_3 are the smallest of all the angles θ_i for neighbouring feature points FP_i of FP_1. Also,

$$\theta_2 < \frac{\pi}{2}, \theta_3 < \frac{\pi}{2} \tag{1}$$

The surface distances of the vertex from these feature points are respectively d_{1P}, d_{12} and d_{13} as shown in the figure. While computing the weight of FP_1 at P, we consider the effect of the presence of the other neighbouring feature points namely FP_2 and FP_3 at P. For this, we compute the following weighted sum d:

$$d = \frac{d_{12}\cos\theta_2 + d_{13}\cos\theta_3}{\cos\theta_2 + \cos\theta_3} \quad (2)$$

Thus, d is the weighted sum of the distances d_{12} and d_{13}. The feature point in a smaller angular distance from the FP_1 is assigned a higher value of weight. If there is only one neighbouring feature point of FP_1 such that $\theta_2<\pi/2$, then d is simply computed as $d_{12}/\cos\theta_2$.

We compute the weight assigned to the point P for the deformation due to movement of FP_1 as:

$$W_{1,P} = \sin\left(\frac{\pi}{2}\left(1-\frac{d_{1P}}{d}\right)\right) \quad (3)$$

or more generally

$$W_{i,P} = \sin\left(\frac{\pi}{2}\left(1-\frac{d_{iP}}{d}\right)\right) \quad (4)$$

Thus, point P has a weight for displacement that is inversely proportional to its distance from the nearest feature point FP_1. This determines the local influence of the feature point on the vertices of the mesh. At the same time, nearer the other feature points (FP_2 and FP_3 in this case) to FP_1, less is this weight according to the equation 2 and 3. This determines the global influence of a feature point on the surrounding region, in the presence of other feature points in the vicinity.

It is possible that a vertex is approached by more than one feature point, during the process of mesh traversal. We compute the weight for this feature point following the same procedure, as long as the angular distance criterion (1) is satisfied, and the *surface distance* $d_{iP}<d$, d as defined in equation 2. This second criterion ensures that the feature points FP_j whose nearest neighbours are nearer to the vertex P than FP_j are not considered while computing the deformation for vertex P. Thus, for the example taken here, weights will be computed for vertex P for the feature points FP_1 as well as FP_2 and FP_3, provided d_{2P} and d_{3P} are less than d. As a result, we have for each vertex of the mesh, a list of control points influencing it and an associated weight.

We tested the algorithm on simple meshes with different values of limits in equation 1, and different weighting functions in equation 2 and 3. The ones giving the most satisfactory results were chosen. In equation 3, we chose *sine* function as it is continuous at the minimum and maximum limits.

2.2 Deformation

Once the weights for the vertices have been computed, the mesh is ready for real-time animation. Note that *Initialization* step is computationally intensive, but carried out only once. The weights computed, take into consideration the distance of a vertex from the feature point and relative spread of the feature points around the vertex. Now, from the displacements of the feature points for animation, we calculate the actual displacement of all the vertices of the mesh. Here, we have to consider the effects caused when two or more feature points move at the same time, influencing the same vertex. We calculate the weighted sum of all the displacements caused at the point P due to all the neighbouring feature points. Let FP_i, $i=1,2,\ldots,N$ be the control points influencing vertex P of the mesh. Then

1. D_i = the displacement specified for the control point FP_i
2. $W_{i,P}$ = the weight as calculated in the *Initialization* for vertex P associated with the control points
3. $d_{i,P}$ = the corresponding distance between P and FP_i.

The following equation gives the resultant displacement D_P caused at the vertex P

$$D_P = \frac{\sum_{i=0}^{N} \frac{W_{i,P} D_i}{d_{i,P}^2}}{\sum_{i=0}^{N} \frac{W_{i,P}}{d_{i,P}^2}} \qquad (5)$$

This operation is performed for every frame during the computation of the animation of the mesh.

3. ADAPTATION FOR MPEG-4 FACIAL MESH

Various muscle based models have been effectively developed for facial animation [13][16][17]. The Facial Action Coding System (Friesen, 1978) defines high level parameters for facial animation, on which several other systems are based. We use MPEG-4 facial animation standard, which defines the face object by locations of specific feature points on the facial mesh. Lavagetto *et al* have described an MPEG-4 compatible facial animation engine using a similar mesh deformation technique [7]. However, the important difference is that the wireframe semantics (the locations and the region influenced by all the feature points) have to be specified *a priori* in their method. MPEG-4 Facial Animation

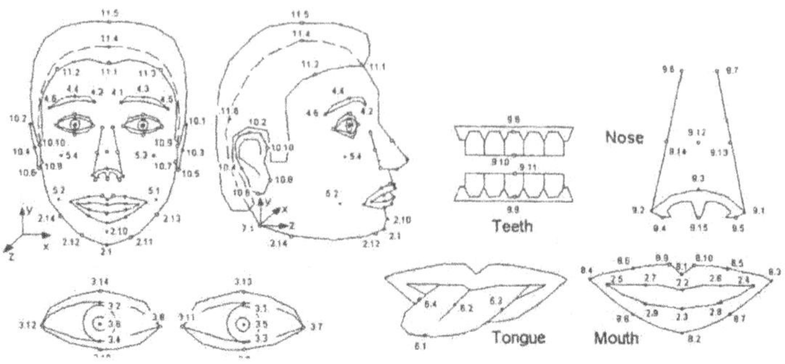

Figure 2. MPEG-4 Facial feature points

The ISO/IEC JTC1/SC29/WG11 (Moving Pictures Expert Group - MPEG) has formulated the new MPEG-4 standard. An efficient coding method has been devised within the framework of the standard for graphics models and their animation parameters specific to the model type. For face models, the Face Definition Parameters (FDPs) are defined by the locations of the feature points (*e.g.* mouth corners, eye corners, eyebrow ends *etc.*) and are used to customize a given face model to a particular face. The Facial Animation Parameters (FAPs) represent a complete set of basic facial actions and allow the representation of most natural facial expressions. All parameters involving motion are expressed in terms of the Facial Animation Parameter Units (FAPU). These correspond to fractions of distances between key facial features (e.g. the distance between the eyes). Figure 2 shows the locations of the feature points as defined by the MPEG-4 standard.

3.1 Mesh Deformation using MPEG-4 Feature Points

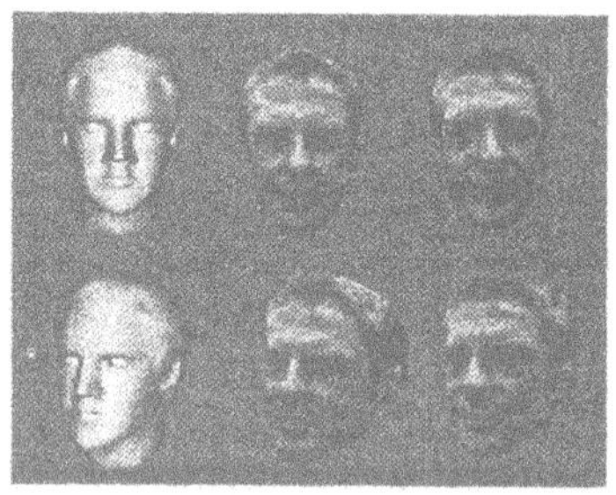

Figure 3. Morphing using deformation

Given a facial mesh, we can define the locations of the MPEG-4 feature points as per the specification, as shown in Figure 2. Also, for each feature point, we have to define the constraints as defined by the mesh deformation algorithm. Once we define this information, the facial mesh is ready to accept any FAPs and animate the face.

We also use the same deformation algorithm to deform the facial mesh in order to obtain a new face from a generic mesh. Figure 3 shows the results in two different views. The face on the left side is a generic facial mesh. The face in the middle is acquired using two orthogonal photographs of a person using the technique described in [8]. In this method, the locations of the feature points are extracted from the images and Rational Free Form Deformation (RFFD) is used to deform the generic face. Appropriate texture mapping is done to add realism. We apply the deformation algorithm explained in the previous section to the same generic face using these MPEG-4 feature points to obtain the face on the right. Thus the deformation algorithm applied for 3D morphing of generic head using MPEG-4 feature points generates satisfactory result.

4. OPTICAL TRACKING FOR ANIMATION

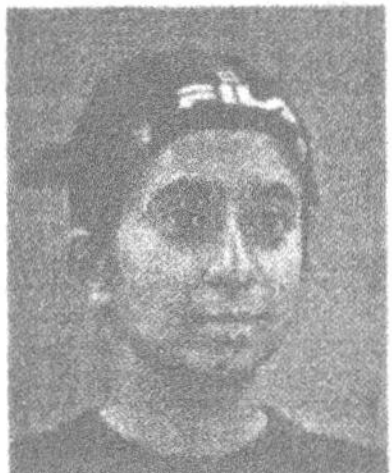

Figure 4. Placement of markers for selected MPEG-4 feature points

Facial feature tracking efforts have ranged from an ordinary video camera with coloured markers to retro-reflective markers and multiple cameras to extract directly the 3D position of the markers. We use one such commercially available system (VICON 8) to track the facial expressions and retarget the tracked features to our facial animation engine to examine the results of the deformation algorithm. We use a subset of MPEG-4 feature points corresponding to the FAP values to track the face and extract the FAPs frame by the frame. The next subsection in brief explains the algorithm for extracting the global head rotation and the calculation of the FAP values with the underlying assumptions. For the capture, we used 6 cameras and 27 markers corresponding to the MPEG-4 feature point locations. 3 additional markers are used for tracking the global orientation of the head. Figure 4 shows the placement of the feature points on the actor's face. We get the 3D trajectories for each of the marker points as the output of the tracking system.

4.1 Extracting Global Head Movements

We use 3 markers attached to the head to capture the rigid head movements (the global rotation and translation of the head). We use the improved translation invariant method [10]. Let (p_i, p_i') be the positions of the points on the surface of the rigid body, observed at two different time instants. For a rigid body motion, the pair of points (p_i, p_i') obeys the following general displacement relationship:

$$p'_i = Rp_i + t \qquad i = 1,2,\cdots,N \tag{6}$$

R is a 3X3 matrix specifying the rotation angle of the rigid body about an axis arbitrarily oriented in the three dimensional space, whereas *t* represents a translation vector specifying arbitrary shift after rotation. Three non-collinear point correspondences are necessary and sufficient to determine *R* and *t* uniquely. With three point correspondences, we get nine non-linear equations while there are six unknown motion parameters. Because the 3D points obtained from the motion capture system are accurate, linear algorithm is sufficient for this application, instead of iterative algorithms based on least square procedure. If two points on the rigid body, p_i and p_{i+1}, undergoing the same transformation, move to p_i' and p_{i+1}' respectively, then

$$p'_i = Rp_i + t \tag{7}$$

$$p'_{i+1} = Rp_{i+1} + t \tag{8}$$

Subtraction eliminates translation t; using the rigidity constraints yields:

$$\frac{p'_{i+1} - p'_i}{\left|p'_{i+1} - p'_i\right|} = R\frac{p_{i+1} - p_i}{\left|p_{i+1} - p_i\right|} \tag{9}$$

The above equation is defined as:

$$\hat{m}'_i = R\hat{m}_i \tag{10}$$

If the rigid body undergoes a pure translation, these parameters do not change, which means the translation is invariant. After rearranging these three equations, we can solve a 3X3 linear system to get R and afterwards obtain t by substitution in equation 6. In order to find a unique solution, the 3X3 matrix of unit $\hat{m}$ vectors must be of full rank, meaning that the three $\hat{m}$ vectors must be non-coplanar. As a result, four point correspondences are needed. To overcome this problem of supplying the linear method with an extra point correspondence, a "pseudo-correspondence" can be constructed due to the property of rigidity. We find a third $\hat{m}$ vector orthogonal to the two obtained from three points attached to the head. Thus, the system has lower dimension, requiring only three non-collinear rigid points. Once we extract the global head movements, the motion trajectories of all the feature point markers are compensated for the global movements, and the absolute local displacements and subsequently the MPEG-4 FAPs are calculated.

5. CONCLUSION AND FUTURE WORK

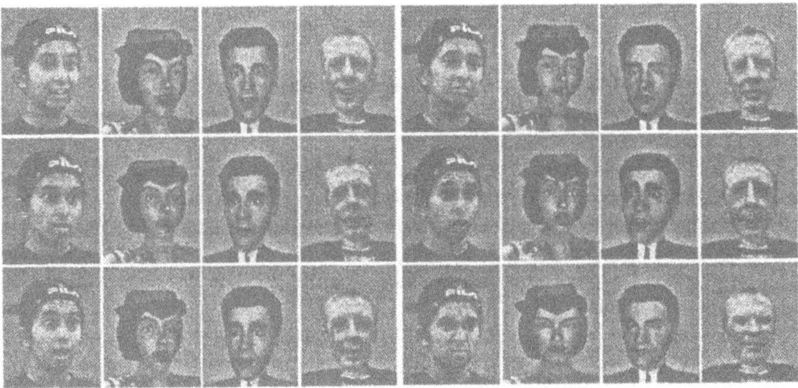

Figure 5. Facial Expressions extracted by Optical Tracking Applied to MPEG-4 Faces

Figure 5 shows the frames of animation depicting different facial expressions on the real face and three different synthetic faces. With the mesh deformation algorithm described here, we obtain a frame rate of 29 frames per second for an MPEG-4 compatible facial mesh with 1257 vertices on a 600 MHz Pentium III PC, with Matrix G400 graphics card using Open GL Optimizer for rendering. Thus, the algorithm is well suited for real time MPEG-4 compatible facial animation. We have assessed the deformation algorithm for realism by extracting the facial features from optical tracking and retargeting them to the synthetic face.

6. ACKNOWLEDGEMENTS

This work is supported by the EU ACTS SONG project. Special thanks are due to Dr. Tom Molet for his help with optical tracking system and to Chris Joslin for proof reading this paper.

REFERENCES

[1] A. Barr, "Global and Local Deformations of Solid Primitives", Computer Graphics, Vol. 18, No. 3, July 1984.

[2] V. Bearle, "A Case Study of Flexible Figure Animation", 3-D Character Animation by computer Course Notes, Siggraph'87.

[3] Y-K. Chang and A. Rockwood. "A generalizad de casteljau approach to 3d free-form deformation" Computer Graphics Proceedings of SIGGRAPH'94, pages 257--260

[4] C. Sabine. "Extended Free-Form Deformation: A Sculpting Tool for 3D Geometric modeling" Proceedings of SIGGRAPH '90, In Computer Graphics, 24, 4, pages 187--196, August 1990.

[5] E. Friesen WV (1978), Facial Action Coding System: A Technique for the Measurement of Facial Movement. Palo Alto, California: Consulting Psychologists Press.

[6] P. Kalra, A. Mangili, N. Magnenat-Thalmann, D. Thalmann, "Simulation of Facial Muscle Actions Based on Rational Free Form Deformations", Proc. Eurographics '92, Cambridge, pp. 59-69.

[7] F. Lavagetto, R. Pockaj, "The Facial Animation Engine: towards a high-level interface for the design of MPEG-4 compliant animated faces" IEEE Trans. on Circuits and Systems for video Technology, Vol. 9, no.2, March 1999.

[8] W. Lee, N. Magnenat-Thalmann, "Fast Head Modeling for Animation", Journal of Image and Vision Computing, Volume 18, Number 4, pp.355-364, Elsevier, 1 March, 2000.

[9] R. MacCracken and K. Joy, Free-form deformation with Lattices of arbitrary topology. Computer Graphics (Proc. of SIGGRAPH'96), pp. 181188, 1996.

[10] W. Martin and J. Aggarwal, "Motion Understanding Robot and Human Vision", Kluwer Academic Publishers, 1988.

[11] L. Moccozet, N. Magnenat-Thalmann, "Dirichlet Free-Form Deformations and their Application to Hand Simulation", Proc. Computer Animation `97, IEEE Computer Society, 1997, pp. 93-102.

[12] Specification of MPEG-4 standard, Moving Picture Experts Group, http://www.cselt.it/mpeg/

[13] F. Parke, "Parameterized Models for Facial Animation", IEEE Computer Graphics and Applications, Vol.2, Nuo. 9, pp 61-68, November 1982

[14] T. Sederberg and S. Parry, "Free Form Deformations of Solid Geometric Models", Computer Graphics, Vol. 20, No. 4, 1986.

[15] K. Singh, E. Fiume, "Wires: A Geometric Deformation Technique", Proc. SIGGRAPH'98, pp 405-414, 1998.

[16] D. Terzopoulos, K. Waters, "Physically Based Facial Modelling, Analysis and Animation", Journal of visualization and Computer Animation, Vo. 1, No. 2, pp 73-90, 1990.

[17] K. Waters, "A Muscle Model for Animation Three Dimensional Facial Expression", Computer Graphics, Vol. 21, No. 4, pp 17-24, July 1987.

A FEATURE-BASED DEFORMABLE MODEL FOR PHOTO-REALISTIC HEAD MODELLING

[†]Yong-Jin Liu, [†]Matthew Ming-Fai Yuen, [‡]Shan Xiong
[†]Hong Kong University of Science and Technology, HK; [‡]Vanderbilt University, USA

Key words: Deformable model; Features; Subdivision surfaces; Facial deformation; Photogrammetry.

Abstract: We propose a feature-based approach for creating photo-realistic textured 3D head model. First, from a discrete data set of human head we generate a generic head model which is feature-based and semi-regular. Then we take a pair of photos of a human subject from two orthogonal directions. After recovering a set of 3D feature points on the head from photos, we build an individualized geometric model level by level. Finally we synthesize the photos into a view-independent texture map and automatically generate the texture coordinates. By mapping the texture onto the geometric model, we can efficiently generate highly photo-realistic head models for individuals.

1. INTRODUCTION

Pioneered by Parke [17], computer-aided modelling of human head has received considerable attentions. We can categorize these approaches into two classes based on how simple the acquisition equipment is: (1) high-cost approaches: in this category high-cost equipments are employed, such as the Cyberware color scanners [2, 15] and the face sculpturing robot system [12]; (2) low-cost approaches: simple low-cost equipments are needed in this category, such as the common CCD or digital cameras [1, 11, 13, 14, 19].

Our approach presented in this paper falls into the category of low-cost approaches. We only use a simple digital camera to capture individual head information which is used to generate photo-realistic head models. The general procedure in all photo-based approaches is similar: first, the 2D features (points, lines) are extracted; then 3D geometric information is recovered from 2D features and furthermore a texture map is generated by blending taken photos; finally, by matching 2D features with predefined features on a 3D geometric model, the texture coordinates are assigned for creating a textured head model.

In our work, we observe that the format of used generic model strongly determines the efficiency of downstream operations, e.g., geometric model deformation and texture coordinates assignment. Based on model format, we briefly review the related work on low-cost approaches. For a detailed survey of this entire field, the reader is referred to the book by Parke and Waters [18] and the references therein.

2. RELATED WORK

Low-cost head modelling approaches can be classified according to the format in which the head models are represented. There are two popular formats widely used for head models: parametric surfaces and polygonal surfaces.

Parametric surfaces describe head models mathematically in parametric equations. Due to the intrinsic parameterisation, it is straightforward to deform the surface and generate texture coordinates. However, it is difficult to model a highly detailed human head using parametric surface, since either the number of control points is increased rapidly, or a network of parametric patches need to be constructed. A typical work using parametric surface for head modelling is presented in [5].

Compared with parametric surfaces, polygonal surfaces are more flexible in modelling fine details. Most of existing low-cost approaches use irregular polygonal mesh for head modelling. However, after specifying a set of feature vertices on a generic model, the applications of polygonal models are confronted by the difficulties of specifications for remaining vertices. Addressing this problem, a number of techniques are proposed: Kurihara and Arai [13] project the vertices into cylindrical parameter plane and use Delaunay triangulation of feature vertices; Ip and Yin [11] look for N nearest feature vertices around each non-feature vertex; Pighin *et al.* [19] and Akimoto *et al.* [1] build a scatter data interpolation function; Lee and Thalmann [14] use a Dirichlet free-form deformation.

With the development of multiresolution techniques, subdivision surfaces have been widely studied [21]. Recent works [8, 10, 22] have extended subdivision surfaces to arbitrary topology and therefore offer a bridge between parametric surfaces and polygonal surfaces. In our work, we use a multi-level displaced subdivision surface for head modelling, which shows advantages in key parts of photo-realistic head modelling, i.e., local and smooth deformation, detail presentation and texture coordinates assignment.

3. FEATURE-BASED SEMI-REGULAR GENERIC HEAD MODEL GENERATION

In our approach, we use a displaced butterfly subdivision scheme to build our generic head model from a discrete data set of a human head.

3.1 Background on Butterfly Subdivision Surface

We follow the notation in Hoppe [10] to describe polygonal model: a mesh M is a pair (K,V), where K is a simplicial complex specifying the connectivity of the vertices, edges, and faces; $V=\{\mathbf{v}_1,\mathbf{v}_2,\cdots\}$, $\mathbf{v}_i \in \mathbf{R}^3$ is a set of vertex position defining the shape of M in $\mathbf{R}^3$.

The butterfly scheme S is an interpolating subdivision scheme for triangle meshes. Given S, one subdivision step carries a mesh $M^i=(K^i,V^i)$ to a mesh $M^{i+1}=(K^{i+1},V^{i+1})$ by $M^{i+1}=SM^i$. The set V^{i+1} can be classified into subsets V_v^{i+1} and V_e^{i+1}, where $V_v^{i+1}=V^i$ is related to the vertices in M^i and V_e^{i+1} is related to edges in M^i. The subdivision surface is then defined by recursively applying the refinement $M^{i+1}=SM^i$ on an initial control mesh M^0. Butterfly scheme is first introduced by Dyn [6, 7], which generates C^1-continuous limit surface on a regular control mesh. Zorin [22] proposes a modified butterfly scheme for the generation of C^1-continuous surfaces of arbitrary topology. Since $V_v^{i+1}=V^i$, we only calculate V_e^{i+1} from V^i. Although we do not iteratively subdivide M^0 infinitely, for each vertex in V^i, $i=0,1,2,\cdots$, its exact tangent plane on the limit surface, spanned by two orthogonal tangent vectors t_1 and t_2, can be computed by analysing the eigen-structure of the local subdivision matrix $\mathbf{S}_n$ [8, 21, 22].

3.2 Discrete Data Preprocessing

Given a discrete data set of a human head $H=\{\mathbf{h}_1,\mathbf{h}_2,\cdots,\mathbf{h}_n\}$ (cf. Fig. 1), we extract its topological information by looking for an implicit function f, such that $f(\mathbf{h}_i)=0$, $\forall \mathbf{h}_i \in H$. We numerically determine the implicit function f based on the sign distance function in [9], as summarized in the following three stcps.

1. Build a Riemannian graph $G=(V,E)$ to estimate normal direction for each data point.

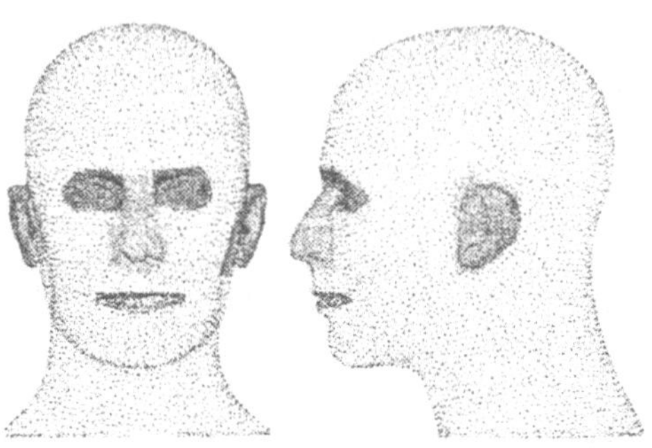

Figure 1. A discrete data set of a human head

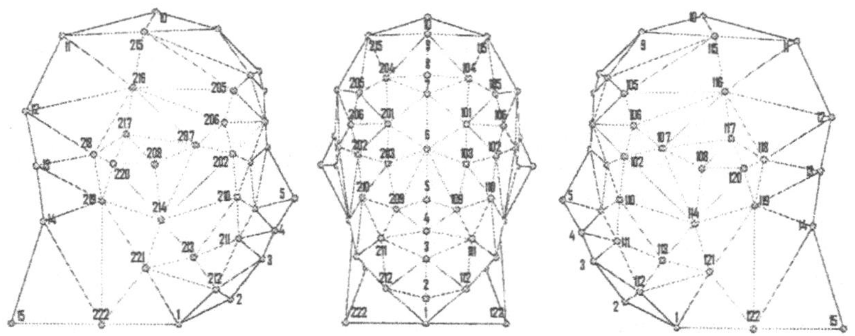

Figure 2. The structure of the predefined 3D feature mesh

2. Extract the minimum spanning tree for graph *G*, which is further traversed in a depth-first search to orient the normal vectors.
3. Use a *k*-nearest-neighbour searching algorithm to numerically determine the value $f(\mathbf{p})$ and the gradient $\nabla f(\mathbf{p})$ for an arbitrary point $\mathbf{p} \in \mathbf{R}^3$.

3.3 Feature Definition

On the human head we define a set of feature points and organize them into a triangular mesh, which we refer to as a *feature mesh* $M^0 = (K^0, V^0)$. Fig.2 illustrates the structure of K^0. The geometric positions of feature points V^0 in $\mathbf{R}^3$ are specified by corresponding points in discrete data. The rules we used to define the ID of feature points are as follows:

- The feature point whose ID number is smaller than 100 lies in symmetry plane.
- The feature point whose ID number is larger than 100 and smaller than 200 lies in left face.

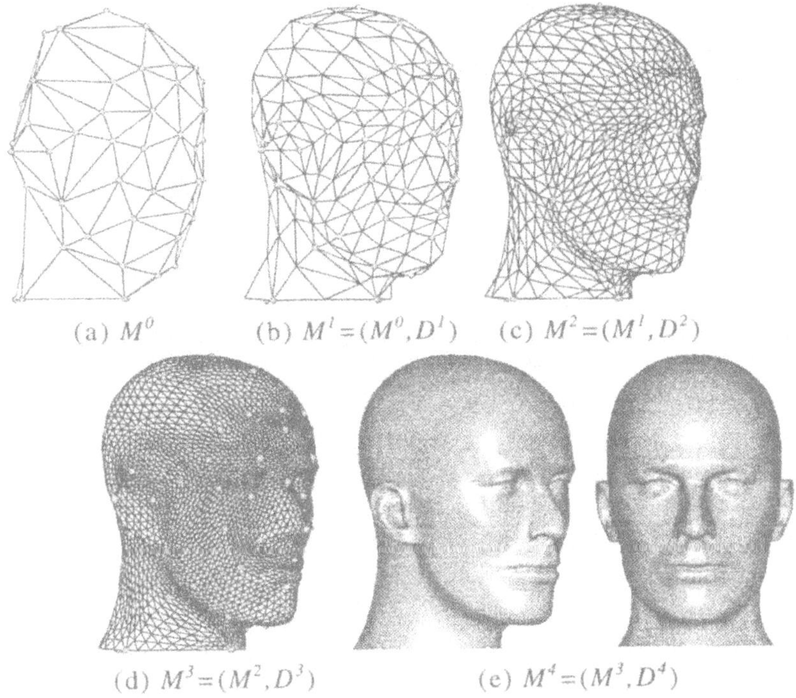

Figure 3. Mesh refinement and its multi-level representation

- The feature point whose ID number is larger than 200 lies in right face, and the feature point 2ij is the symmetrical point of 1ij according to symmetry plane.

3.4 Mesh Refinement

Given a starting mesh M^0, we use a displaced butterfly scheme to refine M^0 to capture full details of the data H. For a given mesh M^i, one refinement step from $M^i=(K^i,V^i)$ to $M^{i+1}=(K^{i+1},V^{i+1})$ consists of two sub-steps: a subdivision step and a displacing step. First, the subdivision step refines mesh $M^i=(K^i,V^i)$ to an intermediate mesh $M^{i+1}=(K^{i+1},V^{i+1})$ using the modified butterfly scheme [22]. For each vertex in V_e^{i+1}, its geometric position and two orthogonal tangent vectors t_1 and t_2 on the limit surface can be calculated using edge and tangent masks. Then in the displacing step $M^{i+1}=(K^{i+1},V^{i+1})\rightarrow M^{i+1}=(K^{i+1},V^{i+1})$, we establish a local frame $\mathbf{F}^{i+1}(j)$ for each vertex $\hat{v}_j^{i+1}\subset V_e^{i+1}$. $\mathbf{F}^{i+1}(j)$ is built up as $\mathbf{F}^{i+1}(j)=(t_1^{i+1}(j),t_2^{i+1}(j),n^{i+1}(j))$, where $n^{i+1}(j)=t_1^{i+1}(j)\times t_2^{i+1}(j)$, $t_1^{i+1}(j)$ and $t_2^{i+1}(j)$ are two unit orthogonal tangent vectors at the position of $\hat{v}_j^{i+1}$. Along the normal direction $n^{i+1}(j)$ in $\mathbf{F}^{i+1}(j)$, we offset each vertex $\hat{v}_j^{i+1}$ to a new position v_j^{i+1}, where $f(v_j^{i+1})=0$.

Starting from M^0, we iteratively perform refinement until we reach the final level 4. As illustrated in Fig. 3, our mesh refinement operation produces a mesh hierarchy M^0, M^1, M^2, M^3, M^4, i.e., our generic head model is semi-regular and is feature-based.

3.5 Multi-Level Displaced Mesh Representation

We represent our feature-based semi-regular head model in multi-levels. Recall that in one refinement step, we first subdivide a mesh $M^i = (K^i, V^i)$ to an intermediate mesh $M^{i+1} = (K^{i+1}, V^{i+1})$ using a modified butterfly scheme S, i.e., $\widehat{M}^{i+1} = SM^i$. $\forall \widehat{v}_j^{i+1} \subset V_e^{i+1}$, $\widehat{v}_j^{i+1} = \mathbf{S}_n V_{mask}^i$, where $\mathbf{S}_n$ is the local subdivision matrix of the scheme S, and $V_{mask}^i \subset V^i$ is a local vertex set in the edge mask of $\widehat{v}_j^{i+1}$. Then in the displacing step, we offset each vertex $\widehat{v}_j^{i+1}$ to v_j^{i+1} along its normal direction $n^{i+1}(j)$ with magnitude $d_j^{\cdot\cdot}$, i.e.,

$$v_j^{i+1} = \widehat{v}_j^{i+1} + d_j^{i+1} n^{i+1}(j) = \mathbf{S}_n V_{mask}^i + d_j^{i+1} n^{i+1}(j) \tag{1}$$

Since local frames $\mathbf{F}^{i+1}(j)$ are self-determined by S and V^i, the vertex set V^{i+1} is fully determined by (S, V^i, D^{i+1}), where D^{i+1} is a detail set D^{i+1} that consists of scalars d_j^{i+1} for each vertex $v_j^{i+1} \subset V_e^{i+1}$, and the topology K^{i+1} is fully determined by (S, K^i). Therefore, our mesh hierarchy can be represented by a feature mesh together with a multi-level scalar detail set, i.e.,

$$M^4 = (M^3, D^4) = (M^2, D^3, D^4) = (M^1, D^2, D^3, D^4) = (M^0, D^1, D^2, D^3, D^4) \tag{2}$$

4. PHOTO-REALISTIC HEAD MODELING

We take a pair of photos of a human subject from the front and side views. We flip the side view photo to obtain one more side view photo. Then we determine a set of 2D features on the photos as follows.

4.1 2D Feature Determination

We organize the vertices in M^0 into seven feature lines. Each feature line has its vision characteristics on photos: the projection of each feature line should be viewable in one or more photos. For each feature line we define several key feature points in it and different feature lines may share common feature points. We first project each feature line onto its viewable photos and interactively determine the corresponding 2D key feature points. We then use the structure snake algorithm [14] to determine the remaining feature point. One example is illustrated in Fig. 4.

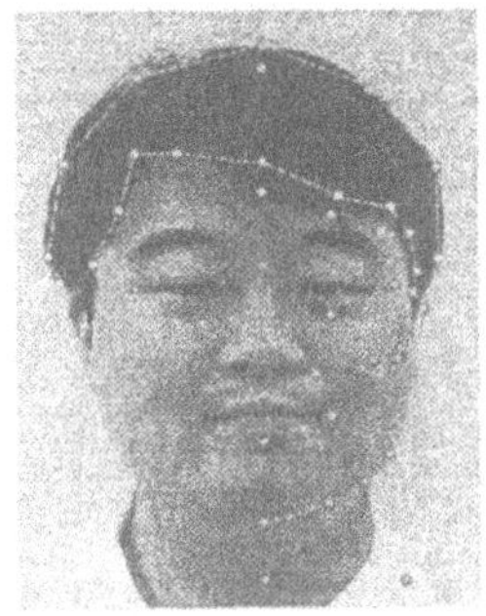
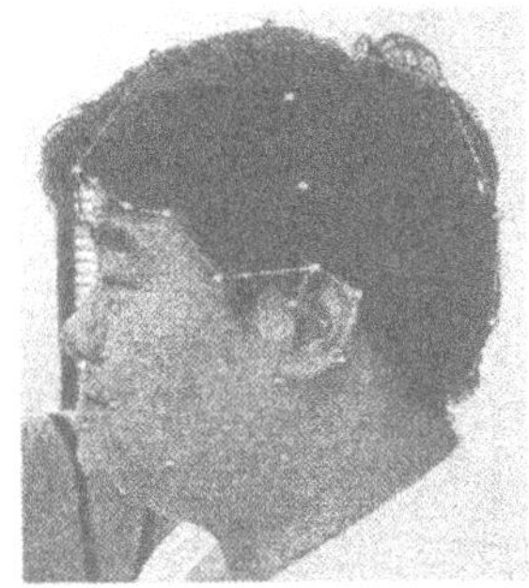

Figure 4. 2D feature determination for individual

To allow more flexibility, we relax the requirement of taking photos from strictly orthogonal directions. We associate a rotation matrix $\boldsymbol{R}$ and a translation vector $\boldsymbol{T}$ to each photo. Using the feature points which are viewable simultaneously on two photos, we calculate $\boldsymbol{R}$ and $\boldsymbol{T}$ for each photo using the structure-from-motion algorithm [20], which is first solved using the Levenberg-Marquardt algorithm [20] and later simplified to a set of linear equations [19].

With $\boldsymbol{R}$ and $\boldsymbol{T}$ for each photo, we recover the 3D coordinates of 2D feature points: if the feature point is viewable in two photos, its exact 3D position can be calculated; if the feature point can only be viewed in one photo, we find its 3D position in the viewing ray nearest to the corresponding vertex in generic model.

4.2 Model Deformation for Individuals

After we specify the 3D position for each vertex in M^0 for individuals, we deform the generic model into a lifelike individualized model using the multi-level representation $(M^0, D^1, D^2, D^3, D^4)$.

Given an individualized feature mesh $\overline{M}^0$, we add back the detail part (D^1, D^2, D^3, D^4) to synthesize an individualized model $\overline{M}^4$. Note that in generic model generation, each scalar detail coefficient d_j^i offsets the vertex v_j^i along the normal direction $n^i(j)$. Starting from $\overline{M}^0$, we first use the same butterfly scheme S to refine a mesh $\overline{M}^i$ to an intermediate mesh $\hat{\overline{M}}^{i+1} = S\overline{M}^i$. We then compute a local frame $\mathbf{F}^{i+1}(j) = (\bar{t}_1^{i+1}(j), \bar{t}_2^{i+1}(j), \bar{n}^{i+1}(j))$ on the fly for each new generated vertex $\hat{\bar{v}}_j^{i+1} \subset \bar{V}_e^{i+1}$ based on $\hat{\overline{M}}^i$ and S. Then along the normal direction $\bar{n}^{i+1}(j)$, we offset each vertex $\bar{v}_j^{i+1}$ with a magnitude d_j^{i+1}. Similar to equation (1), in a mathematic form,

$$\bar{v}_j^{i+1} = \mathbf{S}_n V_{mask}^i + d_j^{i+1} \bar{n}^{i+1}(j) \qquad (3)$$

Now our mesh synthesis process can be described as

$$M^i = (K^i, V^i) \Rightarrow M^{i+1} = (K^{i+1}, V^{i+1}),$$

where $K^{i+1} = SK^i$ and $\overline{V}^{i+1}$ is determined by (S, V^i, D^{i+1}) using equation (3).

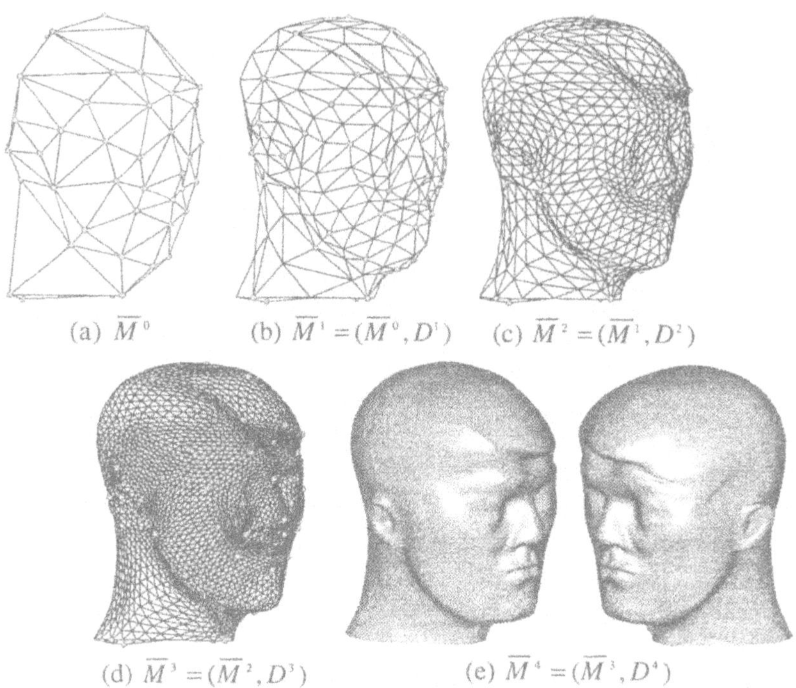

Figure 5. Individualized mesh generation level by level

We synthesize the individualized model level by level based on S and (D^1, D^2, D^3, D^4). See Fig. 5 for an illustration. Since for each level i, every new generated vertex $\bar{v}_j^i$ is offset in its own local frame $F^i(j)$ that build upon a C^1-continuous limit surface, our deformation scheme efficiently guarantees the properties of locality and smoothness.

4.3 Texture Extraction and Texture Coordinates Generation

Generally, there are two types of texture maps used in photo-realistic head modelling: view-dependent and view-independent texture maps. View-dependent texture map blends photos dynamically according to the current viewpoint, and thus, high-frequency details are visible [11, 19]. The price paid for dynamically blending is the need of high memory requirement and low response-speed. Compared with view-dependent maps, the view-independent texture map blends all photos together into a single texture map, and thus, can support rapid display of textured head model from any viewpoints [1, 13, 14]. However, due to the fixed blending weights, the result of view-independent mapping is slightly blurred.

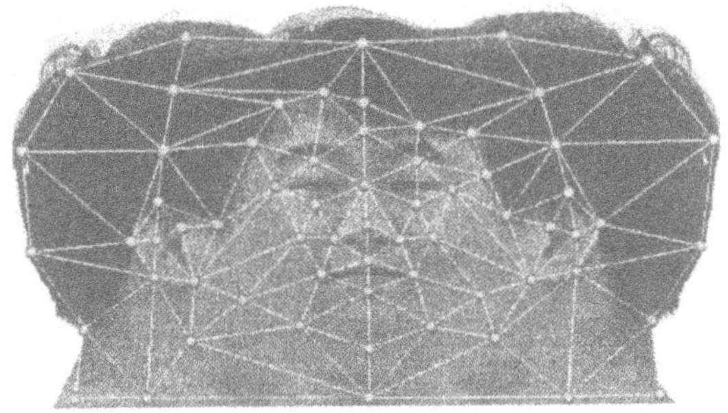

Figure 6. View-independent texture map with the 2D feature mesh

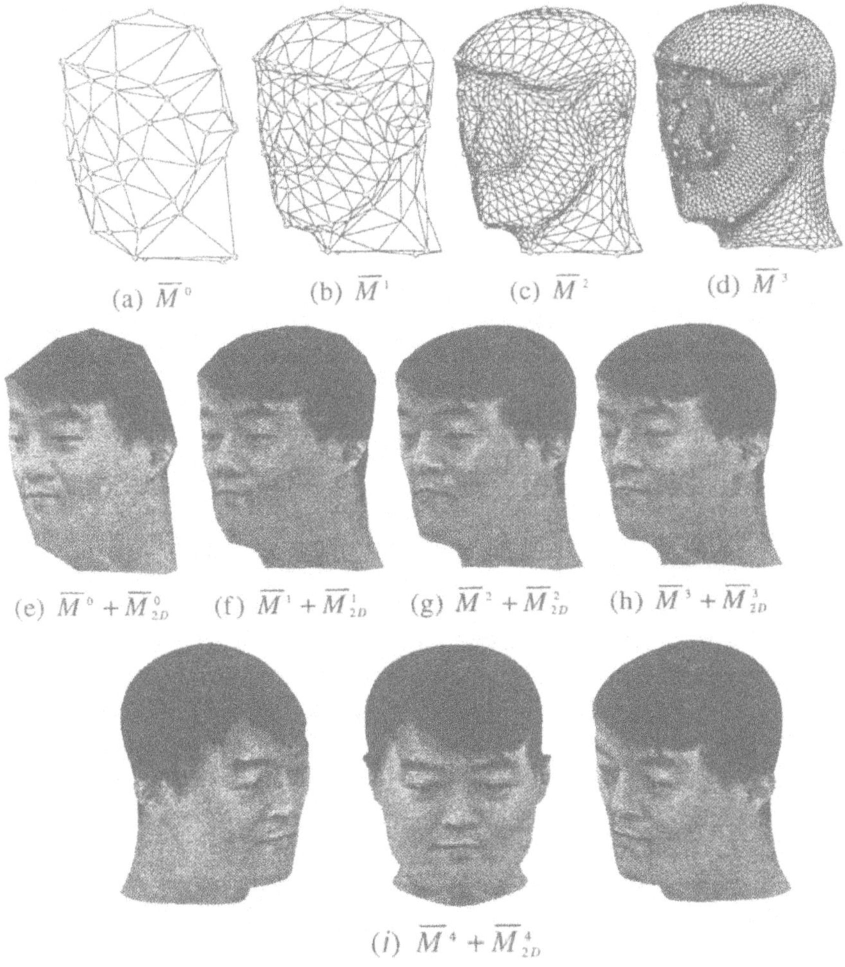

(a) $\overline{M}^0$ (b) $\overline{M}^1$ (c) $\overline{M}^2$ (d) $\overline{M}^3$

(e) $\overline{M}^0 + \overline{M}^0_{2D}$ (f) $\overline{M}^1 + \overline{M}^1_{2D}$ (g) $\overline{M}^2 + \overline{M}^2_{2D}$ (h) $\overline{M}^3 + \overline{M}^3_{2D}$

(*i*) $\overline{M}^4 + \overline{M}^4_{2D}$

Figure 7. Multi-level texture mapping with automatic texture coordinate generation

In our work, we use a view-independent texture map. Based on the set of 2D feature points on each photo, we blend these photos into a view-independent texture map (cf. Fig. 6), which is used for rendering textured head model from any viewpoints. We follow the process in Lee and Thalmann [14] to extract the texture map: photos are first distorted with a predefined index of feature lines, and then, sewed together along feature lines; subsequently a multi-resolution spline technique [3] is applied to remove the boundaries around the sewing regions.

Benefited from our feature-based semi-regular head model, we can automatically assign texture coordinates for the vertices in individualized model $\overline{M}^4$. On the resulting texture map, we build a 2D feature mesh M_{2D}^0, whose vertices are determined by 2D feature points on individual photos. M_{2D}^0 is served as the 2D development of 3D feature mesh $\overline{M}^0$ by splitting it along the feature line 10-11-12-13-14-15 (cf. Fig. 2). We then apply the same butterfly scheme on the 2D feature mesh, i.e., $M_{2D}^{i+1} = SM_{2D}^i$. Thanks to the semi-regular structure of our head model, except the splitting feature line, there is a one-to-one correspondence between the 2D and 3D feature meshes and so hold between the refined meshes $M_{2D}^0, M_{2D}^1, M_{2D}^2, M_{2D}^3, M_{2D}^4$ and M^0, M^1, M^2, M^3, M^4. Note that for $\overline{M}^i$ on each level *i*, every vertex along the splitting feature line 10-11-12-13-14-15 has two separate texture coordinates but identical positions. The 2D meshes M_{2D}^i turned out to be the texture meshes of 3D head models $\overline{M}^i$. To generate a lifelike textured model for individuals, we simply map M_{2D}^i to $\overline{M}^i$ level by level (cf. Fig. 7).

5. CONCLUSION AND FUTURE WORK

In this paper, we propose a feature-based deformable model for photo-realistic head modelling. The key part of our approach is the multi-level displaced representation of our deformable head model. We have demonstrated that using our presented technique, we can generate highly photo-realistic head model for individuals fast and efficiently.

Our feature-based deformable model can be further used in a wide range of applications, which include facial animation, model-based tracking from video, scalar compression for geometry and use of detailed textures for displacements.

REFERENCES

1. Akimoto T., Suenaga Y. Automatic creation of 3D facial models. IEEE Computer Graphics & Applications 1993; 13(5):16-22.

2. Blanz V., Vetter T. A morphable model for the synthesis of 3D faces. Proceedings of SIGGRAPH '99, ACM SIGGRAPH, New York 1999; pp.187-94.
3. Burt P.J., Adelson E.H. A multiresolution spline with application to image mosaics. ACM Transactions on Graphics, 1983; Vol. 2, No. 4, pp 217-36.
4. Catmull E., Clark J. Recursively generated B-spline surfaces on arbitrary topological meshes. Computer-Aided Design 1978; 10(6):350-355.
5. DeCarlo D., Mataxas D., Stone M. An anthropometric face model using variational techniques. Proceedings of SIGGRAPH '98, ACM SIGGRAPH, 1998; pp 67-74.
6. Dyn N., Levin D., Gregory J.A. A 4-point interpolatory subdivision scheme for curve design. Computer Aided Geometric Design 1987; 4:257-68.
7. Dyn N., Levin D., Gregory J.A. A butterfly subdivision scheme for surface interpolation with tension control. ACM Transaction on Graphics 1990; 9(2):160-69.
8. Halstead M. Kass M., DeRose T. Efficient, fair interpolation using catmull-clark surfaces. Proceedings of SIGGRAPH '93, ACM SIGGRAPH, Addison Wesley 1993; pp 35-43.
9. Hoppe H., DeRose T., Duchamp T., Mcdonald J., Stuetzle W. Surface reconstruction from unorganized points. Proceedings of SIGGRAPH '92, ACM SIGGRAPH, Addison Wesley 1992; pp 71-78.
10. Hoppe H., DeRose T., Duchamp T., Halstead M., Jin H., McDonald J., Schweitzer J., Stuetzle W. Piecewise smooth surface reconstruction. Proceedings of SIGGRAPH '94, ACM SIGGRAPH, Addison Wesley 1994; pp 295-302.
11. Horace H.S.I., Yin L.J. Constructing a 3D individualized head model from two orthogonal views. Visual Computer, 1996; vol.12, no.5, pp.254-66.
12. Ko H., Kim M.S., Park H.G., Kim S.W. Face sculpturing robot with recognition capability. Computer Aided Design 1994; 26(11):814-21.
13. Kurihara T., Arai K. A transformation method for modeling and animation of the human face from photographs. Proceeding of Computer Animation '91, Springer-Verlag Tokyo 1991; pp. 45-58.
14. Lee W.S., Magnenat-Thalmann N. Fast head modeling for animation. Image & Vision Computing 2000; 18(4):355-64.
15. Lee Y., Terzopoulos D., Waters K. Realistic modeling for facial animation. Proceedings for SIGGRAPH '95, New York 1995; pp 55-62.
16. Loop C. Smooth subdivision surfaces based on triangles. Master thesis, 1987, Department of Mathematics, University of Utah.
17. Parke F.I. A parametric model for human faces. PhD dissertation, 1974, Univ. Utah.
18. Parke F.I., Waters K. *Computer facial animation*. Wellesley, Massachusetts, 1996.
19. Pingin F., Hecker J., Lischinski D., Szeliski R., Salesin D.H. Synthesizing realistic facial expressions from photographs. Proceedings of SIGGRAPH '98, ACM SIGGRAPH, Addison Wesley 1998; pp 75-84.
20. Szeliski R., Kang S.B. Recovering 3D shape and motion from image streams using nonlinear least squares. Journal of Visual Communication and Image Representation, 1994; 5(1):10-28.
21. Zorin D., Schroder P. Subdivsion for modeling and animation. SIGGRAPH Course Notes, 2000.
22. Zorin D., Schroder P., Sweldens W. Interpolating subdivision for meshes with arbitrary topology. Proceedings of SIGGRAPH '96, ACM SIGGRAPH, Addison Wesley 1996; pp 189-92.

MULTIRESOLUTION MODELING AND INTERACTIVE DEFORMATION OF LARGE 3D MESHES

Jens Vorsatz and Hans-Peter Seidel
Max-Planck-Institut für Informatik

Keywords: Multiresolution, Modeling, Mesh, Deformation

Abstract Due to their simplicity triangle meshes are often used to represent geometric surfaces. Their main drawback is the large number of triangles that are required to represent a smooth surface. This problem has been addressed by a large number of mesh simplification algorithms which reduce the number of triangles and approximate the initial mesh. Hierarchical triangle mesh representations provide access to a triangle mesh at a desired resolution, without omitting any information.

In this paper we demonstrate how a hierarchical structure of a mesh can be derived for arbitrary meshes to enable intuitive and efficient modifications without restrictions on the underlying connectivity. We combine mesh reduction algorithms and constrained energy minimization to decompose the given mesh into several frequency bands and focus on a stabilizing technique to encode the geometric difference between the levels.

Introduction

Modification of complex 3D geometric shapes is a challenging task required for a wide variety of applications, for instance animation and design. Usually, this is done by editing a freeform surface, which represents the outer skin of a solid object. Like their real world equivalent, the surfaces often carry detail information on various scales such as skin wrinkles in the context of animation or e.g. the company sign on an engine hood. Certainly it is desirable to preserve these features while editing the global shape of the surface. During the last years, hierarchical multiresolution representations of geometric shape have become the de facto standard for those purposes.

The basic idea is to separate the high frequency detail from the low frequency shape and encode each detail level relative to a local coordinate

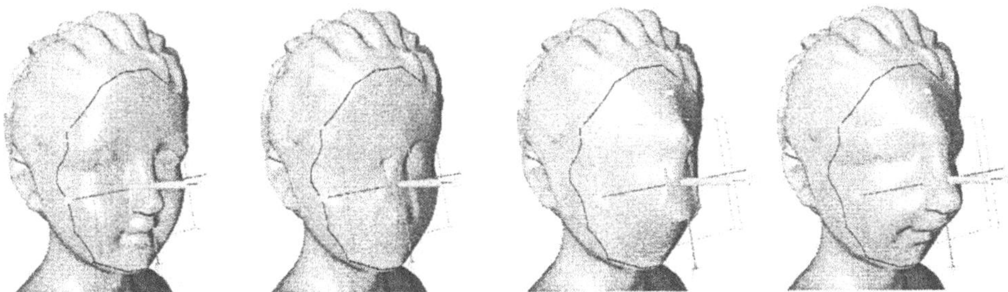

Figure 1 Multiresolution edit: In the area of interest (blue line), the original mesh (outer left) is decomposed into two frequency bands. The geometric difference between the high frequency detail (outer left) and the low frequency shape (center left) is stored with respect to local frames. A designer changes the low frequency shape by shifting the green polygon (center right). Adding the previously stored detail information yields the final result (outer right).

frame induced by the lower frequency shape. That way modifications on a coarser level can be propagated to the finer ones (cf. Fig. 1). More formally, given an arbitrary surface $\mathcal{S}_m$, a multiresolution *decomposition* consists of a sequence of topologically equivalent surfaces $\mathcal{S}_{m-1}, \ldots, \mathcal{S}_0$ with decreasing level of geometric detail. The difference $\mathcal{D}_i = \mathcal{S}_{i+1} - \mathcal{S}_i$ between two successive surfaces is the *detail* on level i which is added or removed when switching between the two approximations. The reconstruction $\mathcal{S}_m = \mathcal{S}_i + \mathcal{D}_i + \ldots + \mathcal{D}_{m-1}$ of the original surface $\mathcal{S}_m$ can start on any level of detail $\mathcal{S}_i$. Multiresolution modeling means that on some level of detail, the surface $\mathcal{S}_i$ is replaced by $\mathcal{S}'_i$. This operation does not have any effect on $\mathcal{S}_0, \ldots, \mathcal{S}_{i-1}$ but $\mathcal{D}_{i-1}$ and hence $\mathcal{S}_{i+1}, \ldots, \mathcal{S}_m$ change since the (unchanged) detail information $\mathcal{D}_i, \ldots, \mathcal{D}_{m-1}$ is now added to the modified base surface $\mathcal{S}'_i$ for the reconstruction of $\mathcal{S}'_m$. In order to guarantee the intuitive preservation of the shape characteristics after a modification on some lower level of detail, this basic setting has to be extended such that the detail information $\mathcal{D}_i$ is encoded with respect to *local frames*. These frames are aligned to the surface geometry of $\mathcal{S}_i$

Fundamental work in this area, based on splines and wavelets, was done by Forsey and Barthels [Forsey and Bartels, 1988, Forsey and Bartels, 1995], Lee et al. [Lee et al., 1997, Lee, 1999], and Gortler and Cohen [Gortler and Cohen, 1995]. Though splines have a straight forward shape control mechanism based on control vertices, it is well-known to be rather complicated to preserve boundary conditions when handling complex geometry.

This is just one of the reasons, why the interest in surface representations in the context of multiresolution editing based on triangular meshes has increased over the last years. Generalizing the patch-based concepts, the wide family of subdivision techniques starts with a coarse base mesh approximating a geometric shape of arbitrary topology and refines it iteratively. An exponential number of vertices is introduced to capture finer detail information, until a prescribed tolerance is reached. This bottom-up approach generates the so-called subdivision-connectivity, which means, that sub-regions of the refined mesh which correspond to a single triangle in the base mesh have the connectivity of regular grids. To separate the high-frequency from the low-frequency, again, one defines decomposition and reconstruction operations. The reconstruction operator is given by the underlying subdivision scheme. To transform a mesh $\mathcal{M}_m$ to the next refinement level $\mathcal{M}'_{m+1} = \mathbf{S}\mathcal{M}_m$ one applies the subdivision operator $\mathbf{S}$ and moves the obtained control vertices by adding the associated detail vectors: $\mathcal{M}_{m+1} = \mathcal{M}'_{m+1} + \mathcal{D}_m$. One can think of the decomposition operator as the inverse of the subdivision operator, i.e. given a fine mesh $\mathcal{M}_{m+1}$ one has to find a mesh $\mathcal{M}_m$ such that $\mathcal{M}_{m+1} \approx \mathbf{S}\mathcal{M}_m$. This can be achieved by solving a minimization problem or more efficiently by discrete fairing [Zorin et al., 1997]. In this case the detail vectors $\mathcal{D}_m := \mathcal{M}_{m+1} - \mathbf{S}\mathcal{M}_m$ become as small as possible.

To achieve the desired multiresolution edit, one shifts a control vertex $\mathbf{p}_i^m$ in $\mathcal{M}_m$. This has influence on several control vertices in the finer levels and causes a smooth bump in the resulting surface while maintaining the high-frequency detail information. The underlying low frequency geometry on each level can be computed by applying the reconstruction operator $\mathbf{S}$ without detail reconstruction ($\mathcal{D}_m := 0$).

One problem which is inherent to multiresolution representations of freeform geometry based on subdivision surfaces is the fixed support of a modification. If control vertices are used as handles to modify the surface on a certain level of detail, the region that actually changes its shape is determined by the support of the associated basis functions. One could simulate more flexibility by moving several vertices at a time, but this annihilates the mathematical elegance of the representation.

Moreover, in practice it is rather unlikely that a mesh with subdivision–connectivity is given as input. For instance 3D acquisition of geometric data with a range scanning device followed by a triangulation or the conversion of CAD data, often result in a triangle mesh with arbitrary connectivity. For this reason sophisticated schemes have been presented to approximate an arbitrary input mesh with one having subdivision–connectivity [Eck et al., 1995, Lee et al., 1998, Kobbelt et al., 1999]. But besides being computationally expensive, the conversion is always a resampling process which gives rise to sampling artifacts. A popular way to avoid the described problem is to build the hierarchical structure the other way around i.e from fine to coarse. For this, techniques which adapt the mesh-complexity to the available hardware resources emerging from another branch in computer graphics can be used . Multiple levels of resolution are produced by incrementally decimating the fine mesh [Garland and Heckbert, 1997, Hoppe, 1996, Kobbelt et al., 1998a, Lindstrom, 2000]. This is often done by applying a decomposition operator, that successively collapses edges and removes the redundant vertices and faces. To capture the detail information, which would be lost otherwise, again, detail vectors have to be stored. For a hierarchical representation, a proper reconstruction has to be ensured. Hence, we need a base point, where the detail vector could be attached to. In contrast to the subdivision scheme, where the base point is predicted by the subdivision operator, no such point exists for the coarse to fine approach, since the mesh-connectivity does not provide the necessary regular structure. For this reason, a vertex removal is split into two steps. First, the original position is altered such that local fairness is achieved. Only recently, a couple of new techniques have been proposed [Taubin, 1995, Kobbelt, 1997, Kobbelt et al., 1998b, Guskov et al., 1999, Schneider and Kobbelt, 2001]. The second step removes the original vertex and encodes the position with respect to its minimized counterpart.

This would require a fairing step for every single vertex. One could also apply the fairing operation to *all* vertices before storing the detail information to lower the computational costs. This would lead to a two-band representation, i.e. a smoothed version, and the original mesh linked by the detail vectors. In practice, a multi-band hierarchy, similar to a level of detail representation would be desirable. This could reflect the multiple scales of features on the surface to stabilize the modeling-process on the one hand and keep down the costs on the other hand.

Hence, to build an appropriate hierarchical structure of a triangular mesh for our modeling purposes, we have to solve two problems. First, we have to choose the right intermediate frequency-bands, such that a modification of a coarser level will lead to reasonable alternation of the finer ones. On the other hand, the detail has to be encoded with respect to a proper base point, to ensure a stable reconstruction. The following sections discuss several approaches for both problems.

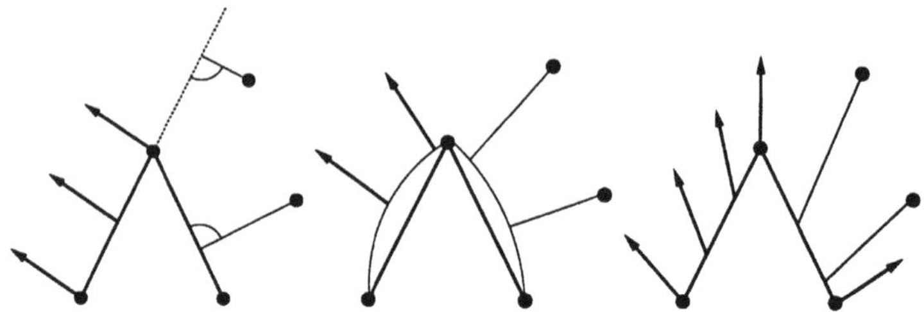

Figure 2 The position of a vertex (loose points) in the original mesh (high-frequency geometry) is given by a base point on the low-frequency geometry plus a displacement in normal direction. There are many ways to define a normal field on a triangle mesh. With piecewise constant normals (left) we do not cover the whole space and hence we sometimes have to use virtual base points with negative barycentric coordinates. The sketch shows, that this can lead to non intuitive reconstructions, if the 'base mesh' is for example flattened out. The use of local quadratic patches and their normal fields (center) somewhat improves the situation but problems still occur since the overall normal field is not globally continuous. Such difficulties are avoided if we generate a Phong-type normal field by blending estimated vertex normals (right).

1. DETAIL ENCODING

As mentioned before, we cannot simply store the detail vectors with respect to a global coordinate system but we have to define them with respect to local frames which are aligned to the low-frequency geometry. This guarantees an intuitive detail preservation under modification of the global shape. Usually, the associated local frame for each vertex has its origin at the location predicted by the smoothing operator (reconstruction operator with suppressed detail). However, in many cases this can lead to rather long detail vectors with a significant component within the local tangent plane. Since we prefer short detail vectors for stability reasons, it makes sense to use a different origin for the local frame. In fact, the optimal choice is to find that point on the low-frequency surface whose normal vector points directly to the original vertex. In this case, the detail is not given by a three dimensional vector $(\triangle x, \triangle y, \triangle z)^T$ but rather by a base point $\mathbf{p} = \mathbf{p}(u, v)$ on the low-frequency geometry plus a scalar value h for the displacement in normal direction. If a local parameterization of the surface is available, the base point $\mathbf{p}$ can be specified by a two-dimensional parameter value (u, v).

The general setting for detail computation is that we have given two meshes $\mathcal{M}_{m+1}$ and $\mathcal{M}'_{m+1}$ where $\mathcal{M}_{m+1}$ is the original data while $\mathcal{M}'_{m+1}$ is reconstructed from the low-frequency approximation $\mathcal{M}_m$ with suppressed detail, i.e. for coarse-to-fine hierarchies, the mesh $\mathcal{M}'_{m+1}$ is generated by applying a stationary subdivision scheme and for fine-to-coarse hierarchies $\mathcal{M}'_{m+1}$ is optimal with respect to some global bending energy functional. Encoding the geometric difference between both meshes requires to associate each vertex $\mathbf{p}$ of $\mathcal{M}_{m+1}$ with a corresponding base point $\mathbf{q}$ on the continuous (piecewise linear) surface $\mathcal{M}'_{m+1}$ such that the difference vector between the original point and the base point is parallel to the normal vector at the base point. An arbitrary point $\mathbf{q}$ on $\mathcal{M}'_{m+1}$ can be specified by a triangle index i and barycentric coordinates within the referred triangle.

To actually compute the detail coefficients, we have to define a normal field on the mesh $\mathcal{M}'_{m+1}$. The most simple way to do this is to use the normal vectors of the triangular faces for the definition of a piecewise constant normal field. This projection can be computed efficiently and works fine, if the resulting coefficient is short compared to the edges of the assigned triangle and if $\mathcal{M}'_{m+1}$ is sufficiently smooth. But since the orthogonal prisms spanned by a triangle mesh do not completely cover the vicinity of the mesh, we have to accept negative barycentric coordinates for the base points if it does not lie within such a prism. This leads to non-intuitive detail reconstruction if the low-frequency geometry is modified (cf. Fig 2).

A technique used in [Kobbelt et al., 1998b] is based on the construction of a local quadratic interpolant $\mathbf{F}$ to the low-frequency geometry. For a vertex $\mathbf{p} \in \mathcal{M}_{m+1}$ it is based on the closest triangle $\mathbf{T} \in \mathcal{M}'_{m+1}$ and its adjacent vertices, which can be found in linear time by a simple local search procedure, starting from $\mathbf{p}$'s corresponding vertex $\mathbf{p}' \in \mathcal{M}_{m+1}$. Since now a local parameterization is given, parameter values (u,v) defining the base point $\mathbf{q}$ can be found by Newton-iteration. We start from the center of $\mathbf{T}$ at $\mathbf{q}_0 = \mathbf{F}(\frac{1}{3}, \frac{1}{3})$, $\mathbf{q}_{n+1}$ is defined by the projection of $\mathbf{p}$ into the tangent plane of $\mathbf{F}$ at $\mathbf{q}_n$. In terms of parameter values (u, v), this leads to the simple update rule $(u_{n+1}, v_{n+1}) \leftarrow (u_n, v_n) + (\triangle u, \triangle v)$, where $(\triangle u, \triangle v)$ is the solution of the linear system

$$\begin{pmatrix} F_u^T F_u & F_u^T F_v \\ F_u^T F_v & F_v^T F_v \end{pmatrix} \begin{pmatrix} \triangle u \\ \triangle v \end{pmatrix} = \begin{pmatrix} F_u^T d \\ F_v^T d \end{pmatrix} \tag{1}$$

with detail vector $\mathbf{d} = \mathbf{p} - \mathbf{q}_n$, which is perpendicular (within a prescribed tolerance) to $\mathbf{F}(u_n, v_n)$ after a few steps. The absolute value of the displacement-coefficient h is set to $\|\mathbf{d}\|$ and has to be multiplied by -1 if $d^T(f_u(u_n, v_n) \times f_v(u_n, v_n)) < 0$. Although this reduces the number of pathological configurations with negative barycentric coordinates for the base point, we still observe artifact in the reconstructed high-frequency surface which are caused by the fact that the resulting global normal field of the combined local patches is not continuous (cf. Fig 2 middle).

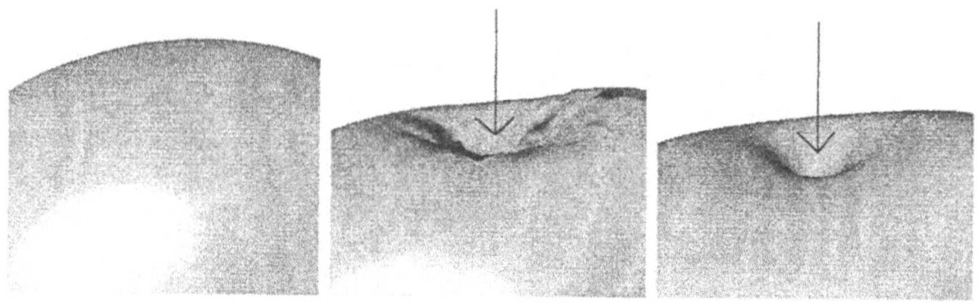

Figure 3 The original shape (left) is modified by pushing a single vertex while minimizing a membrane energy functional. A piecewise linear normal field leads to undesirable mesh artifacts (middle), while storing detail information with respect to a Phong normal field (left) performs a satisfying modification.

We therefore propose a different approach which adapts the basic idea of Phong-shading [Foley et al., 1990] where normal vectors are prescribed at the vertices of a triangle mesh and a continuous normal field for the interior of the triangular faces is computed by linearly blending the normal vectors at the corners. We use the same search procedure as described above and obtain a triangle $\triangle(\mathbf{a}, \mathbf{b}, \mathbf{c})$ with the associated normal vectors $N_{\mathbf{a}}$, $N_{\mathbf{b}}$, and $N_{\mathbf{c}}$. For each interior point

$$\mathbf{q} = \alpha\,\mathbf{a} + \beta\,\mathbf{b} + \gamma\,\mathbf{c}$$

with $\alpha + \beta + \gamma = 1$ we find the associated normal vector $N_{\mathbf{q}}$ by

$$N_{\mathbf{q}} = \alpha\,N_{\mathbf{a}} + \beta\,N_{\mathbf{b}} + \gamma\,N_{\mathbf{c}}.$$

When computing the detail coefficients for a given point $\mathbf{p}$ we have to find the base point $\mathbf{q}$ such that

$$(\mathbf{p} - \mathbf{q}) \times N_{\mathbf{q}}$$

has all three coordinates vanishing. By plugging in the definition of $\mathbf{q}$ and $N_{\mathbf{q}}$ and eliminating $\gamma = 1 - \alpha - \beta$ we obtain a bivariate quadratic function

$$F \; : \; (u, v) \rightarrow \mathbf{R}^3$$

and we have to find the parameter value (α, β) such that $F(\alpha, \beta) = (0, 0, 0)^T$. Again, this can be accomplished by performing several steps of Newton-iteration. Notice that F can be interpreted as a quadratic surface patch in $\mathbf{R}^3$ which passes through the origin. The Taylor-coefficients of F can explicitly be given by

$$\begin{aligned}
F(0,0) &= W + WW \\
F_u(0,0) &= U + UW - W - 2WW \\
F_v(0,0) &= V + VW - W - 2WW \\
F_{uu}(0,0) &= UU - UW + WW \\
F_{uv}(0,0) &= UV - UW - VW + 2WW \\
F_{vv}(0,0) &= VV - VW + WW
\end{aligned}$$

where

$$\begin{aligned}
U &= \mathbf{p} \times N_{\mathbf{a}} \\
V &= \mathbf{p} \times N_{\mathbf{b}} \\
W &= \mathbf{p} \times N_{\mathbf{c}} \\
UU &= N_{\mathbf{a}} \times \mathbf{a} \\
VV &= N_{\mathbf{b}} \times \mathbf{b} \\
WW &= N_{\mathbf{c}} \times \mathbf{c} \\
UV &= (N_{\mathbf{b}} \times \mathbf{a}) + (N_{\mathbf{a}} \times \mathbf{b}) \\
UW &= (N_{\mathbf{c}} \times \mathbf{a}) + (N_{\mathbf{a}} \times \mathbf{c}) \\
VW &= (N_{\mathbf{c}} \times \mathbf{b}) + (N_{\mathbf{b}} \times \mathbf{c})
\end{aligned}$$

This leads to a similar update rule as described in 1. Starting with $(\alpha_0, \beta_0) = (\frac{1}{3}, \frac{1}{3})$, the difference $(\Delta\alpha, \Delta\beta)$ between two consecutive steps can be denoted as follows.

$$\begin{aligned}
\Delta\alpha &= (F_u^T F_v \cdot F_v^T F - F_v^T F_v \cdot F_u^T F)/s \\
\Delta\beta &= (F_u^T F_v \cdot F_u^T F - F_u^T F_u \cdot F_v^T F)/s
\end{aligned}$$

with $s = F_u^T F_u \cdot F_v^T F_v - (F_u F_v)^2$.

In case one of the barycentric coordinates of the resulting point $\mathbf{q}$ is negative, we continue the search for a base point in the corresponding neighboring triangle. Since the Phong normal field is globally continuous we always find a base point with positive barycentric coordinates. Fig. 2 depicts the situation schematically and Fig. 3 shows an example edit where the piecewise constant normal field causes mesh artifacts which do not occur if the Phong normal field is used.

2. HIERARCHY LEVELS

For coarse-to-fine hierarchies the levels of detail are determined by the uniform refinement operator. Starting with the base mesh $\mathcal{M}_0$, the mth refinement level is reached after applying the refinement operator m times. For fine-to-coarse hierarchies there is no such canonical choice for the levels of resolution. Hence we have to figure out some heuristics to define such levels.

In [Kobbelt et al., 1998b] a simple two-band decomposition has been proposed for the modeling, i.e. the high frequency geometry is given

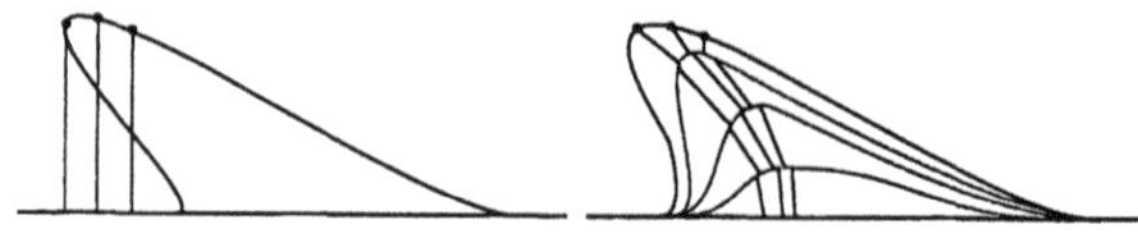

Figure 4 If the high-frequency detail cannot be projected onto the successive level (left), intermediate levels have to be inserted to guarantee a feasible detail reconstruction (right).

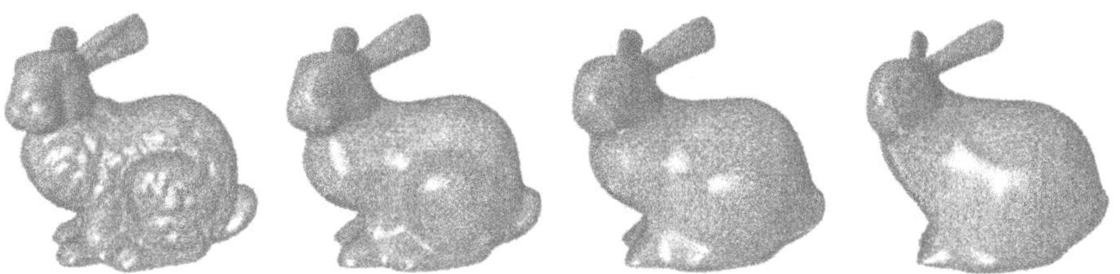

Figure 5 Four versions of the Stanford bunny. The smoother versions are generated by applying mesh decimation down to a certain target complexity and re–inserting the vertices under minimization of some discrete fairness functional. The degree by which geometric detail is removed depends on the coarseness of the base mesh. Notice that all shown meshes share the same connectivity.

by the original mesh and the low-frequency geometry is the solution of some constrained optimization problem. This simple decomposition performs well if the original geometry can be projected onto the low-frequency geometry without self-intersections. Fig 4 schematically shows a configuration where this is not satisfied and consequently the detail feature does not deform intuitively with the change of the global shape.

This effect can be avoided by introducing several intermediate levels of detail, i.e., by using a true multi-band decomposition. The definition of the Phong-type normal field introduced in the last section provides the means to guarantee a stable reconstruction. The number of hierarchy levels has to be chosen such that the $(i+1)$st level can be projected onto level i without self-intersection. Detail information has to be computed for every intermediate level.

Intermediate levels can be generated by the following algorithm (see Fig. 5). We start with the original mesh and apply an incremental mesh decimation algorithm which performs a sequence of edge collapse operations. When a certain mesh complexity is reached, we perform the reverse sequence of vertex split operations which reconstructs the original mesh connectivity. The position of the re-inserted vertices is found

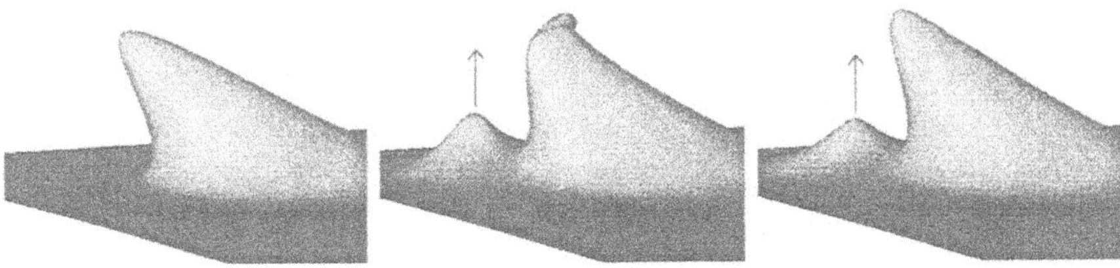

Figure 6 Starting from the original shape (left), a two-band decomposition (middle) can lead to long detail-vectors and hence to exaggerated modifications or even self-intersections for relatively small edits. Multiple levels of detail avoid these artifacts and the modifications behave in a natural fashion (right).

by solving a global bending energy minimization problem [Kobbelt, 1997, Kobbelt et al., 1998b, Guskov et al., 1999, Schneider and Kobbelt, 2001]. The mesh that results from this procedure is a smoothed version of the original mesh where the degree by which detail information has been removed depends on the target complexity of the decimation algorithm.

Suppose the original mesh has n_m vertices, where m is the number of intermediate levels that we want to generate. We can compute the meshes $\mathcal{M}_m, \ldots, \mathcal{M}_0$ with fewer detail by applying the above procedure where the decimation algorithm stops at a target resolution of $n_m, \ldots, n_0$ remaining vertices respectively. The resulting meshes yield a multi-band decomposition of the original data. When a modeling operation changes the shape of $\mathcal{M}_0$ we first reconstruct the next level $\mathcal{M}'_1$ by adding the stored detail vectors and then proceed by successively reconstructing $\mathcal{M}'_{i+1}$ from $\mathcal{M}'_i$.

The remaining question is how to determine the numbers n_i. A simple way to do this is to build a geometric sequence with $n_{i+1}/n_i = \text{const}$ This mimics the exponential complexity growth of the coarse-to-fine hierarchies. Another approach is to stop the decimation every time a certain average edge length $\bar{l}_i$ in the remaining mesh is reached.

A more complicated heuristic tries to equalize the sizes of the differences between levels, i.e., the sizes of the detail vectors. We first compute a multi-band decomposition with, say, 100 levels of detail where we choose $\sqrt[i]{\bar{n}_i} = \text{const.}$. For every pair of successive levels we can compute the average length of the detail vectors (displacement values). From this information we can easily choose appropriate values $n_j = \bar{n}_{i_j}$ such that the geometric difference is distributed evenly among the detail levels.

In practice it turned out that about five intermediate levels is usually enough to guarantee correct detail reconstruction. Fig. 6 compares the results of a modeling operation based on a two-band and a multi-band decomposition.

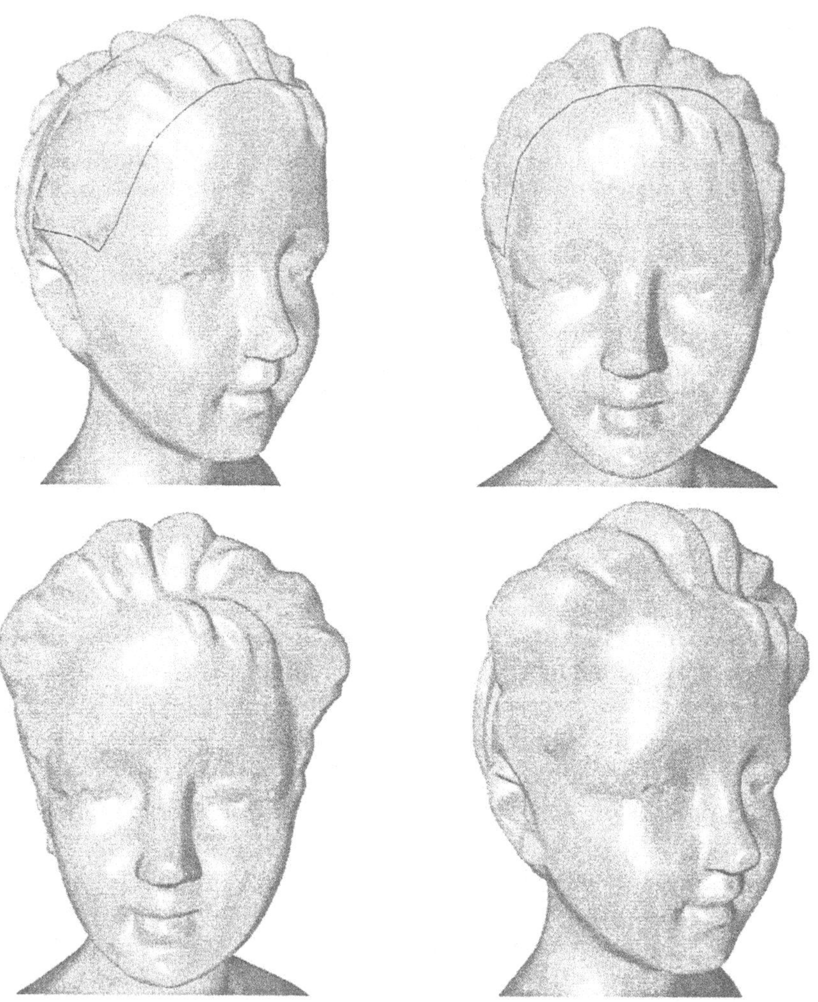

Figure 7 Multiresolution editing of a bust model. The area within the blue line is decomposed into two frequency-bands. The user changes the handle polygon (green) and thus changes the low-frequency surface on top of which the recorded detail based on a Phong-type normal field is reconstructed (lower row).

3. CONCLUSION

We have shown how one can derive a robust hierarchical structure of a triangle mesh with arbitrary connectivity. This enables efficient edits of a complex mesh in an intuitive manner. A designer can apply global deformations without losing detail information inherent to the surface. In particular, we have focused on a method to encode high-frequence detail with respect to a low-frequency base mesh. However, the user can still apply particular edits, where undesirable effects like self intersection of detail vectors during the reconstruction process happen. Moreover, due to the fixed mesh-connectivity, extreme stretches of triangles can occur. We are currently developing a system, which handles changes of the mesh during the modeling process, i.e. insertion of vertices, where the mesh is locally stretched and vertex removal, where the triangle size undergoes a given threshold. We are also keeping track of a promising approach to avoid self intersection without changing the mesh-connectivity.

References

[Eck et al., 1995] Eck, M., DeRose, T., Duchamp, T., Hoppe, H., Lounsbery, M., and Stuetzle, W. (1995). Multiresolution Analysis of Arbitrary Meshes. In *Computer Graphics (SIGGRAPH 95 Proceedings)*, pages 173–182.

[Foley et al., 1990] Foley, van Dam, Feiner, and Hughes (1990). *Computer Graphics*. Addison Wesley.

[Forsey and Bartels, 1988] Forsey, D. R. and Bartels, R. H. (1988). Hierarchical B-spline refinement. In *Computer Graphics (SIGGRAPH 88 Proceedings)*, pages 205–212.

[Forsey and Bartels, 1995] Forsey, D. R. and Bartels, R. H. (1995). Surface Fitting with Hierarchical Splines. *ACM Transactions on Graphics*, 14(2):134–161.

[Garland and Heckbert, 1997] Garland, M. and Heckbert, P. S. (1997). Surface Simplification Using Quadric Error Metrics. In *Computer Graphics (SIGGRAPH 97 Proceedings)*, pages 209–218.

[Gortler and Cohen, 1995] Gortler, S. J. and Cohen, M. F. (1995). Hierarchical and variational geometric modeling with wavelets. In *1995 Symposium on Interactive 3D Graphics*, pages 35–42.

[Guskov et al., 1999] Guskov, I., Sweldens, W., and Schröder, P. (1999). Multiresolution signal processing for meshes. In *Computer Graphics (SIGGRAPH 99 Proceedings)*, pages 325–334.

[Hoppe, 1996] Hoppe, H. (1996). Progressive Meshes. In *Computer Graphics (SIGGRAPH 96 Proceedings)*, pages 99–108.

[Kobbelt, 1997] Kobbelt, L. (1997). Discrete fairing. In *Proceedings of the Seventh IMA Conference on the Mathematics of Surfaces*, pages 101–131.

[Kobbelt et al., 1998a] Kobbelt, L., Campagna, S., and Seidel, H.-P. (1998a). A general framework for mesh decimation. In *Proceedings of the Graphics Interface Conference '98*, pages 43–50.

[Kobbelt et al., 1998b] Kobbelt, L., Campagna, S., Vorsatz, J., and Seidel, H.-P. (1998b). Interactive multi-resolution modeling on arbitrary meshes. In *Computer Graphics (SIGGRAPH 98 Proceedings)*, pages 105–114.

[Kobbelt et al., 1999] Kobbelt, L., Vorsatz, J., Labsik, U., and Seidel, H.-P. (1999). A shrink wrapping approach to remeshing polygonal surfaces. *Computer Graphics Forum, Proceedings of Eurographics '99*, 18(3):119–130.

[Lee et al., 1998] Lee, A., Sweldens, W., Schröder, P., Cowsar, L., and Dobkin, D. (1998). Multiresolution adaptive parameterization of surfaces. In *Computer Graphics (SIGGRAPH 98 Proceedings)*, pages 95–104.

[Lee, 1999] Lee, S. (1999). Interactive multiresolution editing of arbitrary meshes. *Computer Graphics Forum, Proceedings of Eurographics '99*, 18(3):73–82.

[Lee et al., 1997] Lee, S., Wolberg, G., and Shin, S. Y. (1997). Scattered data interpolation with multilevel B-splines. *IEEE Transactions on Visualization and Computer Graphics*, 3(3):228–244.

[Lindstrom, 2000] Lindstrom, P. (2000). Out-of-core simplification of large polygonal models. In *Computer Graphics (SIGGRAPH 00 Proceedings)*, pages 259–262.

[Schneider and Kobbelt, 2001] Schneider, R. and Kobbelt, L. (2001). Geometric fairing of irregular meshes for free–form surface design. *CAGD (to appear)*.

[Taubin, 1995] Taubin, G. (1995). A signal processing approach to fair surface design. In *Computer Graphics (SIGGRAPH 95 Proceedings)*, pages 351–358.

[Zorin et al., 1997] Zorin, D., Schröder, P., and Sweldens, W. (1997). Interactive multiresolution mesh editing. In *Computer Graphics (SIGGRAPH 97 Proceedings)*, pages 259–268.

LOCALLY INTERPOLATING SUBDIVISION SURFACES SUPPORTING FREE-FORM 2D DEFORMATIONS

J. Claes[1], F. van Reeth[2] and M. Ramaekers[2]
[1]University of the Balearic Islands, Spain; [2]Limburg University Centre, Belgium

Key words: free-form deformation, 2D computer animation, subdivision surfaces, Loop subdivision, texture mapping

Abstract: This paper addresses the application of free-form deformations to arbitrarily shaped 2D textured objects, solving specific problems. Based on subdivision surfaces applied in 2D, our method successfully combines the following features: fluid good-looking movement, both general global and precise local control and explicit discontinuities. Moreover we implemented an extension to the approximating subdivision scheme, providing local interpolation and accurate border control.

1. INTRODUCTION

This paper describes a free-form deformation scheme dealing with 2D animated objects. As animations are mostly shown as moving 2D images, it often suffices to decide about the movements in two dimensions only to create convincible animations. This does not work out properly when physically correct movements are needed, but is very suitable to informally deliver creative ideas to a viewer.

The following requirements showed up for free-form deformations suited to accomplish this goal:

- Allow fluid movement, not only at the border, but also at the interior of the animated object, making sure the texture parameterisation of the surface is deformed in a smooth, natural looking way.

- Both global control - needing limited user interaction - and fine local control near specified joints should be integrated into one consistent interface paradigm.
- Allow specific discontinuities; this can be a hole inside the animated object or limbs sticking out from it. E.g. although two feet of a character can be situated close together, usually they should be animated and deformed independently. Moreover, they even might overlap.

In order to cope with all this, we closely examined existing free-form deformation schemes, but unfortunately none of them combined all desired requirements. Therefore we opted to investigate the application of the extensions of the subdivision scheme described in [VanRe01].

The rest of this work is organised as follows. Section 2 describes free-form deformations and explains how they will be used in our application. Section 3 deals with subdivision surfaces with local interpolation. In section 4 the details of our implementation are elucidated, while the next section describes our ongoing future work.

2. FREE-FORM DEFORMATION (FFD) IN 2D

2.1 Existing FFD schemes

Sederberg [Seder86] and Barr [Barr84] were about the firsts to point out possibilities, advantages and implementation schemes of deformations, and more in particular of free-form deformations (FFDs). Many followed this trail, improving and extending their usability for different tasks and requirements.

Sederberg put a 3D B-spline lattice around a selected object, then modified the positions of the vertices of the control lattice, and finally applied that deformation to the object. Coquillart combined Sederberg's lattices to allow more complicated deformations [Coqui90]. In a follow-up paper, she also decoupled the lattice from the object to allow animating the lattice separately or to move the object through a deformed space [Coqui91].

Different representations of the deformation tool were investigated:

- a surrounding control lattice [Seder86],
- combining multiple lattices [Coqui90],
- a lattice build up from subdivision volumes [MacCr96],
- some controlling curves or based on an axis [Barr84],
- control surfaces [Feng96] or
- a scattered set of points [Mocco97].

The type of tool used for the deformation strongly determines which type of deformations are feasible and how easy the user can control them. Each tool can be adequate in its own right, depending on the needs in the specific application.

Most of the work in FFDs is concentrating on 3D deformations, considering 2D deformations as a simplification: just leave out one dimension. Hereby ignoring that when you restrict yourself to 2D deformations, additional goals can be achieved as explained in the introduction (see section 1). One of the people specifically tackling 2D deformations was Sederberg in his Siggraph'93 paper [Seder93], where he describes a method to interpolate between 2 deformed 2D objects. Each object is represented by a polygon. The paper restricts itself to the behaviour of the border, giving no clue about how the interior of the polygons should be deformed.

2.2 Deforming parameterisation and local control

In [Inter97] arguments are given to show the significance of texture mapping for conveying 3D shape, even for non-deformable objects. Moreover, when we only have a flat 2D deformable object that pretends to represent a 3D shape, precise control of the texture mapping becomes extremely important in order to deform in a convincible way.

Zonenschein et al. [Zonen98] studied the texturing of deformable implicit surfaces, indicating texture artefacts ("ghosting") when the objects are deformed. They needed to blend colours and transformations to get a plausible result. We opt for a more exact control of the texture, so we try to avoid blending.

The FFD schemes mentioned in section 2.1 do not specifically take care of the parameterisation (texturing) of the surface: they only concentrate on the general shape. Furthermore, with most of these FFD schemes, local control is not so easy. Local control implicates a denser mesh, but usually this is only possible if the complete mesh is subdivided, which obliges the user to control a huge set of points. Only [Mocco97] and [MacCr96] allow local control, so their approaches needed to be studied closer in view of our application.

We considered the approach of [Mocco97], who organises scattered control points into a Delauney triangulation. Their mesh is not explicitly visible to the user, which has the advantage that the user doesn't need to spend time to create the connections, but has the disadvantage that the user can't make different connections when needed, for example to mimic certain physical connections. As the main goal in [Mocco97] is deforming hands represented by many control points that are positioned relatively close together, a Delauney triangulation forms the most adequate connectivity. When attempting to apply this approach for 2D animation purposes however, with only a limited number of control points, the possibility to create own connections - including explicit discontinuities - turned out to be a necessity. Nevertheless, [Mocco97]'s idea to start out with a Delauney triangulation is also useful in our approach, where we extend the idea with the possibility to re-edit the generated mesh. Unfortunately their scheme to calculate the co-ordinates in the mesh will not be applicable anymore, as it strongly depends on the Voronoi diagrams defined by these triangulations. Furthermore the convex hull property prohibits having the type of discontinuities we need.

MacCracken and Joy's solution to FFDs [MacCr96] is based on subdivision volumes created by 3D lattices of arbitrary topology. We liked their idea to use subdivision, as it is the only FFD approach facilitating arbitrary topologies. Nevertheless - although in theory there is a lot of freedom in manipulating the deformation - their set-up is rather hard to establish and control by a user. Also, their way of subdividing space makes calculating the co-ordinates of a point referring to the deforming mesh less straightforward. In our approach, instead of their 3D subdivision volumes, we apply subdivision surfaces, augmented with adequate control tools.

The system we propose has specific advantages and features when comparing it to the previously described techniques. None of the techniques combines all of these features into one concise interface. The main differences are:

a) We allow both general global local in areas of less interest and simultaneously precise local control where needed. This combined type of control is also possible in [MacCr96], but their 3D lattices are hard to handle and to position precisely, and furthermore they don't allow for local interpolations. [Mocco97] also allows some combination of local and global control, but does not provide discontinuities.
b) None of the FFD techniques described in section 2.1 explicitly cares for what happens to the object outside of the border. Objects are just embedded in a larger space. Everything that would happen with the FFD transformation outside of the border will just be ignored. In our approach however, we want to allow for discontinuities. If the transformation would extend too far outside the border, the effect of an FFD applied to one part will result in an overlap with neighbouring parts of the object. This overlapping complicates making sure the animation of one part does not influence a neighbouring part, for example in the case of two legs. Therefore we provide very precise border control.
c) Most FFD approaches can easily deform an object as a whole, but have problems handling the interior just as easy. The interior is deformed as to minimise distortions, but this can't be guided as fluently as desired by an animator. We solve this by allowing for interpolating points, not only at the border but also at the interior.

3. LOCALLY INTERPOLATING SUBDIVISION SURFACES

3.1 Recursive subdivision schemes

Recursive subdivision schemes have been used to define curves (in 2D or in 3D), surfaces (usually in 3D) and volumes (in 3D) [MacCr96]. Such a scheme starts with a set of control points, and in each subsequent subdivision step, in-between points are introduced and at the same time the points are averaged by their neighbours. Depending on how adequate the averaging scheme is, this process will eventually converge to a smooth curve, surface or volume. It will result in a curve if the points are connected in one linked list (like a polygon), in a surface if the points are connected like a polyhedron and in a volume with points connected in a lattice. A good introduction to recursive subdivision schemes can be found at [Joy96], while [Zorin00] provides an in-depth overview of the state of the art.

3.2 Using subdivision surfaces for FFD

In this paper, we based our FFD scheme on subdivision surfaces, as such a surface can both represent the border and the interior of a 2D object. A subdivision scheme is said to be uniform if the same scheme is applied unchanged to every point. The scheme is stationary if the same rules are used for all subsequent subdivisions. As interesting mathematical and practical properties require the scheme to be both stationary and uniform, people only avoid them if they want to achieve exceptional goals. One of these goals can be coping with boundary conditions, because the ordinary rules for the interior do not work at the border. As we want to describe a 2D surface that does not cover the entire plane, we necessarily need to have surfaces with a border. Luckily the standard rules for borders keep the properties of the otherwise fully uniform Loop scheme intact.

In [Catmu78] a subdivision scheme is described, that became known as Catmull-Clark subdivision surfaces. Their scheme is both uniform and stationary and has been studied extensively. It turned out to be very adequate for practical use and lends itself to extensions like sharp edges, which were used in real productions, like the animated short "Gerry's Game".

The Catmull-Clark scheme is an approximating scheme: the limit surface smoothly approximates the mesh of initial control points, and normally will not interpolate them. On the other hand, also completely interpolating schemes exist, for example the Butterfly scheme, introduced in [Doo78] and later extended, amongst others by [Dyn90] and [Zorin96]. Interpolating schemes have the advantage that all initial points will be interpolated exactly, which gives good control about their position and makes them useful for fitting a set of digitised points. In practice it turned out that they are not so well suited for interactive editing, as they need a larger support area and unwanted bulges and folds are difficult to control. Moreover for the described approximating schemes it can be guaranteed that the bounding box set out by the control points will contain the entire generated surface, and this property is maintained recursively throughout the subdivision process.

[Halst93] describes a way to convert the approximating Catmull-Clark scheme into a scheme interpolating a set of given points, using a global optimisation technique. They calculated a new mesh of control points for which the limit surface will interpolate the original points. In order to make the surface sufficiently fair, not only the initial points but also the points of the first and second subdivision needed to be moved. Hence, the scheme of [Halst93] gets similar drawbacks for interactive editing, as other fully interpolating schemes.

Apart from the Catmull-Clark subdivision surfaces, another approximating scheme got quite popular: Loop's scheme [Loop87]. While Catmull-Clark subdivision is based on dividing the subsequent meshes into quadrilaterals, Loop is purely working with triangles. When looking at our application – deformations – the use of triangles has some advantages over quadrilaterals. For instance, a point inside a triangle can be consistently expressed by a co-ordinate system set up by the 3 points of the triangle, while a quadrilateral needs to be subdivided into 2 triangles to get the same consistency.

Because of the above-mentioned reasons - the ease of editing control and the appropriateness for our application - we chose to work with an approximating scheme based on triangles: Loop's subdivision surfaces.

3.3 Local interpolation, normal and tension control

As we wanted to have better control over the surfaces, we opted to extend Loop's scheme with interpolation on selected points, without losing advantages such as fairness and the convex hull property. [Levin00] also describes a method to make a scheme locally interpolating, but he does this by applying other weights around the points to be interpolated, hereby turning a uniform scheme into a non-uniform one. This causes an implementation to lose many of the benefits of the original scheme, like not having to deal with local exceptions and maintaining the convex hull property.

First, let's have a look at the formulas of Loop's subdivision scheme. Loop surfaces are built up starting from a mesh of triangles. During each subdivision step, first the mesh is split, introducing a new point at the centre of every edge; these points get interconnected to form a new mesh, having each triangle divided into four new triangles. Then all points are averaged in order to become a smooth surface. This process is executed recursively, resulting in a fine subdivided mesh of small triangles, in the limit forming a surface. The moved points at the centre of an edge are called edge points, while the points of the existing mesh are called vertex points. The rule for adding a new edge point E (on the edge between V_1 and V_2 and with Q_1 and Q_2 as immediate neighbours) in the interior of the mesh (see figure 1) is:

$$V_0' = \sum \beta Q_i + (1 - k\beta) V_0 \quad \textit{with} \quad \beta = \frac{1}{k}\left(\frac{5}{8} - \left(\frac{3}{8} + \frac{1}{4}\cos\frac{2\pi}{k}\right)^2\right) \tag{1}$$

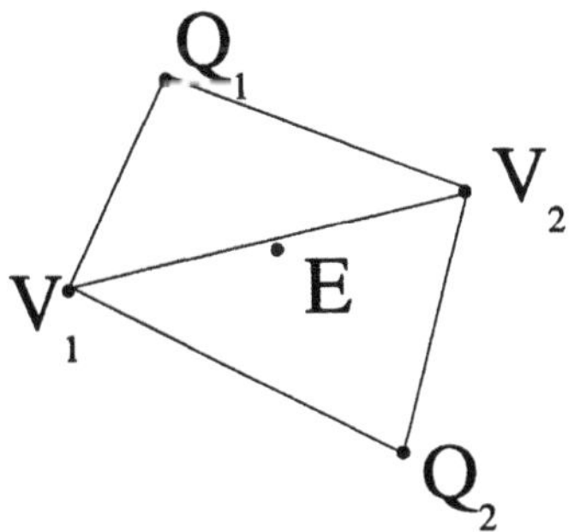

Figure 1. Situation around an interior edge

And the rule for averaging an interior point V_0 (surrounded by k vertices $Q_1 \ldots Q_k$) is the following (see figure 2):

$$E = \frac{3}{8}(V_1 + V_2) + \frac{1}{8}(Q_1 + Q_2) \tag{2}$$

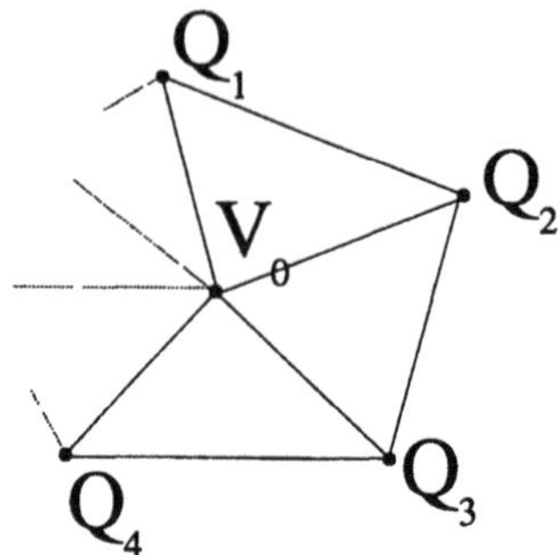

Figure 2. Situation around an interior vertex

The formulas for new edge and vertex points at the border, are simply (see figure 3):

$$V_0' = \frac{3}{4}V_0 + \frac{1}{8}(V_1 + V_2) \quad \text{and} \quad E = \frac{1}{2}(V_1 + V_2) \tag{3}$$

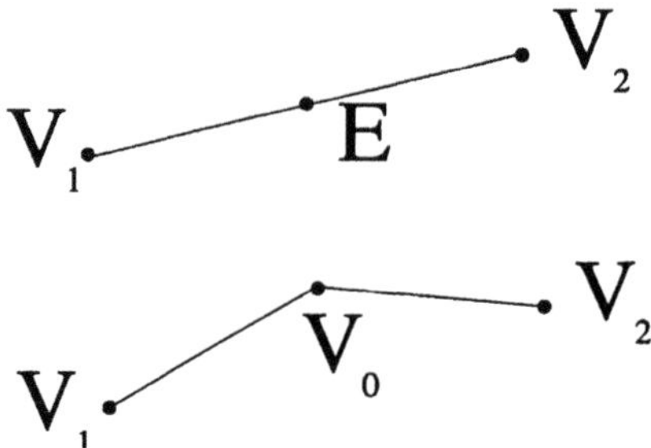

Figure 3. Situation around a border edge and a border vertex

From these formulas it is clear that the border of the Loop surfaces is just a subdivision curve, without influence from interior points. This makes the technique described in [VanRe01] dealing with locally interpolating subdivision curves, valuable for our FFD implementation. Local interpolation is accomplished by extending the control polygon of the curve with ghost points on a line throughout the point to be interpolated. The orientation of this line controls the tangent (thus the normal) at the interpolated point, while the distance between the ghost points affects the tension. Hence, besides local interpolation, the described techniques also provide normal and tension control, without having to revert to a non-uniform scheme. See figure 4 for an example. Extra details can be found in [VanRe01].

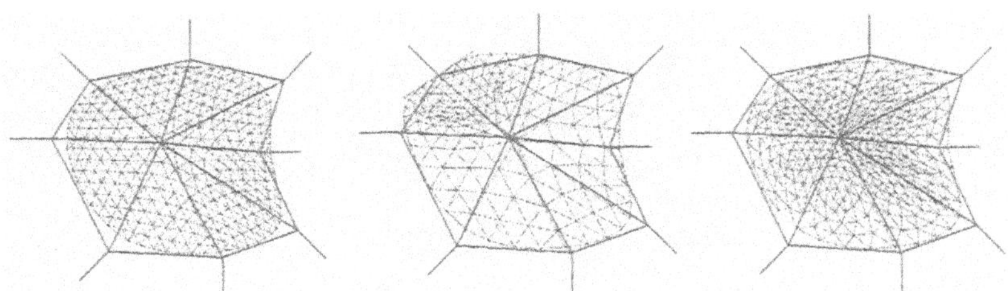

Figure 4. A subdivision mesh, at the left without interpolation, at the centre interpolating a border vertex, and at the right interpolating an interior point (note that for clarity also the normals at the border edges are shown).

The technique described in [VanRe01] can furthermore be extended to the interior of the Loop surfaces. If we want the surface to interpolate an interior control point, the surrounding ghost points should be set up in such a way that their average equals the point to be interpolated. Equation 1 makes sure that if a vertex V_0 is on the given location before the subdivision, it will stay on that same position after the subdivision step. More particularly, the condition to have V_0 being the average of the surrounding vertices can be written as:

$$V_0 = \frac{1}{k}\sum Q_i \tag{4}$$

and substituting this into eq.1 leads to $V_0' = \beta k \frac{1}{k}\sum Q_i + (1-k\beta)V_0$ or $V_0' = V_0$

And thanks to equation 2, the edge points around V_0 will again have V_0 as their average.

$$\frac{1}{k}\sum E_i = \frac{1}{k}\sum\left(\frac{3}{8}(V_0 + Q_i) + \frac{1}{8}(Q_{i+1} + Q_{i-1})\right)$$

or $\frac{1}{k}\sum E_i = \frac{1}{k}\sum \frac{3}{8} V_0 + \frac{1}{k}\sum \frac{5}{8} Q_i$

$$\text{or } \frac{1}{k}\sum E_i = \frac{3}{8}V_0 + \frac{5}{8}\left(\frac{1}{k}\sum Q_i\right)$$

This makes the average of the new edge points equal to V_0 provided that the Q_i also have V_0 as their average. Applying this knowledge in a recursive way will ensure that for all subsequent subdivision steps, the interior vertex V_0 will constantly stay on the same position.

Figure 4 is an example of a mesh with the two sorts of interpolation.

4. IMPLEMENTATION

In our basic approach, we start out with a 2D object to be deformed. The object is represented by a 2D image and can have an arbitrary topology, as it can have holes or limbs sticking out. On this image, the user draws a net of control points. The control points are put both at the interior and near the border. At most places, just an approximating control mesh suffices, but wherever the user needs more control, she can choose to insert an interpolating point (see section 3.3). The user can create some kind of skeleton using this mesh, but this is not a necessity.

Furthermore, special care is taken at the border near places where separate parts that stick out come close together, for example between the upper lip and the nose. In more traditional FFD approaches, at those places the control mesh would be interconnected, forming something like a convex hull. We will draw the discontinuities explicitly, by having the border being continued between them.

When the user finishes setting up the initial mesh, this mesh is frozen to the object, analogous to other FFD approaches. Internally in our program, the mesh will be converted into the triangles belonging to some levels of subdivision. At the corner of each triangle, texture co-ordinates will be generated, mapping the undeformed initial 2D image to this geometry.

In the next stage – also a typical step in FFD – the user can start moving points of the control mesh or even animate them. In the program, the mesh will be subdivided again, the texture co-ordinates belonging to the initial position will be applied and everything will be redrawn, resulting in a deformed object. Typical for our approach, is that apart from moving control points, the user can also manipulate the tension and the normal, giving rise to appealing effects that are hard to establish with other methods. Figure 5 shows a typical example.

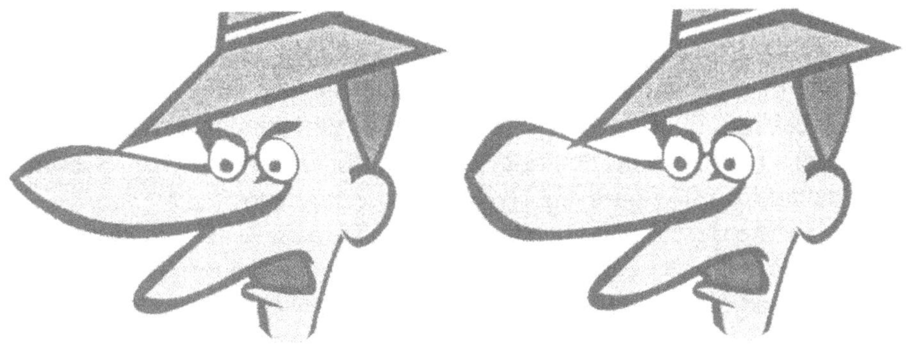

Figure 5. An example of only changing the tension in the border point at the tip of the nose.

An additional advantage of working with the approximating Loop subdivision scheme, is that we can set up a tree of bounding boxes, where each subsequent subdivision level is contained into a bounding box set up by the control points of that level. This enables a quick search for where a point resides into the generated mesh.

Figure 6 refers to a very expressive animation that was created with just a small amount of user input. The animation gives a lot of 3D feeling, while all manipulations are kept strictly 2D.

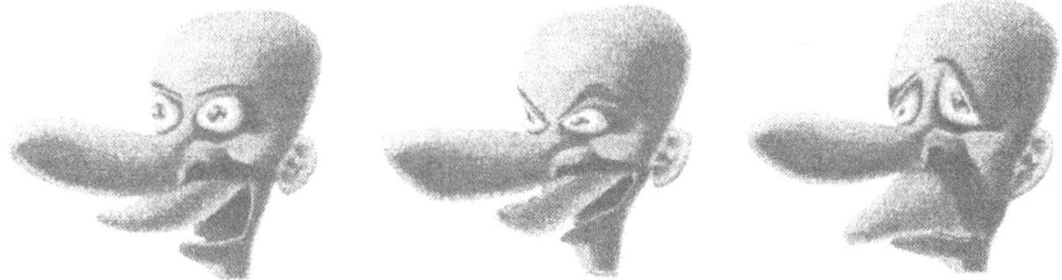

Figure 6. Some frames from an animation created by our system. Interpolating points are used around the eyes, to provide better local control. Between the upper lip and the nose there is an explicit discontinuity to prevent that moving the lip would have undesired effects on the nose.

5. CONCLUSIONS AND FUTURE WORK

In this paper we described a method for deforming 2D images, based on locally interpolating subdivision surfaces with normal and tension control. Our method enables a very smooth movement, explicit discontinuities and both global and local control. None of the other FFD approaches, described in section 2.1 is able to combine all these features into one uniform concept.

In our ongoing future work, we are investigating ways to incorporate higher level editing of the mesh, for example multi-resolution editing. Also we want to have a closer look at combining our methods with physically based modelling techniques and constraint based systems.

Also we are thinking about extending our approach to 3D with keeping in mind the requirements that are also important for 2D deformations. Another track is instead of deforming objects, deforming the space through which the object moves - similar to the ideas presented in [Coqui91].

ACKNOWLEDGEMENTS

The authors are very pleased to acknowledge that this work has been partially funded by the European TMR (Training and Mobility of Researchers) project PAVR (Platform for Animation and Virtual Reality), the European Fund for Regional Development and The Flemish Government. Also the creative input from Luis Gutierrez and Joan Cabot is highly appreciated.

REFERENCES

[Barr84] A. Barr, "Global and Local Deformation of Solid Primitives", Computer Graphics, Vol.18, No.3 (Proc. Siggraph'84), pp. 21-30, 1984.

[Catmu78] E. Catmull, J. Clark "Recursively Generated B-spline Surfaces on Arbitrary Topological Meshes", Computer-Aided Design 10 (Sept. 1978), pp.350–355.

[Coqui90] S. Coquillart, "Extended Free-Form Deformation: A Sculpturing Tool for 3D Geometric Modeling", Siggraph 90, pp.187-196, August 1990.

[Coqui91] S. Coquillart, "Animated Free-Form Deformation: An Interactive Animation Technique", Siggraph 91, pp. 23-26, July 1991.

[DeRose98] T. DeRose, M. Kass, T. Truong, "Subdivision Surfaces in Character Animation", SIGGRAPH 98 Conference Proceedings (July 1998), pp.85–94.

[Doo78] D. Doo, M. Sabin "Behaviour Of Recursive Division Surfaces Near Extraordinary Points", Computer-Aided Design 10 (Sept. 1978), pp.356–360.

[Dyn90] N. Dyn, J. A. Gregory, D. Levin, "A Butterfly Subdivision Scheme for Surface Interpolation with Tension Control." ACM Transactions on Graphics. Vol. 9, No. 2 (April 1990), pp. 160–169.

[Feng96] J. Feng, L. Ma, Q. Peng, "A New Free-Form Deformation Through the Control of Parametric Surfaces", Computers & Graphics, Vol.20, No.4, pp. 531-539, 1996.

[Halst93] M. Halstead, M. Kass, T. DeRose, "Efficient, Fair Interpolation using Catmull-Clark Surfaces", Proceedings of Siggraph 93, pp. 35-44, 1993.

[Inter97] V. Interrante, H. Fuchs, S. Pizer, "Conveying the 3D Shape of Smoothly Curving Transparent Surfaces via Texture", IEEE Transactions on Visualization and Computer Graphics, vol. 3, no. 2, pp. 98-117, April-June 1997.

[Joy96] K. Joy, "On-Line Geometric Modeling Notes", webpages available at http://muldoon.cipic.ucdavis.edu/CAGDNotes/, 1996.

[Levin00] A. Levin, "Surface Design using Locally Interpolating Subdivision Schemes", Journal of Approximation Theory, Vol. 104, No. 1, pp. 98-120, May 2000.

[Loop87] C. Loop, "Smooth Subdivision Surfaces Based on Triangles", Master's thesis, University of Utah, Department of Mathematics, 1987.

[MacCr96] R. MacCracken, K. Joy, "Free-Form Deformations with Lattices of Arbitrary Topology", Siggraph'96, pp.181-188, August 1996.

[Mocco97] L. Moccozet, N. Magnenat Thalmann, "Dirichlet Free-Form Deformations and their Applications to Hand Simulation", Proc. Computer Animation, IEEE Computer Society, pp. 93-102, 1997.

[Seder86] T. Sederberg, S. Parry, "Free-Form Deformation of Solid Geometric Models", Siggraph 86, pp.151-160, 1986

[Seder93] T. Sederberg, P. Gao, G. Wang, H. Mu, "2-D Shape Blending: an Intrinsic Solution to the Vertex Path Problem", Siggraph 93, pp.15-18

[VanRe01] F. Van Reeth, J. Claes, "Interpolatory Uniform Subdivision Curves with Normal Interpolation and Tension Control, Tenerating B-splines of Any Degree", to be submitted to The Visual Computer.

[Zonen98] R. Zonenschein, J. Gomes, L. Velho, L. H. de Figueiredo, M. Tigges, B. Wyvill, "Texturing Composite Deformable Implicit Objects", Proceedings of the XI International Symposium on Computer Graphics, Image Processing and Vision, pp. 346-353, Rio de Janeiro, October 1998.

[Zorin96] D. Zorin, P. Schröder, W. Sweldens, "Interpolating Subdivision for Meshes with Arbitrary Topology", Tech. Rep. CS-TR-96-06, Caltech, Department of Computer Science, 1996.

[Zorin00] D. Zorin, P. Schröder, A. Levin, L. Kobbelt, W. Sweldens, T. DeRose, "Subdivision for Modeling and Animation", course SIGGRAPH 2000.

OBJECT-ORIENTED REFORMULATION AND EXTENSION OF IMPLICIT FREE-FORM DEFORMATIONS

Olivier Parisy, Christophe Schlick
LaBRI, Université Bordeaux 1, 351 cours de la Libération, 33405 Talence, France
(parisy|schlick)@labri.u-bordeaux.fr

Benoît Crespin
LIGIM, Université Lyon 1, 43 bd du 11 novembre 1918, 69622 Villeurbanne, France
bcrespin@bat710.univ-lyon1.fr

Abstract This paper proposes an extension of the *Implicit Free-Form Deformation* technique (IFFD, for short) recently developed by Crespin [Crespin, 1997]. The original formulation of IFFDs is based on a functional paradigm. In this paper, we show that such a functional formulation involves some limitations, especially when efficiency and extensibility are considered. To cancel these drawbacks, an *object-oriented* (OO) reformulation of the technique is proposed, which leads to an efficient implementation and offers a general framework that can be used to express most of existing deformation techniques and develop some original ones.

Keywords: Geometric Modeling, Free-Form Deformations, Implicit Surfaces

1. INTRODUCTION

Since the innovative *warping* technique, introduced by Parent in 1977 [Parent, 1977], geometric deformation techniques have become ubiquitous in Computer Graphics (CG). The basic idea of deformation techniques is to put an indirection between the user and the 3D object he works on. So instead of directly editing the degrees of freedom provided by the geometric model (e.g. vertices for polygonal meshes, control points, knots or weights for spline patches), the user manipulates a *deformation tool* the modification of which are propagated to the model. There are at least three major advantages of deformation techniques over usual edition of 3D objects. First, understanding the meaning of the degrees of freedom provided by the geometric model (that are usually strongly related to its mathematical formulation) is not required. Second, the manipulation of a deformation tool is totally independent of the complexity of the object it is applied on, whereas direct edition of complex objects becomes extremely painful. Finally, as it is disconnected from the geometric model, very intuitive deformation tools can be developed, usually based on a sculpting metaphor.

These impressive features are clearly the reason for which several hundreds of research papers dealing with deformation techniques have been written during the last twenty years. Facing this multitude, a natural trend is to organize, classify and try to find a unifying framework in which all of them can be expressed. A few papers have proposed such a framework [Bechmann, 1994, Blanc et al., 1994, Crespin, 1998]. The goal of this paper is to improve one of these unifying frameworks, namely the functional paradigm, proposed by Crespin in his PhD thesis [Crespin, 1998], and later used to define *Implicit Free-Form Deformations* (IFFD) [Crespin, 1997].

The remainder of the paper will be organized as follows. Section 2 recalls some previous work (free-form deformations, combination of deformations, implicit surfaces) needed to understand the IFFD model. Section 3 describes the original IFFD framework, as presented in [Crespin, 1997], and exhibits some of its limitations. Section 4 proposes an object-oriented reformulation of IFFDs that cancels the previous limitations. Finally, Section 5 presents some results while Section 6 concludes and proposes some directions for future work.

2. PREVIOUS WORK

A general presentation of deformation techniques is out of the scope of this paper (see [Bechmann, 1994, Güdükbay and Özgüç, 1990, Mikita, 1996] for an almost exhaustive survey). This section only aims at exhibiting two of their typical features, the concept of local coordinates to express deformation tools and the idea of building complex deformations by composing simpler ones. Two families of deformations (Free-Form Deformations and Constraint-based Deformations) will be presented for this purpose. The basics of implicit objects will also be recalled, as they are the kernel of the IFFD technique.

2.1. FREE-FORM DEFORMATIONS

Looking at its usage and its numerous derivatives, Sederberg and Parry's Free-Form Deformation (FFD) [Sederberg and Parry, 1986] is probably one of the most successful deformation tool. We will only describe here the original FFD technique, but a whole succession of tools have evolved from this first formulation. It is based on the following mechanism :

1 a lattice (a parallelepipedic network) surrounding the object to deform is defined with a given number of subdivisions following the three coordinates axis (Figure 1, on the left) ;

2 for each point of the object, its local coordinates relative to the lattice (called *lattice coordinates*) are computed ;

3 points of the lattice are then moved by the user ;

4 for each point of the object, its new global coordinates are computed, considering that the set of points of this lattice defines a Bézier volume (using a trivariate tensor product), and that the lattice coordinates have not changed (Figure 1, on the right).

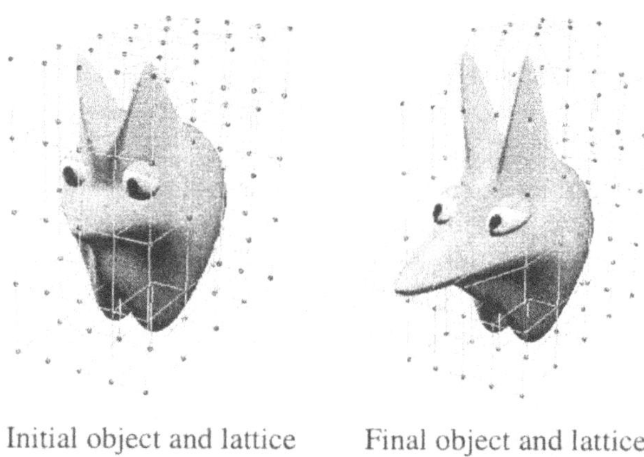

Figure 1 An FFD example

The first step corresponds to the *definition* and the *location* of the deformation tool, the second one to a *freezing* of the coordinates, the third to the *manipulation* of the tool and the fourth to an *unfreezing* of coordinates, resulting in a global-space deformation.

This technique has some very interesting features :

- The fact that the deformation is computed with the hypothesis that the lattice coordinates are frozen leads to a rather intuitive behavior : from a user's point of view, the object seems to be embedded in a transparent jelly (the lattice), which communicates its deformation to the model.
- The freezing step, which is the most computation demanding, is done only once (its result is kept during the whole interaction) whereas the local deformation and the unfreezing, much less expensive, are usually done in an interactive way.
- By moving only a few points of the lattice, a continuous deformation of an arbitrary number of points of the model is obtained. From this point of view, FFD may be referred to as a "high-level" deformation tool.

Note that the freezing step is discrete in nature ; because its result has to be cached, it can only be performed on a finite subset of characteristic points of the object (*cf.* Section 3.2).

2.2. CONSTRAINT-BASED DEFORMATIONS

Another interesting deformation technique was proposed by Borrel and Rappoport [Borrel and Rappoport, 1994] and can be seen as a generalization to continuous deformations of the original *warping* technique developed by Parent [Parent, 1977]. In this approach, a set of n displacement constraints are simultaneously applied to a volume. Each constraint is defined as an ellipsoid C_i ($i \in [1, n]$) with a center $O_i \in \mathbb{R}^3$ and a weighting function $F_i : \mathbb{R}^3 \rightarrow \mathbb{R}$ that is inversely proportional to the distance from O_i.

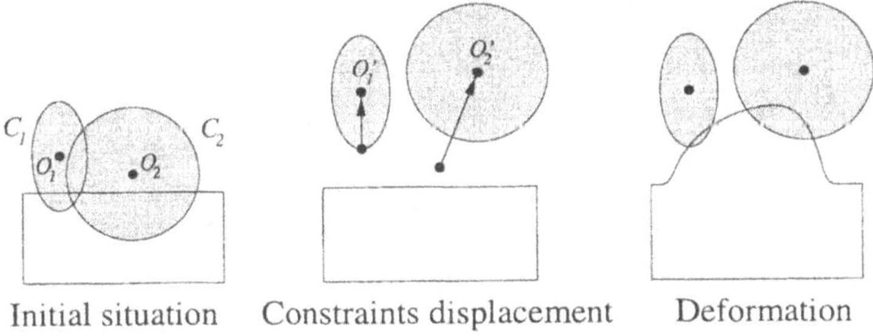

Figure 2 Constraint-based deformation scheme

The first step in the deformation process lets the user place the ellipsoids at their initial location O_i. Once the user has translated one or more ellipsoids to some new locations O'_i, a displacement is applied to any point $M \in \mathbb{R}^3$. This displacement is roughly defined as the sum of the local displacements $\vec{O_iO'_i}$, weighted by the values $F_i(M)$. This process is summarized on Figure 2.

More precisely, the resulting deformation D from $\mathbb{R}^3$ to $\mathbb{R}^3$ is given as a $3 \times n$ matrix D_m which must satisfy Equation 1. D_m is obtained by a pseudo-inversion algorithm depending on the initial positions O_i and the weighting functions F_i.

$$\forall i \in [1, n]\, ,\ O'_i = D(O_i) = D_m \times \begin{bmatrix} F_1(O_i) \\ F_2(O_i) \\ \cdots \\ F_n(O_i) \end{bmatrix} \qquad (1)$$

This approach, called *Scodefs* for "Simple Constrained Deformations", offers an arbitrary combination of global or local deformations, especially because it is not dependent on a particular topology as are traditional FFD. Moreover, Bechmann [Bechmann, 1994] showed that FFD can more or less be reformulated in the Scodefs formalism.

But this technique also has serious drawbacks. First, because the matrix computation is performed *after each displacement of an ellipsoid*, the freezing step of traditional FFD is lost, and this forbids the use of too many constraints. Scodefs are also poorly intuitive when constraints are too close from each other. Finally, specific kinds of deformations such as twisting or tapering are impossible to obtain with Scodefs unless allowing rotation or scaling of ellipsoids in addition of translation ; unfortunately, the computation of the deformation matrix is much more complicated in this case.

2.3. IMPLICIT OBJECTS

The idea of using implicit models in geometric modeling was initially proposed by Blinn [Blinn, 1982] (see [Bloomenthal et al., 1997] for an exhaustive survey). An implicit object is based on a set of primitives P_i where each primitive is the source of a potential field, defined by a *field function* $F_i(x, y, z)$ that maps $\mathbb{R}^3$ to $\mathbb{R}$ (or a subset of $\mathbb{R}$). At a given point $P(x, y, z)$ of the Euclidian space, the fields of all the sources are computed and added together (*blending*), leading to a global field function $F(x, y, z)$:

$$F(x,y,z) = \sum_{i=1}^{n} F_i(x,y,z)$$

A 3D surface can then be defined from this global field function $F(x, y, z)$ by giving a threshold value T and rendering the equipotential surface S for this threshold :

$$S = \{(x,y,z) \in \mathbb{R}^3 \ / \ F(x,y,z) = T\}$$

The advantage of this approach is that union or difference of primitives are then equivalent to sums or differences of their associated potentials, which are straightforward to perform. It is thereof easy to combine an arbitrary number of simple primitives to obtain a complex one. If correct hypothesis on potentials are fulfilled, the resulting surface is continuous and, unlike other models, no intersection computation is needed to generate the global surface.

Though this approach exhibits seductive properties, some trade-off must be highlighted :

- Implicit surfaces are difficult to visualize in an interactive way because the tessellation needed to get hardware rendering is expensive [Bloomenthal, 1994] ;

- Texture mapping is difficult to apply to implicit surfaces as they do not exhibit a natural parameterization.

It must be noticed that these drawbacks only apply if implicit objects are used for geometric modeling. If they are considered as a mathematical model for doing anything else, interactive visualization and texture mapping are not required anymore and only the good side of the model is kept.

3. IMPLICIT FREE-FORM DEFORMATIONS

3.1. MOTIVATION

As noted by Crespin [Crespin, 1998], the weighting approach found in Scodefs is very similar to the *blending* process used in implicit-based modeling. Weighting functions F_i (*cf.* Section 2.2) actually look like usual field functions found in implicit literature, although the authors do not refer to them. Consequently, these functions permit an automatic continuity on the boundary between different deformation constraints, which recalls the continuity provided between blended implicit primitives. Moreover, the results obtained by combining several deformations are often prone to unwanted artefacts (bulges, lost of symmetry, non-commutative combinations, etc.) that can only be reduced by complex and non-intuitive tricks (direct manipulation of control points, use of additional deformations, etc.). An unified tool to express the combination of deformations may be a solution to cancel these artefacts. Hence, he proposed a deformation technique called *Implicit FFD* (*IFFD*) which :

- Allow the combination of different deformation primitives according to some field (or weighting) functions associated to each one. This combination would ideally be simpler than in the Scodef model.

- Provide high-level deformation primitives, based on local coordinates systems, such as FFD tools. Indeed, a 3-step recurrent scheme (freezing, manipulation, unfreezing) can be seen in the way many deformation tools are used. Thus, it seems interesting to formalize these tools so that they may be manipulated in an unified way.

- Re-introduce a freezing step to avoid expensive computations.

3.2. DEFORMATION FUNCTION

In most cases, a deformation function D will be applied to discrete sets of characteristic points (such as vertices of polygonal meshes, control points of spline patches, etc.) which will be represented as a vector $\vec{M}$ of size m (its components M_i being the points). This will abusively be referred to as "points deformation" or "coordinates deformation", though it only defines the translation of each M_i to $M_i' = D(M_i)$. Similarly, we will also often refer to "points" where "coordinates of points" would be more appropriate.

A local space $\mathbb{L}$ can be associated to each deformation tool ; in most cases, it will be $\mathbb{R}^d$, with $d \leq 3$. The global deformation function D can then be decomposed in

- ϕ ($\mathbb{R}^3 \rightarrow \mathbb{L}$) : the (invertible) immersion function ;
- Δ ($\mathbb{L} \rightarrow \mathbb{L}$) : the local space deformation.

Where $D = \phi^{-1} \circ \Delta \circ \phi$ and

$$M_i \xrightarrow{\phi} \tilde{M_i} \xrightarrow{\Delta} \tilde{M_i'} \xrightarrow{\phi^{-1}} M_i'.$$

In this formulation, the superscript "~" means local coordinates and " ′ " means deformed coordinates ; ϕ is the freezing step, Δ the manipulation step and ϕ^{-1} the unfreezing step already described in Section 2.1.

As an example, an FFD with an initial lattice L and a deformed lattice L' can be expressed as follows :

$$(M_i, L) \xrightarrow{\phi} (\tilde{M_i}, L) \xrightarrow{\Delta} (\tilde{M_i}, L') \xrightarrow{\phi^{-1}} (M_i', L'),$$

In other words, we consider the coordinates used by the deformation process as couples composed of a characteristic point M_i and a lattice L.

3.3. DEFORMATION PRIMITIVES

A deformation primitive Π_j is defined as a global deformation fonction D_j associated to a scalar field function F_j of the same kind of those used in implicit objects (see Section 2.3).

When the primitive Π_j is applied on a given point M_i, it defines a couple (d_{ij}, f_{ij}) where $d_{ij} = D_j(M_i)$ (the point after deformation) and $f_{ij} = F_j(M_i)$ (its associated scalar field value).

By applying n primitives Π_j to m points M_i, we define a $m \times n$ deformation matrix $\mathcal{D}$:

$$\mathcal{D} = [d_{ij}] \text{ where } d_{ij} = D_j(M_i)$$

and a $m \times n$ field matrix $\mathcal{F}$:

$$\mathcal{F} = [f_{ij}] \text{ where } f_{ij} = F_j(M_i)$$

3.4. BLENDING FUNCTION

A blending function Ψ is defined to collapse each row of matrix $\mathcal{D}$ into a single value M_i' that represents the final image of M_i. This blending is a n-ary operator that uses the corresponding rows of matrix $\mathcal{F}$ as weighting factors.

A possibility for Ψ that behave nicely (commutative, $I_{\mathbb{R}^3}$ when no primitive is modified) is :

$$M_i' = M_i + \frac{\sum_{j=1}^{n} F_j(M_i)(D_j(M_i) - M_i)}{\sum_{j=1}^{n} F_j(M_i)}.$$

3.5. IFFD

Finally, by collecting all previous components, an IFFD is defined by a set of n deformation primitives and a blending function Ψ. When applied to a point vector $\vec{M}$, the resulting point vector $\vec{M}'$ is defined by :

$$\vec{M}' = \Psi(\mathcal{D}(\vec{M}), \mathcal{F}(\vec{M}))$$

Figures 3 presents an example of a simple IFFD that involves two spherical primitives and a translation of one of them. It is worth noticing that even such simple instances of IFFDs are able to produce effects similar to Barr's classical bend or twist operators [Barr, 1984].

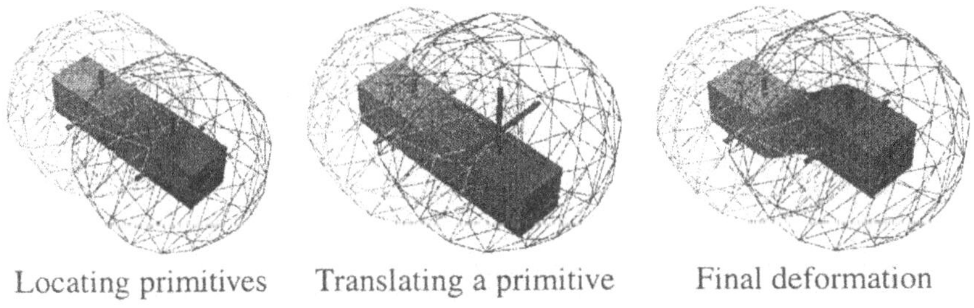

Figure 3 Translation of a primitive

4. OBJECT-ORIENTED FORMULATION OF IFFD

The formulation of the FFD given in Section 3.2 shows that a strictly functional representation, even if expressive enough, may get somewhat bloated. Indeed, as it manipulates couples composed of a point M_i and a lattice L, the lattice has to be duplicated at m occurrences to fulfill the functional paradigm.

Moreover, this formulation is not able to manage two other points of practical interest :

- The freezing step (done once) is clearly distinct from the unfreezing (done at an interactive rate).

- The user has no direct access to the local coordinates (i.e. relative to the deformation tool) which are always internal to the deformation function.

To address all these problems, we propose to reformulate IFFD by using an object-oriented (OO) approach.

4.1. OO REFORMULATION OF DEFORMATIONS

Computations for all components of a point vector $\vec{M}$ can be combined : instead of considering D as a function from $\mathbb{R}^3$ to $\mathbb{R}^3$, and then extending it to point vectors by applying it to each component of this vector, we will now define it as an algorithm taking these vectors as parameters from the start ; this way, more efficient computation may be performed.

More precisely, a deformation can then be defined as a class affording the following methods :

Method	*Parameters*	*Behavior*	*Return value*
freeze	$\vec{M}$	Computes $\tilde{M}_i$	None
manip		Computes $\tilde{M}'_i$	None
unfreeze	None	None	$\vec{M}'$

Note that by using methods, we have dropped the concept of mathematical function, because border effects are now possible. Indeed, the local coordinates $\tilde{M}_i$ (before tool manipulation) and $\tilde{M}'_i$ (after tool manipulation) are now local attributes of the deformation class, so that they can only be manipulated by its methods. The idea here is that because the local space is specific to each deformation tool, hiding them leads to an unified vision (and manipulation) of them.

4.2. EXTENSION TO THE IFFD MODEL

Using the OO-formulation of deformations, so that each primitive Π_j encapsulates objects of this class, IFFD can be reformulated as specializations of the same class :

Method	*Parameters*	*Behavior* ($\forall j$)	*Returns*
freeze	$\vec{M}$	$\begin{cases} \text{Computes } \mathcal{F} \\ \Pi_j\text{.freeze}(\vec{M}) \end{cases}$	None
manip		Π_j.manip()	None
unfreeze	None	$\Pi_j\text{.unfreeze}() \to \mathcal{C}$	$\Psi(\mathcal{C}, \mathcal{F})$

It is interesting to notice that IFFDs themselves can be expressed in the same formalism as the deformations which compose them ; this illustrates their genericity and the adequacy of our formulation.

5. SOME RESULTS

As a proof of concept, and to test IFFDs usability, this OO-framework was implemented as a plug-in for *Maya* (the 3D modeling and rendering software environment developed by Alias|Wavefront [Alias|Wavefront, 2000]). We will present here some meaningful use of this tool.

5.1. BASIC EXAMPLES

The following pictures will illustrate the various degrees of liberty available using IFFDs. In all of them, only simple affine transformations are used for the manipulation of the primitives. But of course, more complex manipulations may be used.

Figure 4 shows two spherical primitives located on a planc ; by applying rotations, translations and scalings to these primitives, the plane is accordingly deformed. Notice how influence of the two primitives blend smoothly in the zone deformed by both primitives (i.e. in the intersection of the balls defining non-null fields). The deformation depends also on the geometry of the field (Figure 5) and of the way it decreases (Figure 6). Finally, a more complete example is presented on Figure 7.

5.2. MORE DETAILED EXAMPLES

More complex objects were modeled to test whether interesting shapes could be achieved. As an example, Figure 8 shows a ship and a little creature (notice the spherical-shaped primitive bending its ear) built by performing various IFFD-based deformations on an initial sphere. Note that for all primitives, the deformation functions used were always combinations of translations, rotations and scalings (as for the examples of Section 5.1). Spherical and conic fields were used and combined to a Blanc-Schlick function [Blanc and Schlick, 1995] to profile their decreasing.

As an illustration, Figure 9 details the ship's noozle hollowing. A single conic primitive was used for this purpose : after the creation and setting of the primitive (left picture), it was translated to the front of the hull, which resulted in the expected hole (right picture).

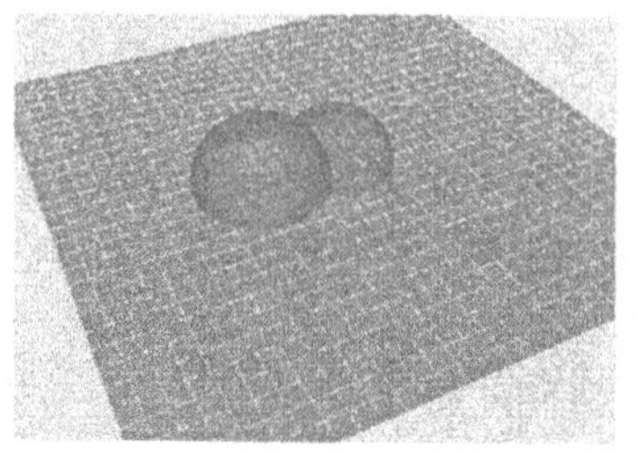
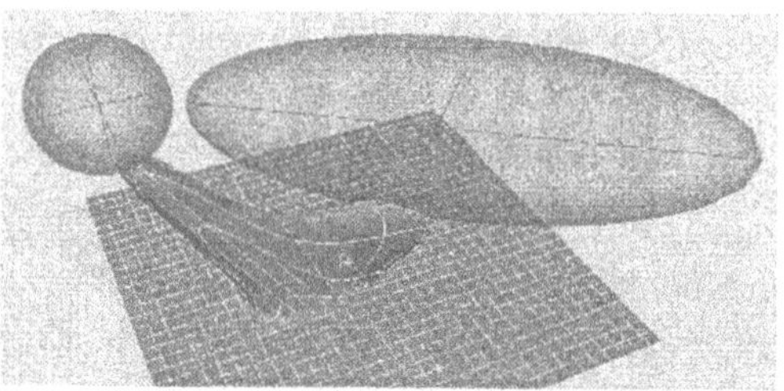

Figure 4 Deforming a plane using two primitives

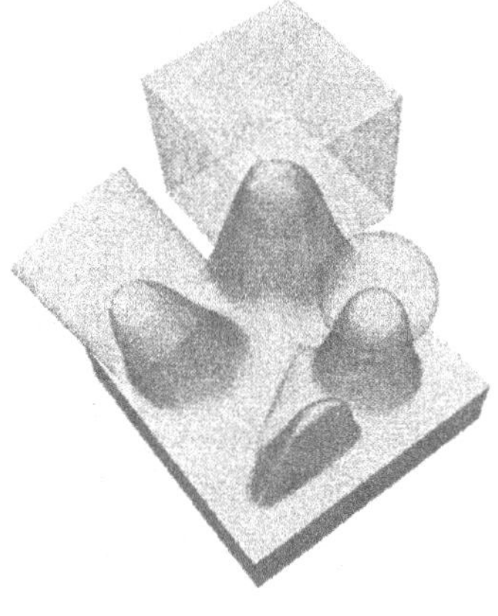

Figure 5 Miscellaneous field shapes

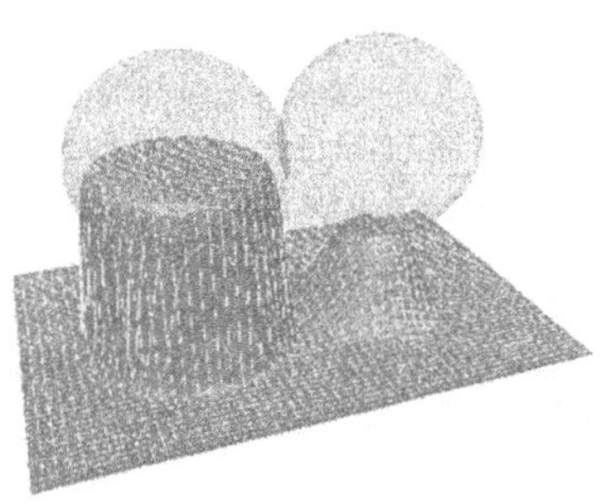

Figure 6 Some field decreasings

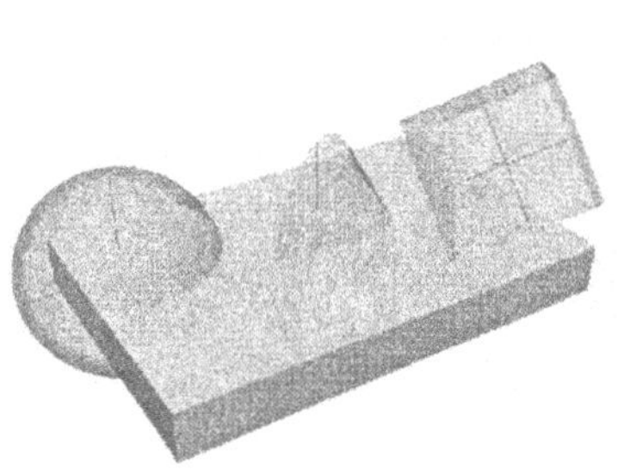
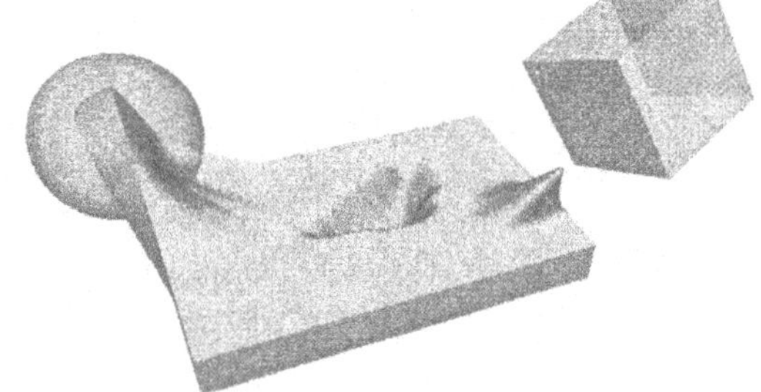

Figure 7 Complete IFFD example

Figure 8 Models designed using IFFDs

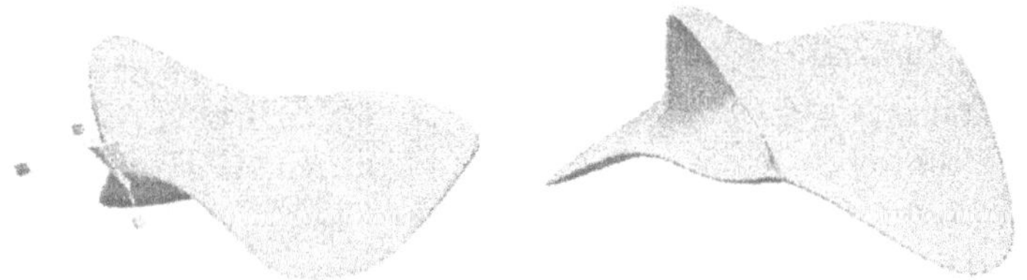

Initial setting of the primitive After primitive translation

Figure 9 Nozzle hollowing using an IFFD

6. CONCLUSION

After a presentation of some interesting trends in free-form deformation and how IFFD unifies most of them, we showed how its object-oriented formulation expresses well their modularity and the way they are used.

This leads to a straightforward implementation in the data flows paradigm of *Maya*, which proved useful even with simple primitives because of the various degrees of liberty permitted by the many field parameters. Interestingly, these can be easily manipulated using a GUI, which enabled the geometric modeling of complex objects as showed in Section 5.2.

A possible extension would be to include more complex scalar fields ; generalized cylinders as an example may be used. Another idea would be to test whether interesting animations could be obtained using fields changing over time or objects moving in those fields, as with AFFD [Coquillart and Jancéne, 1991].

References

[Alias|Wavefront, 2000] Alias|Wavefront (2000). (`http://www.aliaswavefront.com/en/Home/homepage.html`).

[Barr, 1984] Barr, A. (1984). Global and local deformations of solid primitives. *Computer Graphics (SIGGRAPH'84 Proceedings)*, 18(3):21–31.

[Bechmann, 1994] Bechmann, D. (1994). Space deformation models survey. *Comput. & Graphics*, 18(4):571–586.

[Blanc et al., 1994] Blanc, C., Guitton, P., and Schlick, C. (1994). A methodology for description of geometrical deformations. In *Pacific Graphics'94*.

[Blanc and Schlick, 1995] Blanc, C. and Schlick, C. (1995). Extended Field Functions for Soft Objects. In *Implicit Surfaces'95 Proceedings*, pages 21–32.

[Blinn, 1982] Blinn, J. (1982). A generalization of algebraic surface drawing. *Trans. on Graphics*, 1(3):235–256.

[Bloomenthal, 1994] Bloomenthal, J. (1994). An implicit surface polygonizer. In *Graphics Gems*, volume 4, pages 324–349.

[Bloomenthal et al., 1997] Bloomenthal, J., Bajaj, C., Blinn, J., Cani-Gascuel, M.-P., Rockwood, A., Wyvill, B., and Wyvill, G. (1997). *Introduction to Implicit Surfaces*. Morgan Kaufmann.

[Borrel and Rappoport, 1994] Borrel, P. and Rappoport, A. (1994). Simple constrained deformations for geometric modeling and interactive design. *ACM Transactions on Graphics*, 13(2):137–155.

[Coquillart and Jancéne, 1991] Coquillart, S. and Jancéne, P. (1991). Animated free-form deformation: An interactive animation technique". In *SIGGRAPH '91 Proceedings*, pages 23–26.

[Crespin, 1997] Crespin, B. (1997). Implicit free-form deformations. In *Implicit Surface 99 Proceedings*, pages 151–158.

[Crespin, 1998] Crespin, B. (1998). *Modélisation et déformation de forme libre à base de surfaces implicites équipotentielles.* PhD thesis, Université Bordeaux I.

[Güdükbay and Özgüç, 1990] Güdükbay, U. and Özgüç, B. (1990). Free-form solid modeling using deformations. *Comput. & Graphics*, 14(3/4):491–500.

[Mikita, 1996] Mikita, M. (1996). 3d free-form deformation: Basic and extended algorithms. In Purgathofer, W., editor, *Proc. of the* 12th *Spring Conference on Computer Graphics*, pages 183–191. Comenius University, Bratislava.

[Parent, 1977] Parent, R. (1977). A system for sculpting 3-d data. *Computer Graphics*, 11(2):138–147.

[Sederberg and Parry, 1986] Sederberg, T. and Parry, S. (1986). Free-form deformations of solid geometric models. *Computer Graphics (SIGGRAPH'86 Proceedings)*, 20(4):151–160.

SOFT TISSUE MODELLING FROM 3D SCANNED DATA

Jean-Christophe Nebel
Department of Computing Science, University of Glasgow, UK

Key words: Computer graphics, 3D scanners, FEM, soft tissue modelling.

Abstract: Human body 3D scanners are becoming a mature technology that generates accurate static photo-realistic 3D models of real human beings. However the data collected allow only the construction of the outer surface of the body. In this paper we describe how from 3D surface data we generate 3D volumetric meshes of soft tissues suitable for the finite element method (FEM). We then deform these meshes using our implementation of the FEM for 3D volumetric meshes. Finally we present some experimental results of the deformation of a human body and detail a methodology to evaluate the distribution of soft tissue layers from a 3D scan of a specific individual.

1. INTRODUCTION

Human body 3D scanners are becoming a mature technology that generates accurate static photo-realistic 3D models of real human beings. However the data collected allow only the construction of the outer surface of the body. Hence the scans do not have any internal structure and physical properties regarding the skeleton, the skin or the soft tissues of the scanned human. Many works have been done about fitting skeletons in the 3D scans, - segmentation -, in order to allow their animation as articulated figures. However, an other challenging aspect of scan animation is the integration of soft tissue models (skin, muscles, fat...) in these scans for the simulation of the deformation of these soft tissues during motion and interaction within a virtual 3D environment. In order to offer realistic deformations (physically and visually accurate), the modelling of soft tissues should be based on the equations of the mechanics using the physical properties of these tissues. Moreover the 3D models representing individuals, the soft tissue properties should be customised according to the person scanned.

In this paper we present how from 3D surface data we generate 3D volumetric meshes of soft tissues suitable for the finite element method (FEM). We then deform these meshes using our implementation of the FEM. Since the 3D scanned data have an accuracy of about 1mm and represent specific individuals, our aim is to generate soft tissue deformations customised to these individuals. For that reason, we aim to generate deformations as accurate as possible, whatever the computation time needed. In the future, this work will be used in medical applications.

First we give a review of the techniques used for soft tissue modelling and 3D scan deformation, then we show how we generate volumetric meshes from 3D scans, we also describe our implementation of the FEM for 3D meshes. Finally we present some experimental results and detail a methodology to get the distribution of fat layers on a specific body.

2. PREVIOUS WORK

2.1 Soft tissue modelling

Many approaches to soft tissue modelling are based on surface models. Early works restricted themselves to pure geometric deformation [Ko88]. Another approach has been to use models based on implicit surfaces [Ma95], [Mo97] and [Ne98]. These models are composed of a skeletal model upon which parameterised muscles are built up manually and the entire body form is then "skinned," i.e. covered in virtual skin.

However realistic deformations can only be achieved by using physically based models. Surface based models were developed using the finite element method (FEM) for facial animation [Ko98] and surgery simulation [Br96]. They have proved to be very powerful in the context of animation, but they have obvious limitations since they were aimed to show visually convincing deformations.

Two types of volumetric models have been developed depending on the need of interaction with the 3D model. Real time deformations have been demonstrated using models based on the Hooke's law and Lame equation [De99] and [Aubel00] or combining elastic surface and geometric constraints [Tu98]. The most realistic models are based on volumetric mass spring system or FEM simulation. Usually soft tissues are divided in different layers (Skin, fat, muscle...) which have distinct physical properties. The first models were based on mass spring system [Te90] and [Le95] and are still used because they have a lower computational cost [Bi99]. The finite element method imposed itself as the most accurate way of simulating soft tissue deformation since non-linear elasticity and incompressibility can be simulated [La86] and [Ro98].

One of the barriers to using finite element analysis in soft tissue deformation is the generation of the 3D volumetric mesh on which the simulation will be applied. The mesh generation is a critical feature of the pre-processing stage since the accuracy of the numerical results is strongly related to the quality of the underlying meshes.

2.2 3D scan deformation

The most effective techniques for generating 3D static photo-realistic models of real human are called scanning techniques. Several methods can be used: laser beams [Tr00] and Cyberware™, structured light technique [WI00] or photogrammetry [Si00] and [Va00]. Their accuracy is usually sufficient for getting very realistic 3D models, whose accuracy is about 1mm. Moreover colour pictures are mapped on these models what ensures photo realistic appearance. The main difference between the results these full body scanners provide is about the type of data they can capture. Indeed very few of them have short capture time. The scanners, based on laser beams and structured light, have a capture time of about 15 seconds, whereas the ones using photogrammetry, so called 3D imagers, only need few milliseconds. Obviously only the latter type of scanners has the ability to capture subjects which are moving or are in positions which cannot be held for a long time. Hence 3D imagers are unique tools for the investigation of soft tissue modelling.

Whatever the type of scanner used, the data collected allow only the construction of the outer surface of the body, therefor the scans do not have any internal structure and physical properties regarding the skeleton, the skin or the soft tissues of the scanned human.

Many works have been done about fitting skeletons in the 3D scans, segmentation, in order to allow their animation as articulated figures. First that was made by slicing the scans and selecting landmarks manually [Jo95] and [Pa97]. More recently the automatic segmentation of the human body has been investigated too. [Nu97] offered the automatic segmentation of the human body into 6 functional parts (2 arms, 2 legs, a torso and a head). This work was refined by focusing on key landmarks of the human body [De98]. Finally [Ju00] worked on segmenting the human body in 16 parts. Although manual interventions may be still needed, since the segmentation of extremities is not always accurate enough, these latest results are very encouraging.

Once a skeleton has been fitted inside a 3D model, the vertices of the surface have to be connected to the skeleton. This has been done manually in the game industry for years [La94]. [Su99] has demonstrated a technique for mapping automatically each vertex of a 3D scan to a skeleton placed inside the model to enable seamless animation of the 3D model. Since the purpose of their work is real time animation, the deformation of the model is based only on the relationship between vertices and the skeleton and geometrical constraints. The next step is obviously the integration of realistic soft tissues inside these 3D models.

3. THE PROPOSED METHOD

3.1 Principle

The soft tissues, we are interested in our research, consist of three elements: the epidermis, the dermis and the subcutis (see Figure 1). The epidermis is the outermost layer that contains the primary protective structure and the dermis is a fibrous layer that supports and strengthens the epidermis. The subcutis is a subcutaneous layer of fat beneath the dermis that supplies nutrients to the other two layers and that cushions and insulates the body; the subcutis is usually connected to muscles.

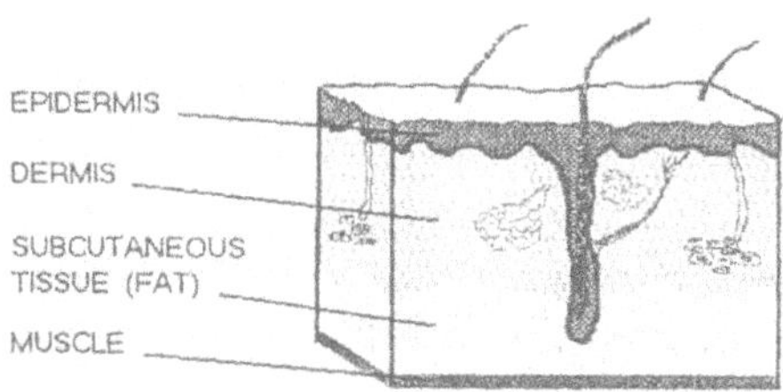

Figure 1. Soft tissue anatomy

Since the anatomy of these soft tissues shows a structure of three layers, volumetric meshes based on this structure are well suited to simulate accurately soft tissues in most parts of the body [Bo00]. However for the fatty parts of the body, e.g. belly and female breasts, another structure should be used: the fatty part should be represented by a volumetric mesh instead of a single layer. We will deal about this case in the next section.

Scanned data obviously provide the surface of the upper mesh of the structure, we can make the assumption that the thickness of the different layers is constant on a small area. Hence we generate the volumetric mesh by selecting an area of a scan and duplicating this surface mesh to generate the frontiers between the three layers. These meshes, placed in parallel according to the layer thicknesses, are then connected to each other. The meshes generated by 3D scanners are supposed to be composed of triangles, or can be easily converted into triangular meshes, so the connections between two parallel meshes of that kind generate a layer of prism elements. Physical properties are then assigned to each prism element accordingly to the layer it belongs to.

Finally the nodes of the lowest frontier of the fat layer are connected to muscles. Since muscles are very hard - compared to the other soft tissues - we assume that they cannot be deformed by realistic and non-destructive external forces. Hence muscles can be deformed only if they move by themselves. Forces are then applied on the exterior of the mesh and deformations are computed using the FEM.

3.2 Fatty part modelling

As mentioned previously, the structure used to model the fatty parts of the body (belly, female breast...) should be slightly different from the one presented in the previous section. The layer structure is kept for the epidermis and the dermis, however the subcutaneous fat cannot be modelled by a layer anymore. It should be represented by a volumetric mesh according to the scan data.

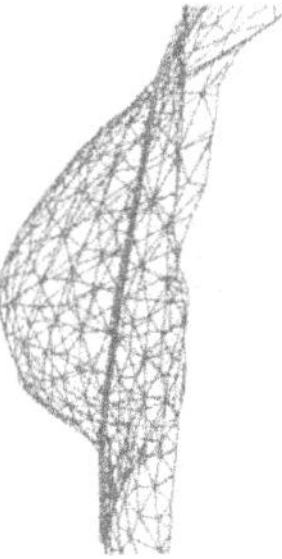

Figure 2. Evaluation of the chest wall

Using the 3D scans, the volume of fat has to be evaluated. In the case of breast simulation we evaluate the position of the chest wall [Mo99] (see Figure 2), we then select the surface defined by the breast and close this surface using a mesh defining the chest wall. The chest wall mesh is generated from the points delimitating the breast surface using a 2D advancing front method. Finally the volumetric mesh modelling the breast fat is generated from the 3D closed surface representing the surface of the breast using a 3D advancing front method [Ho88], [Ge88], [Ca95] and [Fr96]. The volumetric mesh, which is composed of tetrahedral elements, is then scaled down in order to fit inside the two skin layers generated from the surface mesh.

A more general and detailed presentation of the modelling of the fatty parts of the human body will be offered in a future paper.

3.3 Finite element model

The finite element method is a numerical technique that has been applied in many fields. It has become a standard tool in industry and is slowly finding its way into the field of biomechanics.

In this method, the region that is to be analysed is discretised up into sub-regions called elements, these elements are connected at points called nodes. As mentioned previously, our model has to deal with two types of 3D elements: prisms and tetrahedrons. For the time being we consider them as being linear. So their shape functions have standard expressions, N, available in most FEM textbooks, i.e. [En99] [Fa99]. The region is represented by functions defined over each element. This generates a number of local functions that are much simpler than those required to represent the entire region. The next step is to analyse the mechanical response for each element. A stiffness matrix, K, and a force vector, F, are built for each element in the structure, where U is the displacement of each node: $F = KU$

In our model we idealise the soft tissues as elastic, so the standard equation of classical elasticity can be used to express K.

We define the following variables:
ε is the strain of the material
σ is the stress of the material
V is the volume of the element
D is the material property matrix

B is the matrix relating strain to displacement, it depends only on the shape functions, $B = f(N)$.

The governing equations of the model are described as follow:

Strain-displacement relationship: $\varepsilon = BU$

Strain-stress relationship: $\sigma = D\varepsilon$

Force-stress relationship: $F = \int_V B^T \sigma \; dV$

Consequently the expression of K is: $K = \int_V B^T D \; B \; dV$

For an isotropic 3D element where E is the Young's modulus and ν is the Poisson's ratio, the expression of D is:

$$[D] = \frac{E}{(1+\nu)(1-2\nu)} \begin{bmatrix} 1-\nu & \nu & \nu & 0 & 0 & 0 \\ \nu & 1-\nu & \nu & 0 & 0 & 0 \\ \nu & \nu & 1-\nu & 0 & 0 & 0 \\ 0 & 0 & 0 & \frac{1-2\nu}{2} & 0 & 0 \\ 0 & 0 & 0 & 0 & \frac{1-2\nu}{2} & 0 \\ 0 & 0 & 0 & 0 & 0 & \frac{1-2\nu}{2} \end{bmatrix}$$

Once all the element stiffness matrices and force vectors have been obtained they are combined into a structure matrix equation. This equation relates nodal displacements for the entire structure to nodal loads. After applying boundary conditions the structure matrix equation can be solved to obtain unknown nodal displacements. Intra-element displacements can be interpolated from nodal values using the functions that were defined over each element.

4. RESULTS AND DISCUSSION

4.1 Deformation of an upper arm

Since our work is aimed at medical applications, where simulations are limited to specific areas of the body, we demonstrate our method through the deformation of an upper arm on which a force is applied.

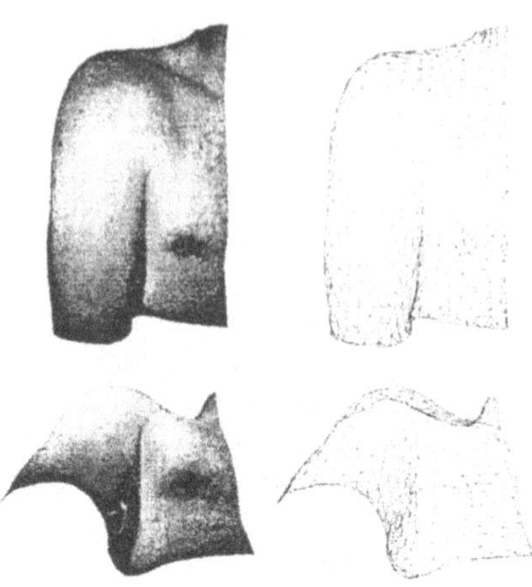

Figure 3. 3D model of a shoulder and upper arm

At first the geometry of the 3D volumetric mesh has to be generated. The 3D surface and the appearance of the right shoulder and upper arm of the author are captured using the C3D imager [Si00] (see Figure 3). A piece of the upper arm is cut out of the generated 3D model (see Figure 4), this mesh is used as a base for the construction of the 3D volumetric mesh.

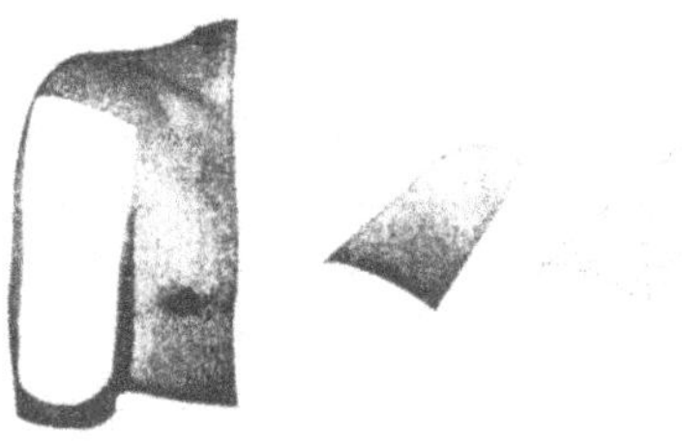

Figure 4. Collection of the 3D surface

We duplicate the surface mesh to generate the three layer volumetric mesh (see Figure 5). The thicknesses of the epidermis, dermis and subcutaneous fat are set respectively, using average values, at 0.2mm, 2mm [Ru66] [Ho74] and 8.9mm [Fr81].

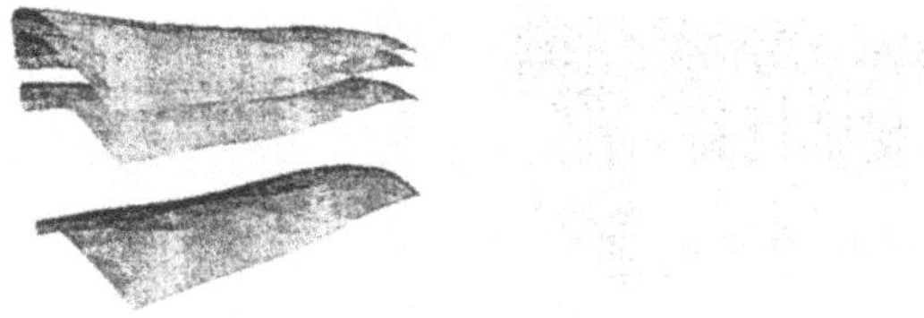

Figure 5. Volumetric mesh (not at scale)

Then we set physical properties to these materials. Since they are incompressible [La87], their Poisson's ratios are set at 0.50. Finally their Young's moduli are set respectively at 90.10^9 N.m^2, 45.10^9 N.m^2 and 30.10^9 N.m^2.

In order to apply the FEM on that volumetric mesh, boundary conditions have to be defined. The lowest layer (fat layer) is fixed to muscles (deltoid, biceps and triceps) and an external force is applied on the mesh (0.15 N). Then the deformation is computed (see Figure 6).

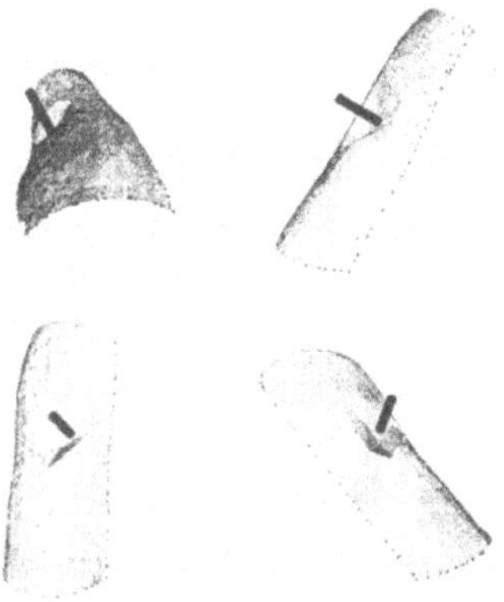

Figure 6. Deformed mesh seen from different view points

Finally the deformed mesh is put back inside the initial 3D model. In Figure 7, we show the initial and final meshes of the shoulder and upper arm without texture and with texture and different illuminations.

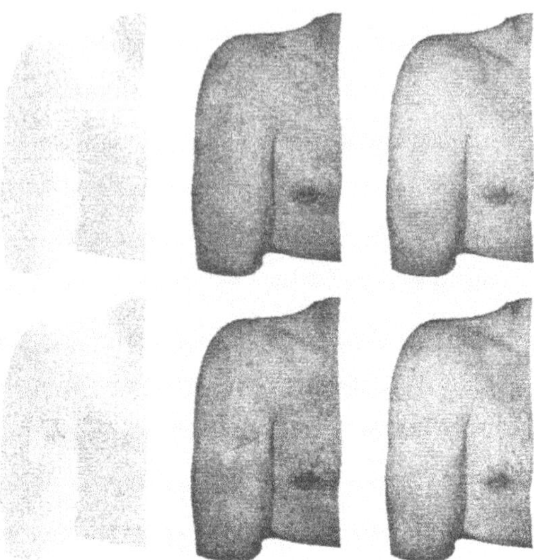

Figure 7. Deformed 3D model

4.2 Discussion

These results demonstrate our method for generating and deforming realistic 3D volumetric mesh. This method is automatic once the area of interest and forces have been specified. Moreover, visually, the deformation looks quite realistic.

Since the data used for the fat layer thickness is an average value, it does not make much sense to compare precisely the simulated deformation with the deformation that similar conditions would generate on the real human. That limitation occurs because of the lack of data to evaluate the distribution of fat layers on a specific individual.

The accuracy of a simulation using FEM depends on the accuracy of the geometry of the mesh representing the soft tissues and the knowledge of the physical properties of these tissues. The physical properties of the human skin and fat are very well known [Da82], [La87]. For example, regional differences of skin thickness have been extensively studied [Ru66], [Ho74]: the two first layers of human skin (dermis and epidermis) varies in thickness from 0.5mm on eyelids to more than 5mm on the middle of the upper back.

However the thickness of fat layers varies a lot depending on the localisation and especially on the individual (few mm to few cm). Its evaluation relies on measurements on the individual. On one hand, the most efficient methods are either invasive or require expensive material (bioelectrical impedance analysis, X-rays, CT and MRI). On the other hand, skin fold measurement is a simple and cheap method for estimation of the depth of the fat layer [Hi79]. The drawback of this method is that it is a manual and tedious task, since hundreds of measurements are needed to get a realistic evaluation of the distribution of fat layers on a specific body.

We can investigate another method that would be more suitable for our application: anthropometric measurements (girths and lengths), is a quick method used to estimate body composition. By measuring 11 sites on a body, calculations of percent body fat [Ho92] and weight [Be74] can be evaluated. Moreover three other indices, the endomorphy (roundness), the mesomorphy (muscularity) and the ectomorphy (lankyness), can be calculated to get a better picture of the physical shape of an individual [Ca91].

Using a set of models whose fat distribution and key indices are known, we should be able to interpolate the fat distribution for any new individual. Since we are currently working on automatic anthropometric measurements on full body scans using segmentation and landmark recognition techniques [De98] and [Ju00] this process of fat distribution evaluation could become fully automatic.

5. CONCLUSION AND FUTURE WORK

We presented a full process allowing realistic deformation of 3D scanned data based on the FEM applied on volumetric meshes. The generation of the volumetric mesh is automatic once the area of interest has been specified. Moreover that technique can be applied on any scanned data since there are no constraints regarding the initial mesh.

Results were demonstrated, the present limitations were discussed and details were given about a way of getting the distribution of fat layers on a specific body.

We are currently working on this specific issue. Once this investigation completed we will be able to evaluate the limitations generated by our linear model for soft tissue deformation.

REFERENCES

[Au00] A. Aubel, D. Thalmann, Realistic Deformation of Human Body Shapes, Proc. Computer Animation and Simulation 2000, Interlaken, 2000

[Be74] A. R. Behnke and J. H. Wilmore, Evaluation and regulation of body build and composition, Prentice-Hall, USA, 1974

[Bi99] D. Bielser, V. A. Maiwald and M. H. Gross, Interactive cuts through 3-dimensional soft tissue, Computer Graphics Forum, 18(3), 1999

[Bo00] L. Boissieux, G. Kiss, N. Magnenat Thalmann and P. Kalra, Simulation of skin aging and wrinkles with cosmetics insight, Computer animation and simulation'00, 2000

[Br96] M. Bro-Nielsen and S. Cotin. Real-time volumetric deformable models for surgery simulation using finite elements and condensation, Computer Graphics Forum, 15(3), pp 57-66, 1996

[Ca91] JEL Carter & BH Heath, Somatotyping: Developments and Applications. Cambridge University Press, New York, 1991.

[Ca95] M. J. Castro Díaz and F. Hect, Anisotropic Surface Mesh Generation, INRIA Research, Report, No 2672, 1995.

[Da82] C. H. Daly, Biomechanical properties of dermis, the journal of investigative dermatology, Vol. 79, pp 17-20, 1982

[De98] L. Dekker, S Khan, E. West, B. Buxton and P. Treleaven. Models for understanding the 3D human body form. Proc. IEEE workshop on model-based 3D image analysis, pp 65-74, Bombay, India, 1998

[De99] G. Debunne, M. Desbrun, A. Barr and M.-P. Cani, Interactive multiresolution animation of deformable models, Computer animation and simulation'99, 1999

[En99] K. M. Entwistle, Basic principles of the finite element method, London : IOM Communications, 1999

[Fa99] M. J. Fagan, Finite element analysis, Longman 1999

[Fr81] J. Frank, A. M. Klidjian and S. J. Karran, The radiological assessment of arm muscle and fat stores in normal and malnourished patients, Clinical radiology, 32, pp 467-470, 1981

[Fr96] P. J. Frey and H. Borouchaki, Delaunay tetrahedralization using an advancing-front approach, in Proceedings of the Fifth International Meshing Roundtable, Pittsburgh, PA, 1996.

[Ga54] S. M. Garn, Fat paterning and fat intercorrelations, Human biology, 26 ,pp 59-69, 1954

[Ge88] P. L. George and H. Borouchaki, Delaunay Triangulation and Meshing Application to Finite Elements, Editions HERMES, Paris, 1998.

[Jo95] R. R. M. Jones, P. Li, K. Brook-Wavell and G. M. West, Format of human body modelling from 3D body scanning, International journal of clothing science, 7(1), pp 7-16, 1995

[Ju00] X. Ju, N. Werghi and P. Siebert, Automatic Segmentation of 3D Human Body Scans, IASTED International Conference on Computer Graphics and Imaging 2000 (CGIM 2000), 19-23 Nov. 2000, Las Vegas, USA.

[Ko88] K. Komatsu, Human skin model capable of natural shape variation, The visual computer, Vol. 3, pp 265-271, 1988

[Ko98] R. M. Koch, M. H. Gross and A. A. Bosshard. "Emotion editing using finite element models." In Proc. Eurographics'98, 1998.

[Hi79] J. H. Himes, A. F. Roche and R. M. Siervogel, Compressibility of skinfolds and the measurement of subcutaneous fatness, Am J Clinical Nutrition, Vol. 32, pp 1734-1740, 1979

[Hi80] J. H. Himes, A. F. Roche and P. Webb, Fat areas as estimates of total body fat, The American journal of clinical nutrition, vol. 33, pp 2093-2100, 1980

[Ho74] K. A. Holbrook and G. F. Odland, Regional differences in the thickness (cell layers) of the human stratum corneum: an ultrastructural analysis.

[Ho88] K. Ho-Le, Finite element mesh generation methods: a review and classification, Computer Aided Design, Vol 20(1), 27-38, 1988.

[Ho92] J. A. Hodgdon, Body composition in the military services: standards and methods, in Body composition and physical performance 1992, pp 55-70, National Academy Press, 1992

[La86] W. F. Larrabee, A finite element model of skin deformation, Laryngoscope, 96, pp 399-419, 1986

[La87] Y. Lanir, Skin mechanics, Chapter 11, in Handbook of Bioengineering, McGraw-Hill, USA, 1987

[La94] J. Lander, Skin them bones: game programming for the web generation, Game developer, May, 1994

[Le95] Y. Lee, D. Terzopoulos and K. Waters, Realistic modeling for facial animation Computer graphics, Vol. 29, pp 55-62, 1995

[Ma95] Magnenat Thalmann N, Thalmann D., Proc.IEEE, Switzerland, 1995. " Digital Actors for Interactive Television ".

[Mo97] L.Moccozet, N.Magnenat-Thalmann, "Multilevel Deformation Model Applied to Hand Simulation for Virtual Actors", VSMM97, Geneva, Switzerland, 1997.

[Mo99] R. A. Moffett, A Prototype 3D Breast Surgery Planning and Assessment Tool, MSc IT, Department of Computing Science, University of Glasgow, Glasgow, October 1999.

[Ne98] L. P. Nedel and D. Thalmann. Modeling and deformation of the human body using an anatomically based approach.

[Nu97].J. H. Nurre, Locating landmarks on human body scan data. International conference of recent advances 3D digital imaging and modelling, pp 289-295, 1997, IEEE NJ, USA

[Pa97] R. P. Pargas, N. J. Staples and J. S. Davis, Automatic measurement extraction for apparel from a 3D body scan, Optics and Lasers in Engineering, 28(2), pp 157-172, 1997

[Ro98] S. H. M. Roth, M. H. Gross, S. Turello and F. R. Carls, A Bernstein-Bezier based approach to soft tissue simulation, Computer Graphics Forum, 17(3), 1998

[Ru66] R. F. Rushmer, K. J. K. Buettner, J. M. Short and G. F. Odland, The skin, Science, 154(3747), pp 343-348, 1966

[Si00] J. Paul Siebert and Stephen J. Marshall, Human body 3D imaging by speckle texture projection photogrammetry, Sensor Review, 20 (3), pp 218-226, 2000.

[Su99] W. Sun, A. Hilton, R. Smith and J. Illingworth, Building layered animation models from captured data, Computer Animation and Simulation'99, Springer Computer Science, pp 145-154, 1999

[Te90] D. Terzopoulos, Physically based facial modelling, analysis and animation, The journal of visualization and computer animation, Vol. 1, pp 73-90, 1990.

[Tr00] R. Trieb, 3D-Body Scanning for mass customized products - Solutions and Applications, International Conference of Numerisation 3D - Scanning 2000, 24-25 May 2000, Paris, France.

[Tu98] R. Turner and E. Gobbetti. Interactive construction and animation of layered elastically deformable characters, Computer Graphics Forum, 17(2), pp 135-152, June 1998.

[Va00] G. Vareille, Full body 3D digitizer, International Conference of Numerisation 3D - Scanning 2000, 24-25 May 2000, Paris, France.

[Wi00] S. Winsborough, An insight into the design, manufacture and practical use of a 3D-Body Scanning system, International Conference of Numerisation 3D - Scanning 2000, 24-25 May 2000, Paris, France.

CONTEXTUALLY EMBODIED AGENTS

Catherine Pelachaud
Department of Computer Science, University of Rome "La Sapienza", Rome, Italy

Key words: embodied agent, face-to-face communication, communicative facial expression, 3D facial model

Abstract: In this chapter we present our work on the elaboration of a contextually embodied agent. We define such an agent as an agent capable of planning what to communicate as well as deciding with which verbal and nonverbal signals to output considering contextual information. We first present our 3D facial model that follows MPEG-4 standard. Then we present our taxonomy of communicative facial expressions. We describe our discourse planner that generate synchronized verbal and nonverbal signals. Our planner takes as input a communicative goal and output a multimodal discourse where nonverbal expressions are modulated based on contextual information.

1. INTRODUCTION

As computers are being more and more part of our world we feel the urgent need of proper user interface to interact with. The use of command lines typed on a keyboard are obsolete, specially as computers are receiving so much attention from a large audience. The metaphor of face-to-face communication applied to human-computer interaction is receiving a lot of attention (André et al., 1998; Cassell, 2000; Poggi et al., 2000; Johnson et al., 2000; Nass et al., 2000). Humans are used since they are born to communicate with others. Seeing faces, interpreting their expression, understanding speech are all part of our development and growth. But face-to-face conversation is very complex phenomenon as it involved a huge number of factors. We speak with our voice, but also with our hand, eye, face and body. Our gesture modifies, emphasizes, contradicts what we say by words. The production of speech and nonverbal behaviors work in parallel and not in antithesis. They seem to be two different forms (voice and body gestures) of the same process (speech). Nonverbal behaviors add information on what will be difficult to express by words. They may have the function of an adverb or adjective to modulate what is being said. For example, they can express emotion, attitude toward the others. One cannot imagine the production of one behavior without the occurrence of the other ones. It is therefore important to consider both verbal and nonverbal behaviors while building an embodied agent. The agent must have the capacity to decide which facial expressions to show, which words to say with which intonation. The choice of the communicative act (word, eye movement, facial expression) to perform is based on whom we are taking to, in which context the conversation takes place. Of course this choice is not a necessarily conscious one. We do not talk in the same way to a child, a foreigner, or to an important person. An impulsive person will not express herself in the same manner as a shy person. Our goal is to create a contextually embodied agent, that is an agent capable of planning what to communicate as well as deciding with which verbal and nonverbal signals to output considering contextual information.

In this paper we first present our 3D facial model. We concentrate on the computation of communicative facial expressions and how these expressions are modulated based on contextual information. We will also present our discourse planner that generate embodied verbal and nonverbal signals.

2. FACIAL MODEL

Our facial model is based on MPEG-4 standard (Doenges et al., 1997). The model uses a pseudo-muscular approach (Pasquariello, 2000). The muscle contractions are obtained through the deformation of the polygonal network around feature points. Each feature point corresponds to skin muscle attachment. The deformation is performed in a zone of influence that has an ellipsoid shape whose centroid is the feature point. The displacement of points within this area of influence obeys to a deformation function that is function of the distance between the points and the feature point (see figures 1 and 2).

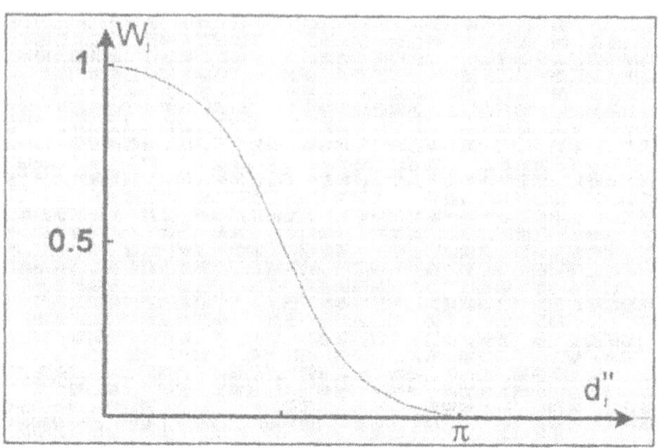

Figure 1: Deformation function

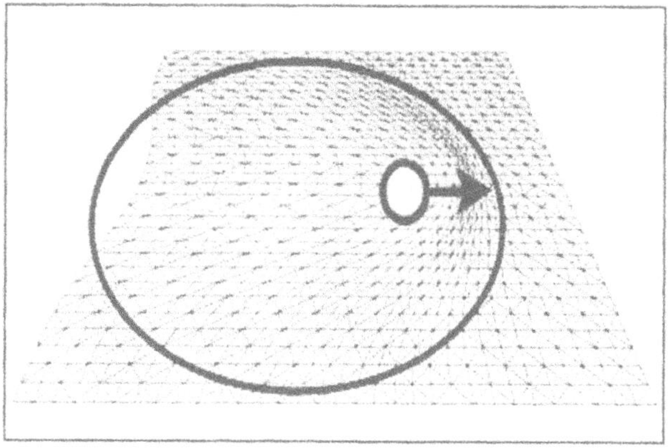

Figure 2: Skin deformation in the area of influence

Two sets of parameters describe and animate the 3D facial model: facial animation parameter set (FAPS) and facial definition parameter (FDP). The FDPs define the shape of the model while the FAPS define the facial actions. When the model has been characterized with FDP, the animation is obtained by specifying for each frame the values of FAPS. The facial model also includes particular features such as wrinkles and furrow to enhance its realism. Brow wrinkles are simulated by discontinuous lines on the forehead and appear when the eyebrows raise (action of the frontalis). They have been implemented using bump mapping technique (see figure 3). Identically frown wrinkles are vertical lines between the two eyebrows and appear under the action of the corrugator. The nasolabial furrow goes from the nose to the corner of the mouth and appears under the action of muscles whose end is around the corner of the mouth. Here bulges and furrows have been modelled using a specialized displacement function that move outward points within a specific area. The points of area A that are affected by muscular contraction will be deformed by the muscular displacement function, while the points of area B (area of the bulge / furrow) will be moved outward to simulate the skin accumulation and bulging (see figures 4, 5 and 6).

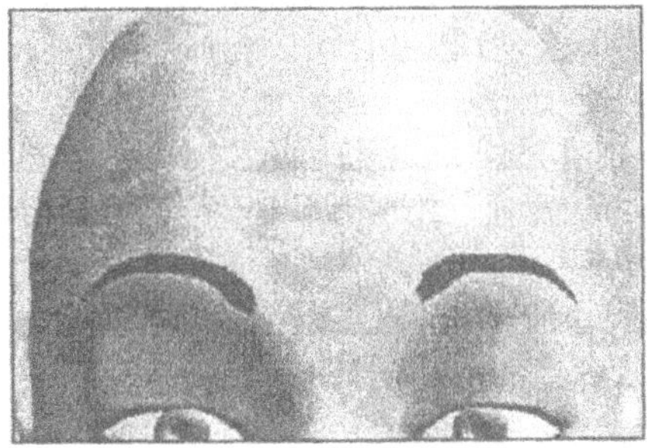

Figure 3: Brow wrinkles

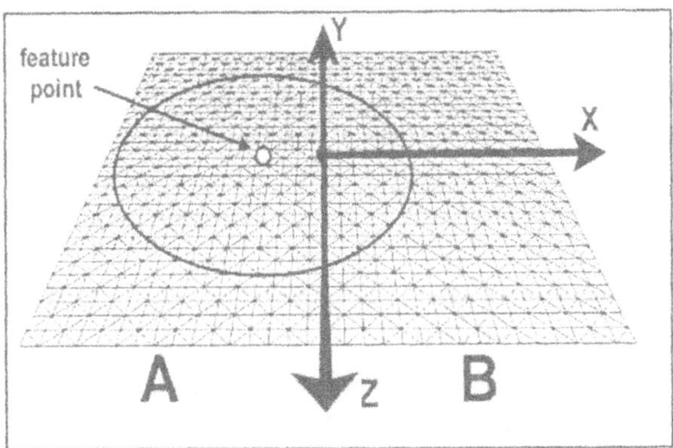

Figure 4: Within the area of influence, the two zones A (muscular traction) and B (accumulation)

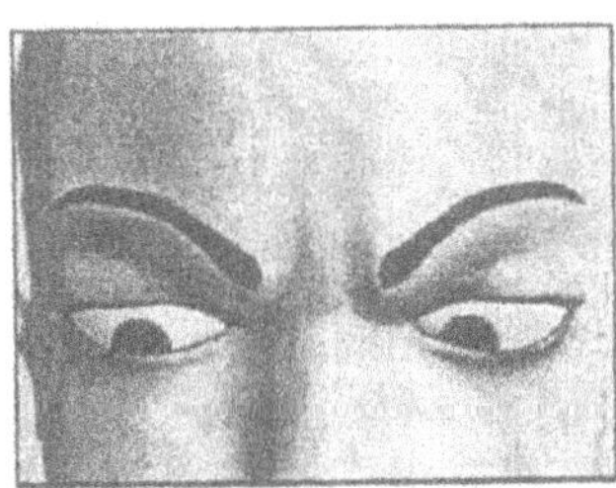

Figure 5: Folds and bulges – frown

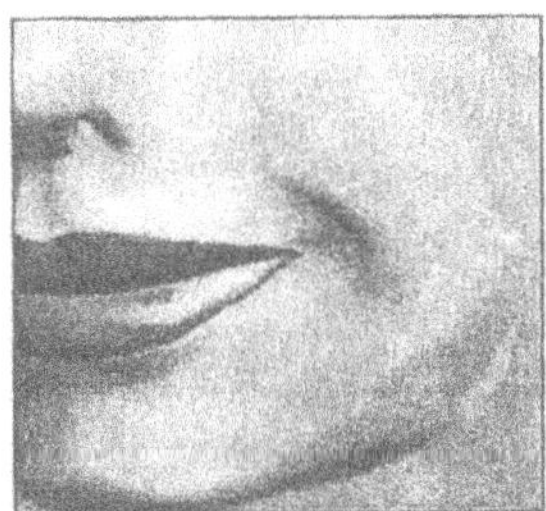

Figure 6: Folds and bulges – smile

3. FACIAL COMMUNICATIVE FUNCTIONS

Faces are an important means of communication and may have several communicative functions. They are used to control the flow of conversation; that is they help in regulating the exchange of speaking turns, keeping the floor or asking for it (Duncan and Fiske, 1985). Actions such as smiling, raising the eyebrows, and wrinkling the nose may accompany the flow of speech and are synchronized at the verbal level, punctuating accented phonemic segments and pauses (Ekman, 1979). Other facial expressions may substitute for a word or string of words, or emphasize what is being said. They can also express attitude toward one own speech (such as irony) or toward the interlocutor (like showing submission). They are also the primary channel to express emotion (Ekman, 1982).

We have decided to consider facial expressions not from the actions involved in the expression (e.g. raising eyebrows) but rather from their communicative functions (Poggi and Pelachaud, 1998). Indeed the same expression may change meaning depending on its place and time of occurrence in the conversation. Raising eyebrows signal surprise but also emphasis of what is being said; they signal question mark, specially in the case of non-syntactically questions but they are also part of the expression used when suggesting something to someone. The expression would vary in their temporal properties (onset and offset values as well as duration of the action) and in the intensity of the actions. Moreover not everybody uses the same expression to carry a given function.

In order to characterize nonverbal communicative functions, we need two information: their meaning and their visual action. The latter ones are described as a list of FAPS parameters that will drive our 3D facial model (see Section 2.). The former ones are represented as a set of goals and beliefs the speaker has the goal to communicate. We therefore differentiate communicative functions in four categories (Poggi et al., 2000):

1. information about speaker's beliefs
2. information about speaker's intentions
3. information about speaker's affective state
4. metacognitive information about speaker's mental state

3.1 Information about speaker's beliefs

In this class we gather functions that provide information on speaker's eliefs. The speaker may be certain or uncertain of what she is saying. She may use words like 'may be', 'perhaps', or use conditional such as 'might', 'could' but she can also raise her eyebrow to mark uncertainty. She may contrast several elements in her speech, she may precise, restate what she just said... This can be done verbally (e.g., 'because', 'but') but also facially (raising eyebrow to show contrast between beliefs). She may also mimic the property of things (abstract entity or real object): squeezing the eyes when mentioning 'a very subtle nuance between 2 concepts' or a tiny pin on her jacket to imitate how little is the difference or how tiny is the pin. Each function in this class gives information on how certain the speaker is of her belief, how she relates several beliefs with each others and how she believes the property of an object is.

3.2 Information about speaker's intention

This class groups several levels of information type.

- **single communicative act**: It can be about information of the intention of one single communicative act: the performative of a sentence. In a previous work (Poggi and Pelachaud, 1998) we have proposed a formalism to represent performative of a sentence as well as to highlight the existing link between performative verbs and facial expressions. Imploring might be expressed with the eyebrow of sadness while giving an order might be indicated with a frown. There exist three main classes of performative: request, inform and ask. Within a main class there exist several performatives. A request may be suggested, advised, implored. We can warn a person to inform her or we can announce her something. We can interrogate or question her to ask her information. The choice of a particular performative is determined by considering the following elements: a) we will consider consciously or unconsciously the type of social relationship that exists between ourselve and the addressee; b) we will evaluate how certain or uncertain we are about what we are going to say, and c) we will establish for whom is the action requested. The latest element will distinguish advise vs command in the request class as well as inform vs warn in the inform class. The degree of certainty of our beliefs determines if we will assure our beliefs or we will suggest them. Finally the type of social relationship will decide if we can order the addressee to perform a given action or if we may suggest it. We also found that some facial expressions are linked to performative (Poggi and Pelachaud, 1999). A person A implores a person B to perform an action a as A knows she can not achieve a without the help of B. A will be sad if B does not help her. When imploring A will display the expression of sadness (inner eyebrows raised). On the other hand A will raise her eyebrow to mark her uncertainty while suggesting something.

- **whole hierarchy of intentions**: Facial expressions are often used to mark new information in a sentence: a raising eyebrow or a head nod and gazing at the addressee usually accompany accented word (Ekman, 1979). These signals emphasize what the speaker makes relevant to the addressee, what she marks as being important in her speech.
- **overall arrangement of discourse**: A conversation is made of an exchange of speaking turns. During a conversation we may encounter situation where participants start talking simultaneously, or on the opposite no interlocutor takes the speaking floor. One may interrupt speaker's talk to start talking without expecting one's speaking turn. Verbal and nonverbal cues help this process. A turn-taking system (Duncan, 1985) refers to how people negotiate speaking turns in a conversation, or any ritual meeting. In giving the speaking turn, the speaker often gazes at the addressee, her arm and hand come to rest... On the other hand just before taking the speaking turn one gazes at the current speaker and starts gesticulation.
- **direct addressee's attention to events**: Gaze or head direction may have a deictic function such as pointing gesture. In some situation a gaze may be more useful to indicate a place, person, object... than a gesture. In a social gathering it might be more preferable to refer to the person we are talking about with a simple gaze. It will be less noticeable than a pointing hand...

3.3 Information about speaker's affective state

Emotions are best expressed with the face. They may be triggered by an event, action, or a person's action (Ortony et al., 1988). Some emotions are triggered by an event and are not directed toward someone (examples are emotion of fear, surprise). One can feel emotion toward another person (such as love, scorn, hate). Ekman and his colleagues have proposed the existence of universal facial expressions linked to six emotions (Ekman, 1982). Of course for each emotion there exists several variants of these facial expressions. We can bite our lips of anger or show our teeth. Moreover the display of the facial expression of emotion will be modulated by our culture, our social environment, to whom we are talking to... In this case, Ekman refers to Display Rules (Ekman, 1979) that is cultural rules that regulates the display of a given expression. We believe (Decarolis et al., 2000 that other rules regulate the display or non-display of an expression: if we are with a very apprehensive person that we like, we will not show our fear not to frighten her. But if we are a very impulsive person we might not consider this fact and just display our emotion.

3.4 Metacognitive information about speaker's mental state

Metacognitive function provides meta-information on what we are talking about. When we are thinking or remembering something we break our eye gaze with the addressee in order to concentrate on our thoughts. But we can also use such an expression to deliberately show we are thinking. At an oral exam we might ostentatiously display such an expression to make people believe we are deeply thinking.

4. NOTION OF CONTEXT

The choice of a communicative act and its display is not part of the speaker's communicative goal from the beginning, but it comes from consideration of context (Poggi and Pelachaud,1998). A speaker decides which specific Performative to use in one's sentence (or other non-verbal communicative act) on the basis of the social situation, the social relationship to the addressee, and of the addressee's cognitive, affective and personality factors. Requesting something to somebody may be performed as an order, a suggestion, an imploration... You will implore somebody if you know that this person has the capacity to get what you want while you can not get it by yourself. On the other hand if you know you have some power over a person you may order him to get what you desire. Each different types of request has an associated facial expression. So the choice of the appropriate signals depends on the situation the conversation takes place and the relation between the speaker and the addressee. Finally the display of a facial expression may be cancelled, masked by another expression, de-intensify or intensify depending on the context (Ekman, 1982). If you just pass a difficult exam but your friend did not you will not show too much your happiness not to make him feel worse.

5. ENRICHED DISCOURSE PLANNER

As our goal is to have an agent capable of planning what to say and with which signals we have built what we call an enriched discourse planner (Decarolis et al., 2000). The system (see figure 7) takes as input a communicative goal, the goal the agent has to communicate. The Plan library elaborates a first plan where the rhetorical relations between parts of the discourse are specified. This plan is then enriched with information about emotion display. As mentioned in section 3.3, an emotion is triggered by an event, action or person. We have implemented C. Elliott's set of rules (Elliott, 1992) that are based on (Ortony et al., 1988) to trigger an emotion.

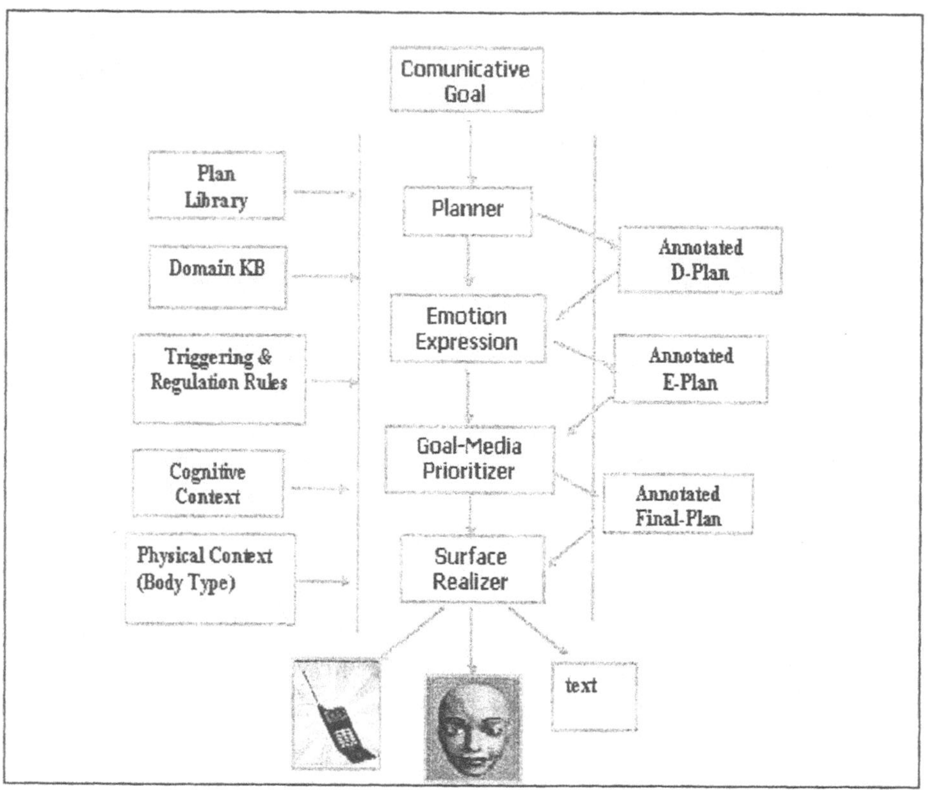

But the display of an emotion is regulated by a set of regulation rules (Decarolis et al., 2000) that are an over set of the display rules introduced by Ekman (1982). These rules take into consideration several elements of the context to decide whether or not an expression should be displayed: personality of the agent and of the addressee, cognitive capacity of the addressee, and relationship between the agent and the addressee. The general structure of the regulation rules is of the type:

IF (Feel Ag e) AND DC-Cond THEN (Display Ag e)

or

IF (Feel Ag e) AND DC-Cond THEN NOT(Display Ag e)

Where *Ag* stands for agent, *DC-Cond* for conditions on the context, and *e* for the given emotion.

Where the regulation rules have been activated, the discourse plan is enriched with these rules. This new plan is then computed as an XML document. For example, such an XML annotated document is:

```
<expr type= "ImThinking">
I have been in
<expr type= "Distress"> jail </expr>
for a very
<expr type= "LargeAdjectival"> long </expr>
period
</expr>
```

The XML tags are then interpreted and translated into FAPS that drive the 3D facial model.

6. CONCLUSION

In this paper we have presented the architecture underlying the creation of a contextually embodied agent. A taxonomy of nonverbal facial and gaze expressions has been elaborated. This taxonomy is based on the meaning of the communicative behaviors. This allows us to represent the communicative act of a speaker as a set of beliefs and goals and to establish a visual signal (facial behavior, gaze) to each of them. The discourse planner we have implemented has been enriched with triggering and regulation rules as well as with contextual information giving the ability to our agent to retain her expression or not. Our agent may become a reflexive agent not only an impulsive agent!

7. REFERENCES

E. André, T. Rist, and J. Mueller. "Integrating reactive and scripted behaviors in a life-like presentation agent." *In Proceedings of the second International Conference on Autonomous Agents*, pages 261--268, 1998.

J.L. Austin. *How to do thinks with words*. Oxford University Press, London, 1962.

J. Cassell. "Embodied conversational interface agents." *Communications of the ACM*, 43(4):70--78, April 2000.

J. Cassell, C. Pelachaud, N.I. Badler, M. Steedman, B. Achorn, T. Becket, B. Douville, S. Prevost, and M. Stone. "Animated conversation: Rule-based generation of facial expression, gesture and spoken intonation for multiple conversational agents." In

Computer Graphics Proceedings, Annual Conference Series, pages 413--420. ACM SIGGRAPH, 1994.

N. De Carolis, C. Pelachaud, and I. Poggi. " Verbal and nonverbal discourse planning." In *Workshop on "Achieving Human-Like Behavior in Interactive Animated Agents workshop"*, Fourth International Conference on Autonomous Agents, 2000.

P. Doenges, F. Lavagetto, J. Ostermann, I.S. Pandzic, and E. Petajan. "MPEG-4: Audio/video and synthetic graphics/audio for mixed media." *Image Communications Journal*, 5(4), May 1997.

S. Duncan and D.W. Fiske. *Interaction Structure and Strategy.* Cambridge University Press, 1985.

P. Ekman. "About brows: Emotional and conversational signals." In M. von Cranach, K. Foppa, W. Lepenies, and D. Ploog, editors, *Human ethology: Claims and limits of a new discipline: contributions to the Colloquium*, pages 169--248. Cambridge University Press, Cambridge, England; New-York, 1979.

P. Ekman. *Emotion in the human face.* Cambridge University Press, 1982.

C. Elliott. *An Affective Reasoner: A process model of emotions in a multiagent system.* PhD thesis, Northwestern University, The Institute for the Learning Sciences, 1992. Technical Report No. 32.

W.L. Johnson, J.W. Rickel, and J.C. Lester. "Animated pedagogical agents: Face-to-face interaction in interactive learning environments." To appear *in International Journal of Artificial Intelligence in Education*, 2000.

C. Nass, K. Isbister, and E.J. Lee. "Truth is beauty: Researching embodied conversational agents." In S. Prevost J. Cassell, J. Sullivan and E. Churchill, editors, *Embodied Conversational Characters.* MITpress, Cambridge, MA, 2000.

A. Ortony, G.L. Clore, and A. Collins. *The Cognitive Structure of Emotions.* Cambridge University Press, 1988.

S. Pasquariello. *Modello per l'animazione facciale in MPEG-4.* Master's thesis, University of Rome, 2000.

I. Poggi and C. Pelachaud. Performative faces. *Speech Communication*, 26:5--21, 1998.

I. Poggi and C. Pelachaud. "Emotional meaning and expression in performative faces." In *International Workshop on Affect in Interactions: Towards a New Generation of Interfaces*, Annual Conference AC'99 of the EC I3 Programme, Siena, October 1999.

I. Poggi, C. Pelachaud, and F. de Rosis. "Eye communication in a conversational {3D synthetic agent." *Special Issue on Behavior Planning for Life-Like Characters and Avatars of AI Communications,* 2000.

ON IMPLICIT MODELING FOR FITTING PURPOSES

Ralf Plänkers
Pascal Fua*
{Ralf.Plaenkers,Pascal.Fua}@epfl.ch
Computer Graphics Lab (LIG)
Swiss Federal Institute of Technology (EPFL)
CH 1015 Lausanne

Keywords: Body fitting, body modeling, implicit surface, metaball

Abstract Tracking and modeling people from video sequences has become an increasingly important research topic, with applications including animation, surveillance and sports medicine. In this paper, we propose a model based 3–D approach to recovering both body shape and motion. It takes advantage of a sophisticated animation model to achieve both robustness and realism. Stereo sequences of people in motion serve as input to our system. From these, we extract a 2.5–D description of the scene and, optionally, silhouette edges. We propose an integrated framework to fit the model and to track the person's motion. Constraints for 3–D points and silhouette edges are presented in detail. We recover not only the motion but also a full animation model closely resembling the subject.

Introduction

Tracking and modeling people from video sequences has become an increasingly important research topic, with applications including animation, surveillance and sports medicine. In this paper, we propose a 3–D approach to recovering both body shape and motion. We obtain stereo- and silhouette-data from synchronized cameras and we fit to it a sophisticated body model. We use it to eliminate erroneous data, to

*The work reported here was funded in part by the Swiss National Science Foundation.

A detailed description of the human body in the form of an animated layered model is at the root of our work. It provides *a priori* information about the shape, and the allowable motions of the human body. This is essential for interpreting noisy data and solving the resulting ambiguities. The model we use is made of volumetric primitives attached to an articulated skeleton (Thalmann et al., 1996). This implicit surface formulation has several advantages, among them a lower number of parameters and a 3–D distance measure that is differentiable and fast to compute.

As input to our system we use image sequences of people in motion. Multiple synchronized and calibrated cameras are used to extract stereo information. Because cameras are relatively cheap and disparity maps such as the ones we use can be acquired at frame rate on ordinary computers (Konolige, 1997), this is not a major limitation for many applications. Also, stereo works well both on textured clothes and on bare skin. Silhouette edges can be included when available. Stereo and silhouettes are complementary sources of information: Stereo works well where the surface faces the camera but fails where the surface slants away. Silhouettes, on the other hand, provide information exactly there, at the occluding contour.

We have developed an extensible least squares framework that we use to fit the body model to the different types of input data, with minimal human intervention. To initialize the process, the user simply clicks on the approximate location of a few key-points in one image pair. The recovered shape and motion parameters can then be used to reconstruct the original motion, to display it from a different viewpoint or to make other animation models mimic the subject's actions.

Recently, techniques have been proposed to track human motions from video sequences. They are fairly effective but use very simplified models of the human body, such as ellipsoids or cylinders, that do not precisely model the human shape. The recovered motion can indeed be applied to other models. However, a model of the filmed person that would be sufficient for a truly realistic animation is not obtained. The interested reader is referred to the recent surveys in (Gavrila, 1999; Moeslund and Granum, 2001) for further references.

Automatic (Hilton et al., 1999) and semi-automatic (Lee et al., 2000) systems for 3–D model acquisition from orthogonal photographs have been developed recently. They work fairly well for the intended applications like populating virtual worlds. However, most of the realism is due to texture mapping while the geometry is only a crude approximation.

While laser scanning technology provides a fairly good surface description of a static object, using video sequences allows us in addition to measure and track the person in motion and, thus, to recover the positions of the articulations inside the skin surface.

1. Body Model

The animated body model we use is made of volumetric primitives called *metaballs* attached to an articulated skeleton. Each one generates a potential field and the skin is taken to be an isosurface of the combined potential (Thalmann et al., 1996).

1.1. State Vector

Our goal is to use video-sequences to estimate our model's shape and derive its position in each frame. Let us therefore assume that we are given N consecutive video frames and introduce position parameters for each frame.

Let B be the number of body parts in our model. We assign to each body part a variable length and width coefficient. These dimensions change from person to person but we take them to be constant within a particular sequence. This constraint could be relaxed, for example to model muscular contraction.

The model's *shape* and *position* are then described by the combined state vector

$$\Theta = \{\Theta^w, \Theta^l, \Theta^r, \Theta^g\} \ , \tag{1}$$

where we have broken Θ into four subvectors which control the following model components:

- Shape.
  - $\Theta^w = \{\theta_b^w \mid b = 1..B\}$, the width of body parts.
  - $\Theta^l = \{\theta_b^l \mid b = 1..B\}$, the length of body parts.
- Motion.
  - $\Theta^r = \{\theta_{i,f}^r \mid j = 1..J, f = 1..N\}$, the rotational degree of freedom of joint j of the articulated skeleton for all frames f
  - $\Theta^g = \{\theta_f^g \mid f = 1..N\}$, the six parameters of global position and orientation of the model in the world frame for all frames f

The size and position of the metaballs is relative to the segment they are attached to. A length parameter not only specifies the length of a skeleton segment but also the shape of the attached metaballs in the direction of the segment. Width parameters only influence the metaballs' shape in the other directions.

Motion paramaters Θ^r are represented in terms of Euler angles. We can constrain joint motions to anatomically valid ranges by defining an allowable interval for each of the degrees of freedom. Other methods for describing rotations, such as quaternions or exponential maps, can be used as well.

1.2. Metaballs

Metaballs are defined by a set of points that are the sources of a potential field. Each source is defined by a *field function* $F_i(x, y, z)$ that maps $\mathbb{R}^3$ to $\mathbb{R}$. At a given point $\mathbf{x}(x, y, z)$ of the Euclidean space, the fields of all sources are computed and added together, leading to the global field function

$$F(x, y, z) = \sum_{i=1}^{n} F_i(x, y, z) \ . \tag{2}$$

Choosing a threshold value T then allows us to define the implicit surface

$$\mathbf{S} = \{(x, y, z) \in \mathbb{R}^3 \mid F(x, y, z) = T\} \ . \tag{3}$$

We take the field function F_i to be

$$F_i(x, y, z) = f_i(d_i(x, y, z)) \ , \tag{4}$$

where d_i is a *distance function* that maps $\mathbb{R}^3$ to $\mathbb{R}^+$, and f_i is a *potential function* which maps $\mathbb{R}^+$ to $\mathbb{R}$ (Blanc and Schlick, 1995). The function d_i characterizes the distance between a given point $\mathbf{x}(x, y, z)$ and the source point of a metaball. The most obvious choice is the Euclidean distance, but several other functions have been proposed in the literature.

In this work, we take d_i to be an algebraic ellipsoidal distance:

$$d_i(x, y, z) = \left(\frac{x - \theta_i^w c_{x,i}}{\theta_i^w l_{x,i}}\right)^2 + \left(\frac{y - \theta_i^w c_{y,i}}{\theta_i^w l_{y,i}}\right)^2 + \left(\frac{z - \theta_i^l c_{z,i}}{\theta_i^l l_{z,i}}\right)^2 \ , \tag{5}$$

where $L_i = (l_{x,i}, l_{y,i}, l_{z,i})$ are the radii of ellipsoid i, i.e. half the axis length along the principal directions and $C_i = (c_{x,i}, c_{y,i}, c_{z,i})$ is the primitive's center. Coefficients θ_i^l and θ_i^w from the state vector Θ control relative *length* and *width* of a metaball. They are shared among groups of metaballs according to segment assignment. For simplicity's sake, in the remainder of the paper, we will omit the i index for specific metaballs wherever the context is unambiguous.

We use ellipsoidal primitives because they are simple and, at the same time, allow accurate modeling of human limbs with relatively few primitives because metaballs result in a smooth surface, thus keeping the number of parameters low. Using algebraic distances for fitting purposes can result in overfitting in the high-curvature regions in some cases (Sullivan et al., 1994). For our specific application, however, the ellipses only have limited degrees of freedom and are rigidly attached to a skeleton structure. Their shape is controlled by higher level width and length parameters, and, thus, such problems do not occur.

To permit an effective fit of our implicit surface model to the data we use an exponential field function:

$$f_i = \left(\frac{1}{e^{d_i}}\right)^2 = exp(-2d_i) \ . \tag{6}$$

Function f_i is differentiable over the whole domain and it has a long range effect because it approaches zero slowly. In the context of model fitting these two properties are very important as will be discussed in Section 2.

2. Fitting the Models to Image Data

From a fitting point of view, the body model embodies a rough knowledge about the shape of the body and can be used to constrain the search space. Our goal is to derive its degrees of freedom so that it conforms as faithfully as possible to the image data.

Here we use motion sequences such as the ones shown in Figure 2. Silhouette information can be added when available, as shown in 1. Thus, the expected output of our system is a state vector that describes the shape of the metaballs and a set of joint angles corresponding to their positions in each frame.

2.1. Least Squares Framework

In standard least-squares fashion, we use the image data to write *nobs* observation equations of the form

$$y_i(S) = obs_i - \epsilon_i \ , 1 \leq i \leq nobs \ , \tag{7}$$

where S is the state vector of Eq. 1 that defines the shape and position of the limb and ϵ_i is the deviation from the model. We will then minimize

$$v^T P v \Rightarrow Min \ , \tag{8}$$

where $v = [\epsilon_1, \ldots, \epsilon_{nobs}]$ is the vector of residuals and P is a weight matrix associated with the observations. P is usually introduced as diagonal.

Our system must be able to deal with observations coming from different sources that may not be commensurate with each other. Formally we can rewrite the observation equations of Equation 7 as

$$y_i^{type}(S) = obs_i^{type} - \epsilon_i \quad, 1 \leq i \leq nobs \quad , \tag{9}$$

with weight p_i^{type}, where *type* is one of the possible types of observations we use. In this paper, *type* can be object space coordinates or silhouette rays. However, other information cues can easily be integrated.

The individual weights of the different types of observations have to be homogenized prior to estimation according to:

$$\frac{p_i^k}{p_j^l} = \frac{\left(\sigma_j^l\right)^2}{\left(\sigma_i^k\right)^2} \quad , \tag{10}$$

where σ_j^l, σ_i^k are the a priori standard deviations of the observations obs_i, obs_j of type k, l.

Least-squares estimation means finding the joint minimum

$$\sum_{type=1}^{nt} v^{type} P_{type} v^{type} \Rightarrow Min \quad , \tag{11}$$

where nt is the number of observation types. It yields the well-known normal equations which need to be solved using standard techniques.

Since our overall problem is non-linear, the results are obtained through an iteration process. We use an implementation of the Levenberg-Marquardt algorithm (Press et al., 1986) that can handle the large number of parameters and observations we must deal with.

2.2. 3–D Observations

Each 3–D point reconstructed using stereo or similar techniques is introduced as one observation into the system. The point has to lie on the surface of the model in order to be explained by the model. It's objective function, i.e. the error in the model and thus the distance between point and model, has to be minimized. We use the value of the implicit field function as algebraic distance and minimize it instead of a geometric distance. Please refer to (Plänkers and Fua, 2001) for a description of how to compute the Jakobians.

2.3. From Silhouette Data to Observations

Contrary to 3–D edges, silhouette edges are typically 2–D features since they depend on the viewpoint and cannot be matched across images. However, they constrain the surface tangent. Each point of the silhouette edge defines a line, the camera ray, that goes through the optical center of the camera and is tangent to the surface at its point of contact with the surface. The points of a silhouette edge therefore define a ruled surface that is tangent to the surface to be modeled.

3–D position of silhouette edges The main difficulty is to find the metaball surface point X where the constraint applies. In practice, we take this point to be the point on the camera ray which minimizes the implicit formulation of the model, Eq. 6. This point depends on the position of the model and we have to adjust the Jakobian of the constraint in order to account for the model dynamics.

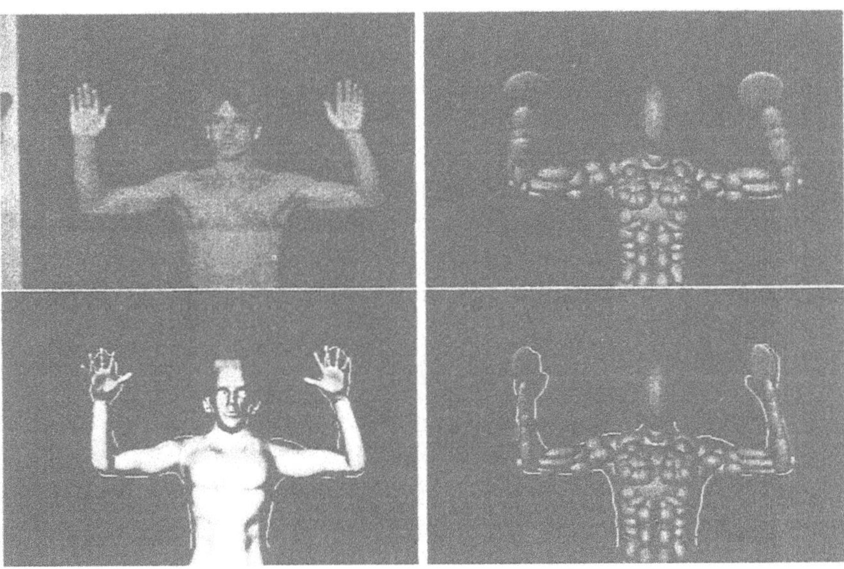

Figure 1. The importance of silhouette information for shape modeling. The original image is shown in the upper left. In the upper right no silhouette constraints were used and the fitting puts the model is too far away from the cloud. This is compensated by enlarging the primitives. The silhouettes provide stricter constraints for the model. The lower row shows the result of the fitting with and without skin rendered.

The importance of using silhouette information is demonstrated by Figure 1. Here, we allowed for changes in the model's posture and the shape parameters of the arms. In the upper row of Figure 1 only the

3–D information is used. The fitting tends to move the model further away from the cloud and to compensate by inflating the arms to keep contact with the point cloud. The noisy stereo data is too ambiguous to sufficiently constrain the model. The silhouettes are needed to constrain it, as shown in the lower row of Figure 1 where we fitted to both stereo and silhouette information.

3. Combining Articulated Structure and Implicit Surfaces

3.1. The Modular Approach

We combine metaballs and articulated skeleton by defining the observation $\mathbf{x} = [x, y, z]^T$ as being a function of the skeleton structure. This way, the derivatives wrt. to the parameters of the articulated structure and those local to the metaballs can be separated by simple application of the chain rule. Following is a description of deriving derivatives for the common Euler-Angle formulation of rotational joints. Here, a joint can only have a rotation around a single fixed axis. More complicated joints can be modeled by several single-DoF joints sharing the same position but having different orientations.

Euler-Angles. For some distance function $d(\mathbf{x}, \theta^r)$ with $\mathbf{x} = [x, y, z]^T$ being the observation in local coordinates of joint j and $\theta^r = \{\theta^r_j\}$, $j = 1..J$ the rotational joint parameters of the object we can write the jacobian entries wrt. to each DoF θ^r_j as

$$\frac{\partial d}{\partial \theta^r_j} = \frac{\partial d}{\partial \mathbf{x}} \cdot \frac{\partial \mathbf{x}}{\partial \theta^r_j} \quad . \tag{12}$$

The first term $\frac{\partial d}{\partial \mathbf{x}}$ only depends on the chosen distance function. The second term $\frac{\partial \mathbf{x}}{\partial \theta^r_j}$ expresses the change induced by the rotation at joint j. Decomposing a rotational joint into a directional axis $\mathbf{a}$ and an angle value θ^r_j, i.e. the amount of rotation around this axis, we can rewrite the second term as

$$\frac{\partial \mathbf{x}}{\partial \theta^r_j} = \mathbf{a}_j \times \overrightarrow{\mathbf{O}_j\mathbf{O}_E}(\theta^r_j) \quad . \tag{13}$$

with $\overrightarrow{\mathbf{O}_j\mathbf{O}_E}$ being the vector from the joint j's reference frame to the end-effector under the current rotation θ^r_j. All vectors are expressed in global coordinate frames. In the case of an observation the vector needs to be inverted to yield $\overrightarrow{\mathbf{O}_{obs}\mathbf{O}_j}$. For proof we refer the interested reader to (Baerlocher and Boulic, 1999). For Euler-Angles this Eq. 13 can directly be used by repeating it for each axis that allows a rotation $(omega, phi, kappa)$.

Metaball Parameters. Local metaball parameters, like size or position which are independ of the skeleton posture are derived as follows. For some distance function $d(\mathbf{x}, \theta^m)$ with $\mathbf{x} = [x, y, z]^T$ being the observation and $\theta^m = \{\theta_i^m\}$, $i = 1..I$ the local metaball parameters of the object we can write the jacobian entries wrt. to each DoF θ_i^m as

$$\frac{\partial d}{\partial \theta_i^m} \tag{14}$$

This means the skeleton structure remains constant and $\mathbf{x}$ can simply be used as already transformed into joint local coordinates, according to the current skeleton configuration. The derivation becomes straightforward.

3.2. Discussion

Separability of the single modules is a clear advantage when it comes to implementation of the method described above. Code reuse and simplicity of functions greatly increase reliability and ease of testing. However, the use of this technique becomes more problematic when combined influences need to be addressed. How do we formulate complex derivatives that describe the interplay of parameters of different types? This problem arises when integrating 2–D silhouette constraints in our 3–D fitting framework. The point on the 3–D silhouette ray that is closest to the model, i.e. the point of intersection with the real-world object, moves along the ray when posture and metaball paramters change. This is much easier to model when using a combined formulation. A sketch of a definition of an alternative formulation that retains the modularity but allows for more complex modeling had been presented during the workshop. A description of this can be found in (Plänkers and Fua, 2001).

4. Results

The sequence in Figure 2(a) shows complex movements of a naked upper body, taken with a camera set up in front of the subject. Three cameras in an L configuration were taking interlaced images at 20 frames/sec with an effective resolution of 432 × 288 per half-frame. Our stereo al-

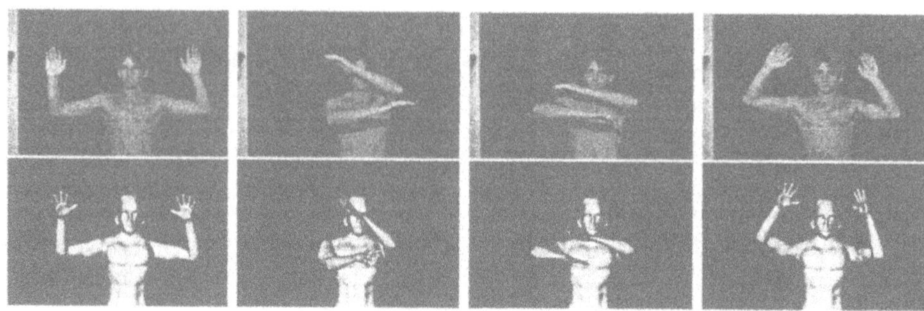

Figure 2. In the top row (a) is the original sequence of the upper body motion. Frames 10, 50, 60 and 90 out of 100 are shown. Results of the tracking and fitting with the animation model are shown in the bottom row with.

gorithm (Fua, 1995) produced very dense point clouds with about 4000 3–D points on the surface of the subject, even without textured clothes. To increase the frame rate and, thus, reduce the difference in posture between frames we used both halves of the interlaced images and adjusted the camera calibration accordingly.

The result of the tracking process is shown in Figure 2(b). The fitting step, using a more detailed model, produced slightly better postures, an adapted skeleton and resized metaballs (Fig. 2(c)). The head of this model was generated from a single video sequence of the subject by using the system of (Fua, 1999).

5. Conclusion and Future Work

We have presented a technique for fitting a complete animation model to image data and tracking complex 3–D motions. The model and the constraints it imposes are used to overcome the inherent noisiness of the data. We recover both motion and body shape from stereo video sequences. The corresponding parameters can be used to recreate realistic 3–D animations. Such a capability should be of great use in the area of human animation since it could also be used to analyze and visualize human motion for medical and training purposes. A more thorough description of our technique can be found in (Plänkers and Fua, 2001).

In future work, we intend to further exploit our strong model, for example the model can help to identify occlusions and decide whether to let the data guide the fitting or to let the prediction change the posture where no data is available. The model could also be used to derive an automatic and robust silhouette extraction algorithm, even with cluttered background.

Baerlocher, P. and Boulic, R. (1999). Inverse kinematics report. Technical report, EPFL–DI–LIG.

Blanc, C. and Schlick, C. (1995). Extended field functions for soft objects. In *Eurographics Workshop on Implicit Surfaces 95*, pages 21–32, Grenoble, France.

Fua, P. (1995). Reconstructing Complex Surfaces from Multiple Stereo Views. In *International Conference on Computer Vision*, pages 1078–1085, Cambridge, MA.

Fua, P. (1999). Using Model-Driven Bundle-Adjustment to Model Heads from Raw Video Sequences. In *International Conference on Computer Vision*, Corfu, Greece.

Gavrila, D. (1999). The Visual Analysis of Human Movement: A Survey. *Computer Vision and Image Understanding*, 73(1).

Hilton, A., Beresford, D., Gentils, T., Smith, R., and Sun, W. (1999). Virtual People: Capturing Human Models to Populate Virtual Worlds. In *Computer Animation*, Geneva, Switzerland.

Konolige, K. (1997). Small Vision Systems: Hardware and Implementation. In *Eighth International Symposium on Robotics Research*, Hayama, Japan.

Lee, W., Gu, J., and Thalmann, N. M. (2000). Generating animatable 3d virtual humans from photographs. In *Computer Graphics forum, Eurographics*, volume 19, pages C1–C10, Interlaken, Switzerland.

Moeslund, T. and Granum, E. (2001). A Survey of Computer Vision-Based Human Motion Capture. *Computer Vision and Image Understanding*, 81(3).

Plänkers, R. and Fua, P. (2001). Articulated Soft Objects for Video-based Body Modeling. In *International Conference on Computer Vision*, Vancouver, Canada.

Press, W., Flannery, B., Teukolsky, S., and Vetterling, W. (1986). *Numerical Recipes, the Art of Scientific Computing*. Cambridge U. Press, Cambridge, MA.

Sullivan, S., Sandford, L., and Ponce, J. (1994). Using Geometric Distance Fits for 3–D. Object Modeling and Recognition. *IEEE Transactions on Pattern Analysis and Machine Intelligence*, 16(12):1183–1196.

Thalmann, D., Shen, J., and Chauvineau, E. (1996). Fast Realistic Human Body Deformations for Animation and VR Applications. In *Computer Graphics International*, Pohang, Korea.

INTERACTIVE MODELLING OF MPEG-4 DEFORMABLE HUMAN BODY MODELS

Hyewon Seo, Frederic Cordier, Laurent Philippon, Nadia Magnenat-Thalmann
MIRALab, University of Geneva, CH-1211 Geneva, Switzerland

Key words: Deformation, simplification, MPEG-4 BDP, seamless body, animation ready model.

Abstract: Acquisition of various human body models is useful in many cases. In this paper, we present some of our recent work on body creation tools. Our goal is to enable rapid creation of various body models that are immediately usable for animation. In doing so, we aim to carry out realistic deformations on the human body models as well as make its usage simple. Our system is composed of several modules: (1) Skin attachment to an H-Anim skeleton is carried out first in order to get deformation in skeletal shape modification as well as in animation. (2) Volumetric deformation module deals with the volumetric scale of body parts such as breast, belly and bottoms. These deformation operators, together with the skeletal deformation allow the automatic adaptation of the body model to different sizes and proportions to accommodate anthropometrical variations. (3) Surface optimization is used to simplify the model in consideration of not only geometric features but also the animation aspect of it. (4) Finally, the BDP generation module describes the geometry of the model as well as how to animate it according to the MPEG-4 BDP specifications.

1. INTRODUCTION

In recent years, human characters have become more and more important in computer animation, virtual reality, entertainment, e-commerce and many other areas. Amongst many of the relevant techniques, model acquisition of the human character model has been attracted considerable attention from many researchers. In practice, it is the first step of the pipeline that encompasses addition of props, face and body animation, coordination along with stages or virtual environments, and synchronization with other media such as sound.

In general, human character modeling techniques are classified by the creative approach and the reconstructive approach. A variety of modeling methods, such as plaster modelling [11], sculptor [3], meatballs [14], free-form deformations [1] fall into the former approach. Within these methods, we often differentiate them according to whether they deal with the skeleton and the skin surface only (surface model) or they contain intermediate layers which simulate the muscle, bone, fat tissue, etc. (multi-layered model). While allowing an interactive design of human bodies either from scratch or by modify existing model, they however require considerable user intervention and thus suffer from a relatively slow production time and a lack of efficient control facilities.

Lately, much work has been devoted to the reconstructive approach. Some of them rely on stereo [4, 16], structured light [11] or 3D scanners [10]. Some systems use 2D images either from video sequences [5] or from photos [6, 7, 8, 9]. In the latter case, modifying existing model tends to be popular due to the expenses of recovering 3D geometry. Based on adding details or features to an existing generic model, these approaches concern mainly the individualized shape and visual realism using a high quality textures. While they are effective and visually convincing in the cloning aspect, these approaches hardly give any control to the user; i.e., it is very difficult to modify these meshes to a different shape as the user intends.

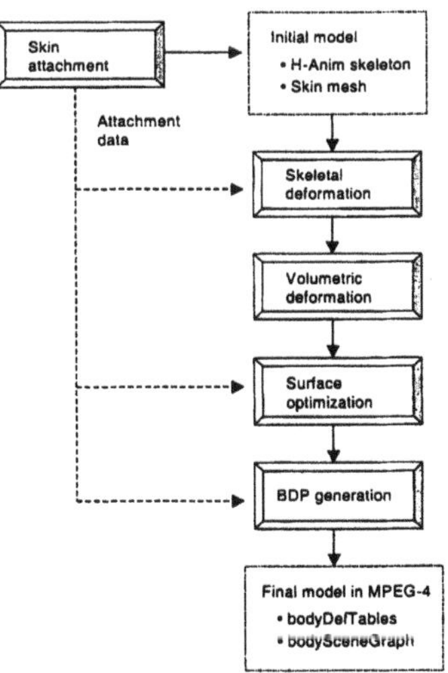

Figure 1. Overview of the creation process

In this paper, we present our approach to create various human body models that are immediately usable for animation. A number of deformers are introduced for each part of the body to automatically adapt the body model to different sizes and proportions. We also discuss geometric optimization and standard support aspects of our system. Our system is composed of several modules working in a pipeline. Figure1 gives an overview of the pipeline.

The rest of this paper is organized as follows: Our design specification is briefly introduced in Section 2. Section 3 describes the generic body model we have chosen to use. Section 4 explains the skeletal deformation used to achieve the variation of limb lengths of the body model. Section 5 details deformations used to modify the shape and volume of different parts of the body. The optimization and standard support issues will be briefly discussed in Section 6 and Section 7 respectively. Section 8 concludes this paper and describes our plans for future work.

2. DESIGN SPECIFICATION

Human morphology has a high variability depending on gender, age, occupation, etc. The description of the body can be defined by many ways. In this work, we focus on the structural measures or static size of the body such as height, breadth and width. We have chosen a set of anthropometrical measurements that correspond to the industrial standards:

- Size of the feet, hands, legs, arms and the neck.
- Width of legs, arms and the neck.
- Width of the waist, breast and hips.

Apart from the shape design, we aim to feature the system with the following aspects:

- Various levels of control: The user can simply type the measured values to drive automatic adaptation on the body or interactively add details.
- Animation ready model: Generate not only the geometric model but also information on how to deform it.
- Performance: Optimize the surface geometry with its deformation aspect considered.
- Standard support: Describe the resulting body model and animation information in MPEG-4 BDP format.

3. BODY MODEL

We have worked on a generic model, which is composed of a skin mesh and a skeleton. For the skin surface mesh, we use body models that have been developed at EPFL and University of Geneva [14].

The skeleton hierarchy we have chosen to use is H-Anim Level of Articulation(LoA) 2 one [15]. This is important, as one of our goals is to make the resulting models MPEG-4 compatible. Figure2 illustrates the generic model for women and skeleton hierarchy excluding hand joints. Including the hierarchy or skeletal description of the body brings two practical advantages. Firstly, it enables an intuitive way of skeletal deformation. Skeletal deformation will be discussed later in this paper (Section 4). Secondly, this information is essential to define the animation ready body. The description of the body into MPEG-4 format (BDP) is described in Section 7.

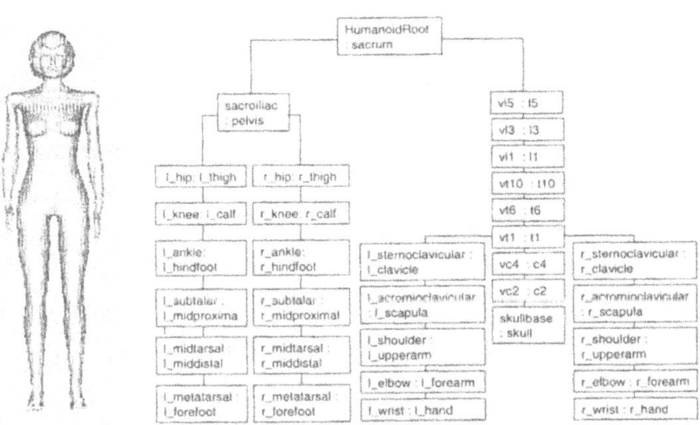

Figure 2. Generic body model: The skin surface model for a woman(left). The skeleton hierarchy excluding hands(right)

4. SKELETAL DEFORMATION

4.1 Skin Attachment

A proper skin attachment is essential to skeletal deformation as well as BDP exportation. The attachment is considered as assigning for each vertex of the mesh its affecting bones and corresponding weights. To say that a vertex is "weighted" with respect to a bone means that the vertex will move as the bone is rotated in order to stay aligned with it. At 100 percent weighting, for instance, the vertex follows the bone rigidly. This method combines for each vertex the transformation matrix of the bones in accordance to their weight. Using the attachment data, the position P_v of the skin vertex v is defined by

$$P_v = \sum_i (M_i \cdot K_i \cdot O_i)$$

where M_i is the transformation matrix of ith affecting bone, K_i is its weight and the offset O_i is the distance from v to the bone.

In order to speed up this process, we have defined a generic attachment data that can be used for every other model. We have explored several existing tools for the attachment [18]. On top of the chosen attachment tool, we have developed an importer/exporter in order to fully automate this process by reusing the once-done generic skin attachment data.

4.2 Skeletal Deformation

Once the skin is properly attached to the skeleton, transformation of the bone automatically derives transformation of the skin mesh. We provide two different levels of control to the user: At the highest level, the user simply types in the measure of these parameters instead of tedious selection and manual deformation. These parameters are then translated into modifications on the skeleton; the size of each bone is adapted to the new measurements. In case the user wants detailed and direct control, s/he can manipulate the skeleton directly in the rendering window using mouse.

This is useful especially to change the length or volume of the limbs. Figure 3 shows the modification of the limb volume and length we obtained by skeletal deformation.

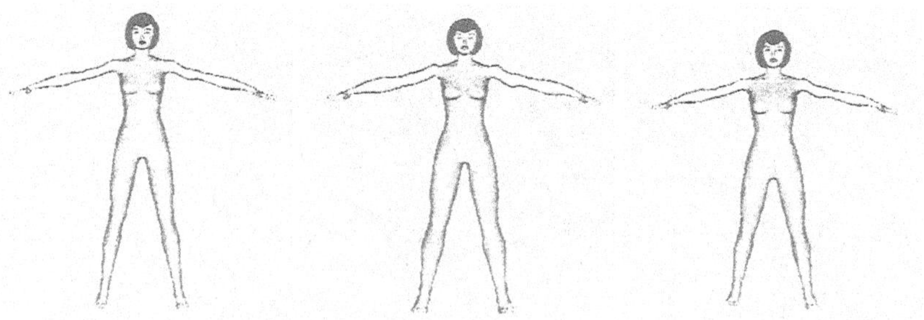

Figure 3. Skeletal deformation: Change of the limb volume and the limb length

5. VOLUMETRIC DEFORMATION

For some parts of the body that concerns the volume measurements, deformation means more than simple transformation of associated bones. Breast or chest, belly, and hips are such examples. As the generic model is based on characteristic lines or contours and thus naturally forms a grid, we use parametric curves to deform these parts locally and smoothly.

5.1 Breast

Being represented as a regular grid, the breast region of the mesh forms a 20 x 23 array. The deformation takes place in the two directions as shown in Figure 4: one along the vertical direction and the other along the horizontal one.

Figure 4. The deformation on the breast using NURBs

Along the vertical lines, we sensibly select 6 points as B-spline control points. The first and the last points are not moved in order not to create discontinuities on the surface. The second and the fifth point as well are just present to give a regular aspect to the surface, i.e. a curve that grows gradually. The third and the fourth point undergo a translation of factor F, as shown in Figure 5. All the other points in the line are sampled using the Boor Cox algorithm.

Along the horizontal direction, the points should be located in such a way that it preserves the shape of the breast. The translations of the control points form a function f, whose evolution takes the forms the shape of the breast. (See Figure 5.) In other words, the value of the factor F will depend on the column for which the deformation is applied, multiplied by the degree of displacement desired by the user. Whenever the user increases or decreases the size via the user interface, s/he will have the resulting measurement value. Figure 6 illustrates some of the results we obtained.

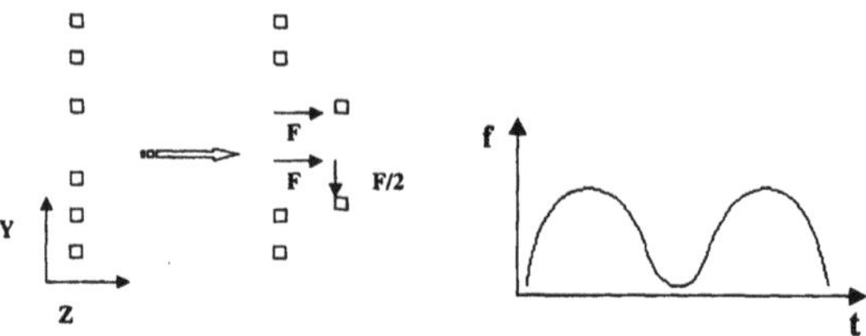

Figure 5. Translation of control points along the vertical direction (left) and function of displacement factor along the horizontal direction (right)

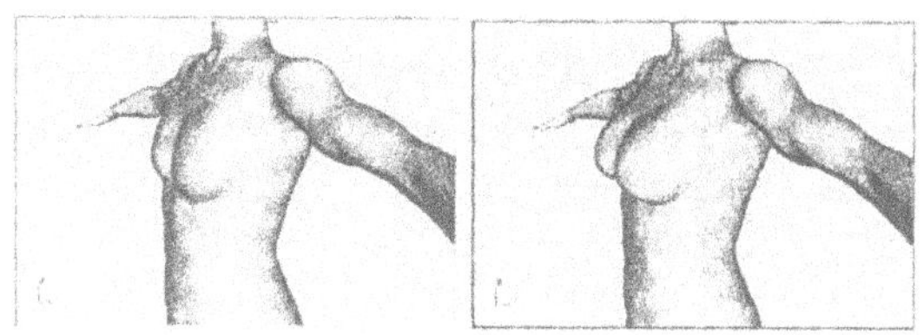

Figure 6. Deformation of the breast

5.2 Belly

The principle of the deformation for the belly is similar to that of the deformation for the breast except that we use Bézier curve in this case. We store the points of the body corresponding to the belly in a matrix of 20 by 25. On the 20 points in the vertical direction, we select 4 points which will correspond to the control points of the Bézier curve (Figure 7).

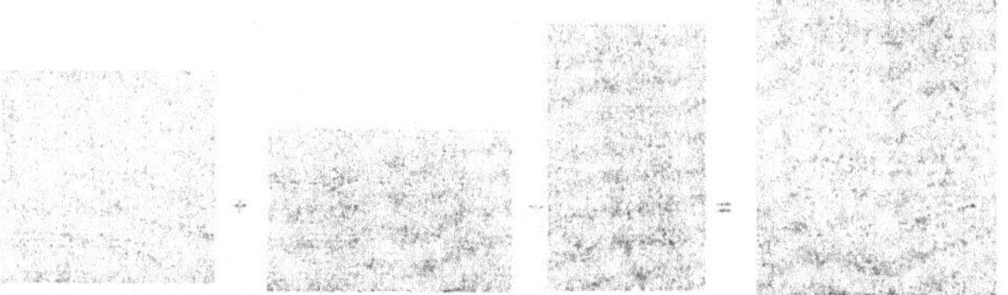

Figure 7. The belly deformation using Bézier

The two control points in the center are put forward along the Z axis by the factor F, coupled with a factor which corresponds to the position of the column the deformation is working. Once these 4 control points are placed at good positions, we sample the curve to position all the other points on it using the De Casteljau algorithm. The displacement factor along the horizontal direction takes the form of the belly as shown in Figure 8, which is followed by the resulting modified shapes in Figure 9.

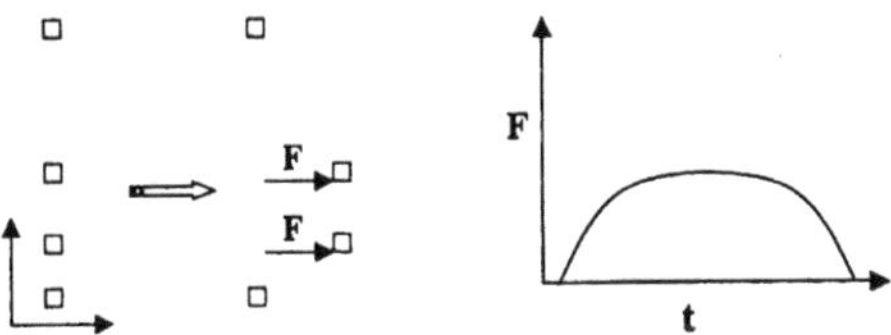

Figure 8. Displacement of control points (left) and function of displacement factor (right)

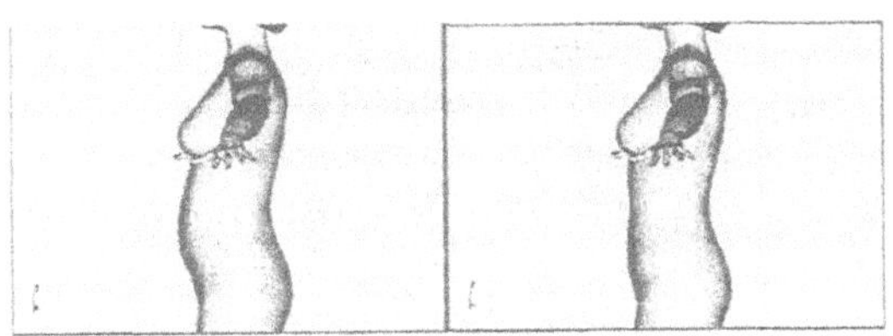

Figure 9. Deformation of the belly

5.3 Bottom

A simple method of deformation based on the FFD (Free Form Deformation) is used for the bottom. The bounding box of the bottom is regularly sampled to obtain 4x4x4=64 control points of the Bézier volume. As we move any of the control points, the enclosed surface will be deformed accordingly.

In most of the cases, only certain points of the volume are necessary. We thus get the differently sized bottoms by simultaneously moving these points, which are the four central points of the back face of the Bézier volume.

6. OPTIMIZATION

Traditionally, simplification techniques have dealt mainly with static objects. These methods focus on preserving visually important features of the model such as sharp edges, high curvatures, and silhouettes during the simplification [2, 13]. When it comes to animated character models however, the direct use of these methods does not make much sense. Apart from the geometric characteristics of the surface, we need also to consider the animation aspect of the model or more specifically, the skin-to-bone attachment information. By assigning higher priority to those vertices that have more influencing bones, we can keep more vertices near joints so that the deformation during animation appears as natural as possible. In this work, we took a simple vertex decimation method with the following evaluation function:

$$\text{Eval}(v) = W_b \times (W_0 \times \text{distance} + W_1 \times \text{normalDeviation} + W_2 \times \text{curvature})$$

where W_b is the number of bones which the vertex v is attached to, W_0 is for the distance between the old vertex and the average plane of the simplified polygon, W_1 for the normal deviations of a vertex and thus sharp features of the mesh, and W_2 for high curvature regions. Each of the weights, when it has a high value compared to the other weights, preserves different characteristics of the mesh.

Some of the results we obtained are shown in Figure 10.

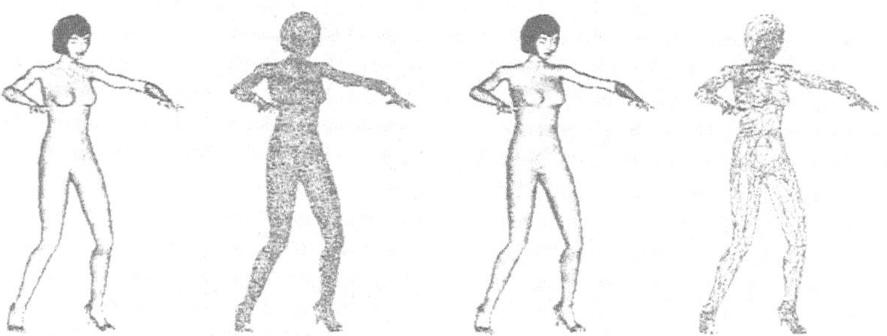

Figure 10. Different Levels of Detail description of the body surface: Full description with 13389 vertices and 25853 faces(left). Simplified model with 4726 vertices and 8578 faces (right).

7. STANDARD SUPPORT

This section explains our work to describe the body model according to the MPEG-4 BDP specifications. The 'Body' node in MPEG-4 organizes definition and animation of a body [17]. Our system in this frame mainly concerns the BDPs, which by definition (Figure 11) gives geometrical description of a body model along with the information on how to animate it. Here, the animation means a skin deformation when given a set of joint angles.

```
BDP {
exposed Field MFNode bodyDefTables NULL
expoed Field MF3Dnode bodySceneGraph NULL
}
```

Figure 11. The BDP node definition in MPEG-4.

The 'bodySceneGraph' is strongly based on VRML H-Anim 1.1 specification [15]. The H-Anim specifies a standard way of representing humanoids in VRML97. The human body consists of a number of 'Segments', which are connected to each other by 'Joints'. The full H-Anim hierarchy is composed of 94 skeleton joints and 12 skin segments including the head, hands and feet.

Algorithm segmentation :

foreach face f

  $W(f, B_i) = 0.0$;

  foreach vertex v

    foreach bone B_i it is dependent

      $W(f, B_i)$ += $W(v, B_i)$;

    end foreach

    Choose the bone B_{max} for which $W(f, B_{max})$ is maximum;

    Add this face to the segment of B_{max};

  end foreach

end foreach

Figure 12. Segmentation algorithm

As mentioned earlier, our choice of the skeleton hierarchy is H-Anim compatible. The remaining work is to segment the skin mesh and locate each of them into the skeleton hierarchy as a proper child node of corresponding joint. Our segmentation algorithm is described in Figure 12. After the segmentation, each skin part is saved in the local coordinate system and is connected to a 'Joint' as a 'Segment' child node.

The bodyDefTables field defines how the segmented mesh of the Segment node in the bodySceneGraph is modified or deformed based on sets of BAPs. Each bodyDefTable contains a list of BAPs, and a list of vertices and their displacements in the bodySceneGraph that are affected by these BAPs. Following are the features of our bodyDefTables generator.

- A number of key postures are provided by default.

- The user can then add a new posture or remove any of the registered postures.
- When confirmed, all the listed postures are transformed into sets of BAPs and the accordingly deformed segments into displacements.

8. CONCLUSION AND FUTURE WORK

In this paper, we have introduced our on-going work on a methodology for creating and scaling bodies and discussed various relevant issues. Our approach provides an efficient way of creating bodies and the resulting models are directly usable for web application. With its support for MPEG-4 which is an industrially recognized format, the resulting model enables efficient and immediate animation for various applications: virtual fashion try on, for instance.

Our plans for future work focus on ways to improve the quality of the model in terms of the accuracy and texture. We also plan to integrate our work with face models for further extensions into a crowd generation system.

The ultimate goal of this research is to enable rapid creation of various body models immediately usable for animation. By doing so, we would like to extend the area of human character modelling to encompass the animation, rendering performance, standard, and other various practical considerations.

9. ACKNOWLEDGEMENTS

This work is supported by SoNG, funded by the European Community.

10. REFERENCES

1. Chadwick, J., Haumann, D.R. and Parent, R.E., "Layerd Construction for Deformable Animated Characters", Computer Graphics, *In Computer Graphics(Proc. SIGGRAPH '89)*, pp.234-243, ACM Press, 1989.
2. Cohen,J. Varshney,A., Manocha,D., Turk,G. and Weber,H., "Simplification Envelopes", *In Computer Graphics(Proc. SIGGRAPH '96)*, pp.119-128, ACM Press, 1996.
3. DeRose T., Kass M., Truong T., "Subdivision Surfaces in Character Animation", *In Computer Graphics (Proc. SIGGRAPH '98)*, ACM Press, pp. 85-94, 1998.
4. Devernay F., Faugeras O.D., "Computing Differential Properties of 3-D Shapes from Stereoscopic Images without 3-D Models", *In Proc. Of Computer Vision and Pattern Recognition*, pp.208-213, 1994.

5. Fua P., "Human Modeling from Video Sequence", *Geomatics Info Magazine*, 13(7): 63-65, July 1999.
6. Gu J., Chang T., Mak I., Gopalsamy S., Shen H., and Yuen M., "A 3D Reconstruction System for Human Body Modeling", *In Modelling and Motion Capture Techniques for Virtual Environments (Proc. CAPTECH'98)*, pp.229-241, Springer, 1998.
7. Hilton A., Beresford D., Gentils T. and Smith R. and Sun W., "Virtual People: Capturing human models to populate virtual worlds". *In Computer Animation (Proc. Computer Animation'99)*, pp.174-185, 1999.
8. Kakadiaris A. and Metaxas D., "3D Human Body Acquisition from Multiple views", *In Proceedings of the Fifth ICCV*, pp.618-623, 1995.
9. Lee W.-S., Gu J., Magnenat-Thalmann N., "Generating Animatable 3D Virtual Humans from Photographs", *Proc. Eurographics 2000*. pp.1-10, 2000.
10. Lee Y., Terzopoulos D., and Waters K., "Realistic Modeling for Facial Animation", *In Computer Graphics (Proc. SIGGRAPH' 96)*, ACM Press, pp. 55-62, 1996.
11. Magnenat-Thalmann N., Thalmann D., "The direction of Synthetic Actors in the film Rendez-vous à Montreal", *Computer Graphics and Applications*, IEEE Computer Society Press, 7(12): 9-19, 1987.
12. Proesmans M., Van Gool L., "Reading between the lines - a method for extracting dynamic 3D with texture", *In Proceedings of VRST*, pp. 95-102, 1997.
13. Schroeder,W., Zarge, J. and Lorensen,W., "Decimation of Triangle Meshes", *In Computer Graphics(Proc. SIGGRAPH '92)*, Volume 25, No. 3, pp.65-70, ACM Press, 1992.
14. Shen J., Thalmann D., "Interactive Shape Design Using Metaballs and Splines", *In Proc. of Implicit Surfaces '95*, Grenoble, pp.187-196.
15. Specification for a Standard Humanoid, Appendix A: Suggested Body Dimensions and Levels of Articulation. http://www.H-Anim.org
16. http://www.turing.gla.ac.uk/turing/copyrigh.htm
17. International Organization for Standardization Organization International Normalization ISO/IEC JTC 1/SC 29/WG 11. Coding of Moving Picture and Audio (N2739 subpart2), 1999.
18. Physic and Skin modifier, 3D Studio max, Kinetix.

EFFICIENT MUSCLE SHAPE DEFORMATION

Amaury Aubel and Daniel Thalmann
Computer Graphics Lab, Swiss Federal Institue of Technology (EPFL), CH 1015 Lausanne, Switzerland

Key words: Shape deformation, muscle modelling, artistic anatomy, physically-based deformation.

Abstract: In this paper we extend previous work [Aubel00] and propose a muscle model suitable for computer graphics based on physiological and anatomical considerations. Muscle motion and deformation is automatically derived from an action line that is deformed using a 1D mass-spring system. The resulting model is fast and can accommodate most superficial human muscles.

1. INTRODUCTION

The basic function of the skeletal muscles is to generate movement. Upon contraction, the fibres, which make up the muscle, contract and slide across each other. As a result, the length of the whole muscle diminishes, so the bones to which the muscle is attached are pulled towards each other. A side effect is that the muscle changes shape during contraction, which impacts the shape of the outer skin. This is well known among painters and sculptors who study the anatomy of the human body to improve their work. Rather surprisingly, commercial modelling packages overwhelmingly ignore muscle modelling as an essential part of body modelling. The most widespread technique for skin deformation in the industry remains *skinning* which amounts to binding each skin vertex to one or more underlying bones. The displacement of a skin vertex during animation is then the result of a weighted combination of the displacements of the bones to which it is bound. The influence of muscles on the skin surface shape is not taken into consideration or restricted to simple geometric primitives that push the skin outwards. In this paper we detail a muscle model that is fast and yet realistic enough for a computer graphics use.

1.1 Related work

Existing muscle models can broadly be classified into two categories: purely geometric models and physically-based ones. We successively review these two approaches.

1.1.1 Geometric Deformations

Geometric models tend to use the ellipsoid as the basic building block. It is a natural choice because an ellipsoid approximates fairly well the appearance of a fusiform muscle. In addition, its analytic formulation lends itself well to inside/outside tests and volume preservation constraints. Thus, several researchers use a volume-preserving ellipsoid for representing a fusiform muscle [Scheepers97, Wilhelms97a]. Others approximate muscles by an implicit surface extracted from a set of ellipsoids [Turner93,Thalmann96]. Finally, multi-belly muscles e.g. the pectoral muscle can be represented by a set of ellipsoids positioned along two spline curves [Scheepers97]. In all these works, muscle flexing and bulging is simulated by binding the degrees of freedom (scaling and possibly translation and/or rotation) of each ellipsoid to the degrees of freedom of the underlying skeleton joints.

Despite its simplicity and attractiveness, the ellipsoid model cannot capture most muscle shapes. In more recent work [Wilhelms97b], Whilhelms et al. use a generalised cylinder made up of a certain number of cross-sections that consist in turn of a fixed number of vertices. Volume variation of the muscle during deformation is reduced by scaling each cross-section so as to preserve its area. Similarly, Scheepers and his colleagues provide a general muscle model that consists of tubularly-shaped bicubic patches [Scheepers97]. Exact volume preservation remains possible as muscles shapes still have an analytic description. Interestingly, they also provide the user with scaling and tension parameters to simulate isometric contractions as well.

1.1.2 Simulation models

One of the first physically-based models is due to Chadwick et al. [Chadwick89]. The muscle is embedded in a FFD lattice [Sedeberg86]. Muscle deformation is achieved by simply deforming the embedding space. The FFD control points are moved by treating them as nodes interconnected by ideal hookean springs. Diagonal springs help to maintain the initial geometric configuration. One of the potential problems is that the FFD box may not approximate the muscle shape very tightly. The FFD control points have moreover no physical reality. As a consequence, the distribution of the muscle mass over the nodes is likely to be problematic. From a more biomechanics oriented point of view, Chen et al. simulate muscle contraction using the Finite Element Theory [Chen92]. However, their work only shows single muscles working in isolation.

Porcher-Nedel and Thalmann introduced the idea of abstracting muscles by an action line (a polyline in practice) representing the force produced by the muscle on the bones, and a surface mesh deformed by an equivalent mass-spring network [Porcher-Nedel98]. An elastic relaxation of the surface mesh is performed for each animation frame thus yielding a collection of static postures. In order to smooth out mesh discontinuities, they employ special springs termed *angular springs* that tend to restore the initial curvature of the surface at each vertex. If the mesh is somewhat coarse, angular springs also help to control volume deformation though not in an exact mathematical manner. However, angular springs cannot deal with local inversions of the curvature. Also, the authors do not explicit how they constrain the surface mesh to follow the action line when it consists of more than one segment.

Ng-Thow-Hing relies on the B-spline solid as the basic primitive for modeling individual muscles in animals and humans [Ng-Thow-Hing00]. The mathematical formulation of the B-spline solid can accommodate multiple shapes of muscles (fusiform, triangular, bipennate, etc.) and various sizes of attachments. Muscular deformation is achieved by embedding a mass-spring-damper network in the B-spline solid. In practice, the network does not coincide with the B-spline's control points but with spatial points of maximum influence since physical characteristics such as mass are best specified at real locations of the muscle. Varying force magnitude in the network results in non-uniform physical effects. In contrast to most previous approaches that solve a sequence of static equilibrium problems only, inertially-induced oscillations can take place here thus enhancing the visual realism. Muscle-muscle and muscle-bone collision forces are also added as reaction constraints [Platt88]. Yet, trying to simulate every muscle-muscle and muscle-bone interaction seems unrealistic. For example, no solution is given as to how multiple collisions[1] between muscles are to be handled.

1.2 Overview

The remainder of this paper is organised as follows. Section 2 exposes some important considerations borrowed from the artistic anatomy, as well as physiological notions that guided us in developing a generic muscle model. In the following section we detail the muscle model. Lastly, section 4 presents our conclusions and possible future work.

2. ARTISTIC ANATOMY

The muscle layer is the main contributing factor to the surface form. Muscles account for half of the total mass of the body and fill in almost completely the gap between the skeleton and the skin [Richer81]. Anatomists distinguish three types of muscles: skeletal muscles, smooth muscles and the heart. They have different functions but exhibit the same fundamental mechanical and constitutive properties [Maurel98]. We shall only consider the skeletal muscles because the other kinds barely influence the surface form.

Skeletal muscles produce the motion of the bones. Structurally, they consist of a contractile central part called *belly* and of tendinous extremities or *aponeurosis* that connect the belly to the bones. In constitutive description, the belly is made up of bundles of elastic contractile fibres. The bundles are wrapped into a single envelope called *fascia*. The belly's fibres are responsible for producing the contraction of the whole muscle. Tendons, which are hardly elastic, act as transmitters and help to move the weight away from the limbs' ends. In general, muscle tissues are several orders of magnitude more elastic than tendons [Fung81].

Upon *isotonic contraction*, the volume of the belly increases thus amplifying its influence on the shape of the skin, whereas the total length of the muscle diminishes so that the bones to which the muscle is attached are pulled towards each other. Upon *isometric contraction*, the shape of the belly alters but the length of the muscle does not change, so no skeletal motion is produced. In a relaxed state, the belly undergoes the action of gravity and hangs somewhat loosely. Finally, muscles vary greatly in shape depending on their location: long fusiform muscles are found mainly in the

[1] A multiple collision occurs for example when a muscle A collides with a muscle B, which in turn collides with a muscle C within the same time step because of the displacement due to the first collision.

limbs; short muscles appear around joints; large flat muscles cover the back [Richer81].

3. MUSCLE MODEL

We believe the real difficulty with muscles lies more with the animation than with the modelling. It is very complex to automatically derive the appropriate position and deformation of a muscle in any possible posture. Note that in our approach, as almost always the case in computer graphics, the motion of the skeleton induces the muscular deformations contrary to what occurs in reality.

Our approach consists of decomposing the muscle into two layers: an action line and a surface mesh. The action line, represented by a polyline with any number of vertices, is moved for each posture using a predefined behaviour and a simple physically-based simulation. It is then used as a skeleton for the surface mesh and the deformations are produced in a usual way [Sun99]. In order to avoid possible confusion, we shall use in the following the term "node" when referring to a vertex of the action line and "vertex" when speaking of a vertex of the muscle surface mesh.

3.1 Action line

First of all, the user specifies a default behaviour for each node of the action line: the node is mapped to a specific bone and its motion is defined with respect to a given number of joints. Then, a 1D mass-spring-damper system is constructed from the polyline. It is used for automatically determining new positions of the nodes. Currently, all nodes are given an equal mass. The user may choose at any time to deactivate the dynamic behaviour of a node, in which case the predefined behaviour takes over. An elastic relaxation is performed for each posture. The physical simulation can be advanced rapidly by relying on an implicit integration scheme since it yields an easily invertible tridiagonal[2] matrix [Kass93]. We add attractive and repulsive implicit force fields (currently ellipsoids and ellipsoidal metaballs) to constrain the action line. Repulsive force fields prevent gross interpenetration while attractive fields help to refine the trajectories of the action line.

[2] A nine-diagonal matrix in fact as each force vector has three entries.

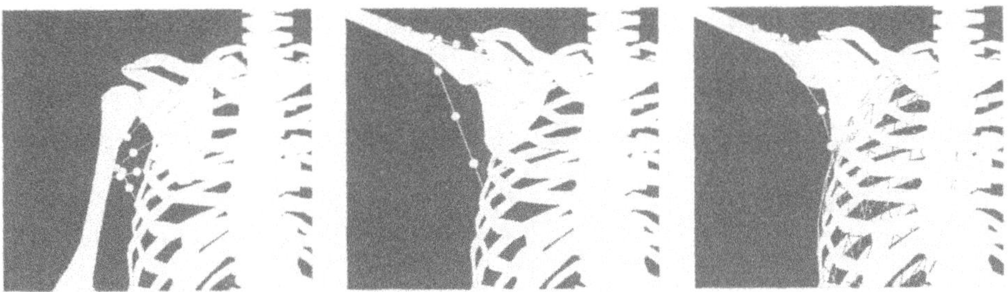

Figure 1. Action lines of the pectoral muscle during shoulder abduction. Right picture shows the use of two attractive force fields (solid and wireframe ellipsoids)

In practice, non-dynamic vertices correspond to the insertion and origin of the tendons. The action line can wrap itself around joints providing that the number and location of vertices is well chosen. Nearly rigid portions of the muscle such as tendons can easily be simulated because the stiffness of each spring is under user's control. The implicit integration easily handles these stiff segments. Analogously, increasing the number of vertices and fine-tuning the stiffness of the created springs can roughly approximate non-linear elasticity.

3.2 Local frames

The positions of the action line nodes provide information as to how the surface mesh will expand or shrink over time. Yet, the orientation of the mesh cannot be inferred from these positions only. A local frame needs to be constructed for each node of the action line. This is an involved operation. We start by computing the Z-axis at each node as depicted in Figure 2: Z is set to the normal of the bisecting plane for every in-between node (V_1, V_2) and to the tangent for the end nodes (V_0, V_3). We then proceed to compute the X-axis. Note that the Y-axis is ultimately found by completing the right-handed co-ordinate system.

The X-axis is first computed for the non-dynamic nodes[3]. We take, in a rest posture, the local frame of the joint (X and Y solid arrows in Figure 2) to which the non-dynamic node is bound and rotate it so as to bring its X, Y, or Z axis in alignment with the node's Z axis. The selected axis is the one that leads to the minimal rotation. In Figure 2 for instance, X yields the smallest rotation. The resulting frame (dashed arrows in Figure 2) is then expressed and saved in the joint's co-ordinate system. During any

[3] Non-dynamic nodes have their motion driven by a predefined behaviour (cf. Section 3.1). They usually (but not necessarily) correspond to the end nodes (V_0 and V_3 in fig. 2).

subsequent animation, this frame is transformed by the joint's current coordinate system, then rotated again so as to be aligned with the node's new Z axis. This rotation is usually quite small because we initially chose the smallest rotation in the rest posture. Thus, the local frame of every non-dynamic node is smoothly updated as the action line moves and deforms itself.

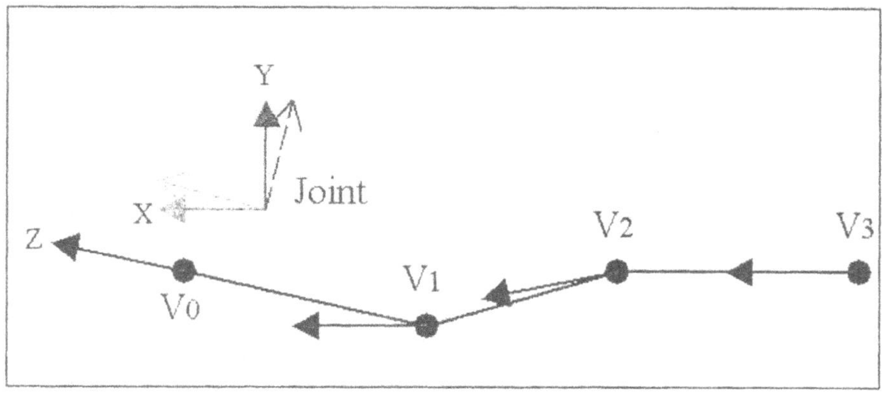

Figure 2. Z axis is set using the bisecting plane. The joint frame is initially rotated so as to align one of its axis (here the X-axis) with axis Z of end node V0.

Figure 3. Left: propagating first node's orientation upwards; Right: Resulting frame interpolation for in-between nodes.

There remains to compute the X-axis for the dynamic nodes in between. It is no use interpolating the two end orientations directly using the commonplace spherical linear interpolation because the two end orientations may be quite different from each other. As spherical linear interpolation picks the shortest path on the quaternion unit sphere, the frame orientation at a node may flip from one animation frame to the next. Besides, direct interpolation does not guarantee the interpolated frames will be aligned with the Z-axis already computed. Our method consists in propagating the X-axis direction of each end frame to the in-between nodes. As Z axis are readily computed using the method described above, we already have, for each node V_i, a plane P_i normal to Z_i in which the remaining X_i and Y_i axis must lie. Starting from axis X_0 at end node V_0, we estimate the axis X_1 in the plane P_1 by sampling the trigonometric circle and finding the minimal deviation from X_0. As we sample the entire circle, we do not get stuck into local minima. We then iterate the process to compute X_{i+1} by minimising its deviation from X_i. We thus propagate the orientation of each end frame to the other end node. Note that Figure 3. shows only the upwards propagation but the inverse downwards propagation is also carried out. Finally, we perform a linear interpolation of the two X axis computed at each node using a ratio that is related to the distance from the in-between node to the two end nodes along the polyline (Figure 3 right).

3.3 Muscle Mesh

We automatically map each surface vertex to the two closest delimiting planes that pass trough an action line's node as in [Sun99]. Vertices positions are later found by linear interpolation of the position and orientation of the enclosing local frames. Isotonic contraction is simulated by scaling each surface vertex orthogonally to the action line. The scaling factor is individually computed based on the action line. We compute the elongation – defined as the current length divided by the initial length – for every segment of the action line (it is computed anyway when evaluating the spring's elastic force). We interpolate these discreet measurements with a cubic spline curve. Thus we obtain a smooth, individual elongation value for each muscle vertex that we use as the scaling factor squared root: $scaling = \sqrt{elongation}$. Though this empirical formula does not ensure volume preservation, we experimentally measured for various muscle shapes a maximal volume variation of 6% when the muscles shorten by 30%, which corresponds to the maximal physiological compression rate [Richer81].

4. CONCLUSION

We presented a two-layered muscle model suitable for computer graphics applications. An action line is used for driving the motion and deformation of the outer layer. As the model makes use of a 1D mass-spring system, muscle deformation can be performed in real-time. Figure 4 shows the deformation of the brachial muscle as an example.

We plan to extend our 1D muscle model to large flat muscles as those in the back for example. Our idea is to use a 2D "action grid", essentially a surface, with nodes interconnected by ideal hookean springs. Then, a surface mesh would be wrapped around the action grid using the same method as that described in this paper. We plan to extend our 1D muscle model to large flat muscles as those in the back for example. Our idea is to use a 2D "action grid", essentially a surface, with nodes interconnected by ideal hookean springs. Then, a surface mesh would be wrapped around the action grid using the same method as that described in this paper.

We are also considering covering the muscles with a deformable skin mesh. Our idea is to deform the skin mesh using a two-stage process. A *skinning* process would be used for roughly positioning each skin vertex. We plan to decouple the degrees of freedom of a 3-DOF joint (e.g. the shoulder) into a swing motion on the one hand and a twist motion on the other. This should prove useful because the skin does not completely follow the skeleton when twisting one's limbs. In the second stage the skin vertices would be pushed and attracted by the underlying muscles.

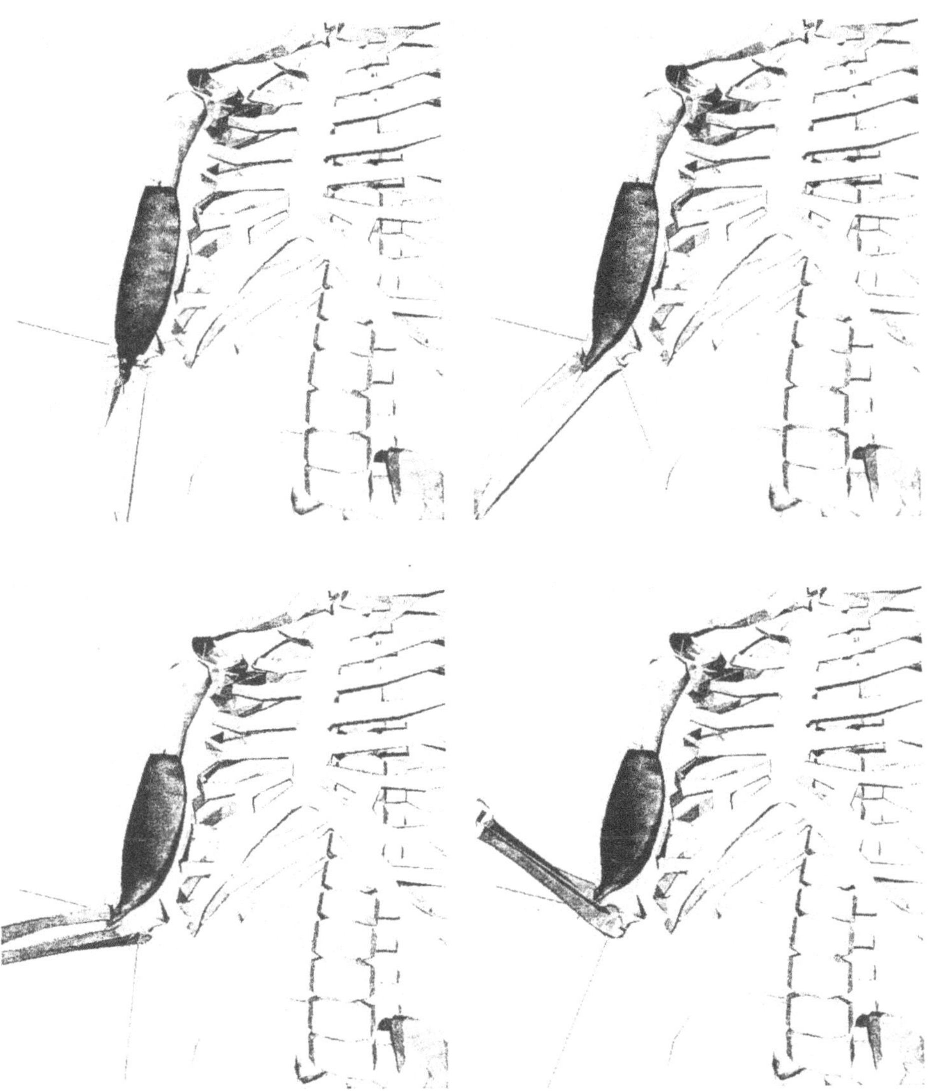

Figure 4. deformation of the *brachialis* muscle (volume variation remains under 3%)

REFERENCES

[Aubel00] A. Aubel, D. Thalmann, "Realistic Deformation of Human Body Shapes", Proc. Computer Animation and Simulation 2000, Interlaken, August 2000, pp. 125-135.

[Chadwick89] J. Chadwick, D. Haumann, R. Parent, "Layered construction for deformable animated characters", Computer Graphics (SIGGRAPH '89 Proceedings), pp.243-252.

[Chen92] D. Chen, D. Zeltzer, "Pump it up: Computer animation of a biomechanically based model of muscle using the finite element method", SIGGRAPH '92 Proceedings, pp.89-98.

[Fung81] Y.C. Fung "Biomechanics: Mechanical Properties of Living Tissues", Springer-Verlag, 1981.

[Kass93] M. Kass, "Introduction to Continuum Dynamics for Computer Graphics", SIGGRAPH Course Notes 60, 1993.

[Maurel98] W. Maurel, Y. Wu, N. Magnenat Thalmann, D. Thalmann, "Biomechanical Models for Soft Tissue Simulation", Springer-Verlag, Berlin/Heidelberg 1998.

[Ng-Thow-Hing00] V. Ng-Thow-Hing, "Anatomically-Based Models for Physical and Geometric Reconstruction of Humans and Other Animals", Ph.D. Thesis, Department of Computer Science, University of Toronto, 2000.

[Platt88] J.Platt, A. Barr, "Constraint Methods for Flexible Models", Computer Graphics (SIGGRAPH '88 Proceedings), pp. 279-288.

[Porcher-Nedel98] L. Porcher-Nedel, D.Thalmann, "Real Time Muscle Deformations Using Mass-Spring Systems", Proc. CGI '98, IEEE Computer Society Press, 1998.

[Richer81] P. Richer, "Artistic Anatomy", Watson-Gutpill Publications, New York, 1981.

[Scheepers97] F. Scheepers, R. Parent, W. Carlson, S. May, "Anatomy-Based Modeling of the Human Musculature", Computer Graphics (SIGGRAPH '97), pp. 163-172.

[Sederberg86] T. Sederberg, S. Parry, "Free-From Deformation of Solid Geometric Models", Computer Graphics (SIGGRAPH '86 Proceedings), pp.151-160.

[Sun99] W. Sun, A. Hilton, R. Smith, J. Illingworth, "Layered Animation of Captured Data", 10th Eurographics Workshop on Animation and Simulation '99, pp.145-154.

[Thalmann96] D. Thalmann, J.Shen, E. Chauvineau, "Fast Realistic Human Body Deformations for Animation and VR Applications", Computer Graphics International'96, Pohang, Korea, June, 1996.

[Turner93] R. Turner, D. Thalmann, "The Elastic Surface Layer Model for Animated Character Construction", Proc. Computer Graphics International '93, Lausanne, Switzerland, Springer-Verlag, Tokyo, pp. 399-412.

[Wilhelms97a] J. Wilhelms, "Animals with Anatomy", IEEE Computer Graphics And Applications, Vol. 17, No. 3, May 1997, pp.22-30.

[Wilhelms97b] J. Wilhelms, A. Van Gelder, "Anatomically Based Modeling", Computer Graphics (SIGGRAPH '97 Proceedings), pp. 173-180.

TOWARDS THE ULTIMATE MOTION CAPTURE TECHNOLOGY

Bradley Stuart, Patrick Baker and Yiannis Aloimonos
Computer Vision Laboratory
Center for Automation Research
Department of Computer Science and
Institute for Advanced Computer Studies
University of Maryland
College Park, MD 20742
{brad,pbaker,yiannis}@cfar.umd.edu

Abstract Recent developments in camera and computer technology have made multiple-camera systems less expensive and more usable. Using such systems, we can generate 3-D models of human activity for use in surveillance, as avatars, or for 3-D effects generation. Some approaches to model generation are voxel coloring, space carving, silhouette intersection, and the combination of multiple stereo reconstructions.

Our attempt to overcome various shortcomings of the above approaches has led to the use of image derivatives and motion to determine the shape and motion of the activity in view. Direct computations of the gradient directions and the image motion normal to the gradient provide the information to generate a 3D + motion model consistent with all the image data. Data structures encode visibility information from each of the cameras surrounding the scene, allowing efficient determination of the subsets of measurements to be combined in a modified space-carving system.

The main contributions of this paper are the following: the development of a system for combining multiple image gradient measurements to determine the 3-D iso-brightness direction and its consistency, a system for combining multiple normal flow measurements to determine the motion normal to the iso-brightness direction, and a data structure based on the rays passing through the centers of projection and the image pixels, forming an unbounded projective grid through the space of the scene and allowing efficient determination and updating of scene point visibility.

Reconstructions of human motion using twenty cameras are presented. The resulting 3D dynamic models of human action can be used: (a) directly as avatars performing specific activities, (b) for creating large libraries of human action models that can be used for animation, and (c) for further statistical/geometric processing that will yield sophisticated models of generic action.

1. PREVIOUS WORK

The question of how to generate new views of a three-dimensional (3-D) scene or object has been addressed in a number of different ways. The methods used fall into three rough categories, depending on whether the method uses only two-dimensional (2-D) data, builds a 2-D depth map ($2\frac{1}{2}$-D sketch), or generates new views from a full 3-D model of the scene.

1.1. VOXEL CARVING

Much recent work has concerned the integration of a large number of views into a single 3-D object model. In the technique called space carving or voxel coloring, space is broken up into small cells (volume elements, or voxels) and the images of these cells are checked for consistency. Cells with inconsistent images are removed from the set of cells which constitute the object [2] [7] [10].

The issue of cell visibility can be addressed in a variety of ways. In [10], the camera configuration is controlled so that voxels are visited in near-to-far order. The space carving technique [7] allows arbitrary camera placement, but cameras are not used until they are passed by the plane sweeping through the scene. Generalized voxel coloring [2] maintains a "layered depth image" to store visibility information, and efficiently determine which voxels are revealed by the carving operation.

Different criteria for voxel consistency have also been used. The technique of volume intersection (shape from silhouettes) uses the logical AND of bit mask images to define consistent voxels. Seitz develops a color consistency test which is based on hue.

1.2. MORPHING

Other approaches to the problem of generating new views from a given set of views are image interpolation and morphing. In image interpolation, interposed frames are created by smoothly varying pixel values between two or more source frames. Interpolation gives unsatisfactory results unless the source frames are very close together.

Morphing improves on this technique by imposing a mesh on the source frames, and moving control points on this mesh smoothly between the frames. Intermediate frames are generated by texture mapping each mesh cell as it moves, and varying the cell texture maps smoothly between the source frames. Defining the mesh requires the establishment of correspondences between points in the source images. Both image interpolation and morphing are strictly 2-D techniques; they do not perform well in the presence of occlusions and 3-D structure in the scene.

1.3. STEREO TECHNIQUES

Stereo techniques use two or more images to compute 3-D structure in the scene. The epipolar constraint is used along with some technique (such as correlation) to find corresponding points on epipolar lines. Additional constraints are added to speed searching or deal with ambiguities. Examples of these are ordering constraints, inter-line constraints and depth smoothness constraints [13]. Once correspondences has been determined, the distance to a point in the scene is then an inverse function of the disparity in the image coordinates. Stereo techniques work well only with a limited range of camera separations. If the cameras are too close, images are too similar, disparities are small, and accuracy suffers. If the cameras are too widely separated, correspondences become difficult to find and the additional constraints employed to find them start to be violated more and more. Narayanan et al. [8] demonstrate techniques combining multiple stereo pairs and filling in the holes that appear behind a single depth map. In [12], optical flow values are back-projected onto these models and 3-D flow values are inferred. Alternately, the optical flow values can be used to augment incomplete 3-D models to make them more accurate.

1.4. STRUCTURE FROM MOTION

Structure-from-motion techniques use the relative motion between camera and scene to determine the depth of points in the scene [11]. The technique is based on motion parallax; when the camera translates relative to the scene, points near the camera have a greater apparent motion than points far away. This translational flow is compounded with the apparent motion due to rotation of the camera. This rotation gives no depth information, but its confusion with the translation makes the structure-from-motion problem considerably more difficult. Structure-from-motion techniques can be based on either optical flow or normal flow. Either way, the technique assumes that flows are due only to the motion of the camera; independent motion in the scene is not allowed. Furthermore, inaccuracies in the determination of camera motion lead directly to inaccuracies in the resulting depth map.

2. CAMERA SETUP AND IMAGE FORMATION

Up to sixteen cameras are installed on each of four walls, for a total of sixty-four cameras. Sixteen of these cameras are single-ccd RGB filtered color cameras; the rest are standard gray-scale cameras. All cameras send 8 bits per pixel of digital data at 640x480 pixels and 60 frames per second. Frame rates up to 85 fps are possible with a restricted region of interest. Data is fed from each camera to a dedicated video capture card; four such cards are installed in each of 16 Pentium II PC's. Each PC has one gigabyte of RAM to allow real-time capture of 3000 uncompressed frames per computer [3]. Projection matrices are computed by nonlinear optimization on up to 25 points of a large calibration object, or more accurately by the method detailed in [1].

3. RAY CARVING

The process of voxel carving typically begins with the division of space into cubes of some fixed size. This introduces restrictions on the shape and size of the space that can be carved, as well as restrictions on the resolution of the cameras that can be usefully employed.

3.1. VOXELS OR RAYS

Instead of splitting the scene arbitrarily with a regular grid, we base our division of space on the rays which pass through the pixels in each camera. Each camera defines a pyramid-shaped bundle of rays passing through the scene. Saito and Kanade [9] define a grid based on the rays from two selected cameras. Here, we do not define any special cameras, using the rays from all cameras equally. Furthermore, we use a continuous (floating point) rather than discrete representation of the intervals on the ray which are solid or transparent. Each filled interval is represented by a pair of numbers, the distances to the endpoints of the interval. These distances are adjusted as portions of the scene are carved away.

The carving method of Seitz [10] restricts the camera positions to be "occlusion compatible." This means that it must be possible to separate the scene from the cameras by a flat or concave surface, and sweep the surface out, processing voxels from near to far. Cameras which violate this ordering can be excluded until they are passed by the sweep surface. One of any pair of cameras which can "see" each other must be excluded until the sweep surface passes the line joining their centers. The asymmetries induced by excluding one camera can be alleviated by sweeping in multiple directions.

One chief advantage of the ray representation is that it provides a compact description of visibility. A point on a ray is visible if its distance is less than or equal to the distance to the beginning of the ray's first filled interval. Rays can be processed in arbitrary or random order; it is not necessary to sweep a surface through the scene.

3.2. COMPUTING DISTANCES ALONG RAYS

Carving efficiently using ray information requires the ability to convert image positions along the ray into 3-D distances and positions. All projective transformations of a line can be defined by specifying the transformations of only three points on that line. Using this fact, we can specify the transformations back and forth among 3-D coordinates along a ray, 2-D image coordinates in any other camera's view of that ray, and 1-D line coordinates of distance along the ray.

The visibility information for the ray is supplemented with the information needed to render the ray into all of the other views. This is analogous to the rendering of epipolar lines needed to determine stereo correspondences. The projective mapping between the ray in 3-D and its images in all the other views is completely determined by defining the mapping for three distinct points on the ray. The camera center is one such point, selected because it is shared by all rays in one image. For a 3×4 projection matrix $\tilde{\mathbf{P}} = [\mathbf{P}\tilde{\mathbf{p}}]$, where $\mathbf{P}$ is a 3×3 matrix and $\tilde{\mathbf{p}}$ is a 3×1 vector, Faugeras [4] gives its position as

$$\mathbf{C} = \mathbf{P}^{-1}\tilde{\mathbf{p}}. \tag{1}$$

The second point selected is the vanishing point for the given ray — the vector parallel to the ray. Again from Faugeras, for homogeneous pixel coordinate $\mathbf{x}$ this direction is the homogeneous vector $\left[\mathbf{D}^{\mathsf{T}} 0\right]^{\mathsf{T}}$, where

$$\mathbf{D} = \mathbf{P}^{-1}\mathbf{x}. \tag{2}$$

The third point $\mathbf{U}$ is taken at a unit distance from the camera center, in the direction of the vanishing point. In homogeneous coordinates,

$$\mathbf{U} = \begin{bmatrix} \mathbf{C} \\ 1 \end{bmatrix} + \begin{bmatrix} \mathbf{D} \\ 0 \end{bmatrix}, \tag{3}$$

where $\mathbf{D}$ has been scaled so that $||\mathbf{D}||_2 = 1$.

By projecting these three points into each of the other images, we are able to convert positions along the image of the ray directly into 3-D distances along the ray itself. Specifically, we define projectivities between the homogeneous image coordinates in the ith camera $\mathbf{c} = \tilde{\mathbf{P}}_i\mathbf{C}$, $\mathbf{d} = \tilde{\mathbf{P}}_i\mathbf{D}$, and $\mathbf{u} = \tilde{\mathbf{P}}_i\mathbf{U}$, and the homogeneous line coordinates $[0,1]^{\mathsf{T}}$, $[1,0]^{\mathsf{T}}$ and $[1,1]^{\mathsf{T}}$, respectively. This projectivity will also map a point $\mathbf{x} = \tilde{\mathbf{P}}_i\mathbf{X}$ lying on the line to the line coordinate $[x_1, x_2]$, where $\frac{x_1}{x_2}$ is the distance from the camera center $\mathbf{C}$ defining this ray to $\mathbf{X}$. This projectivity is defined by the matrix product

$$\mathbf{L} = \begin{bmatrix} s_1 & 0 \\ 0 & s_2 \end{bmatrix} \begin{bmatrix} \mathbf{c} \times \mathbf{n} \\ \mathbf{n} \times \mathbf{d} \end{bmatrix}. \tag{4}$$

The second matrix in this definition ensures that the points **c** and **d** map correctly, while the first defines the scale so that **u** maps to the point $[1, 1]$. The vector **n** in the second matrix is an arbitrary vector defining the null-space of the matrix L. For pointsx $= \tilde{\mathbf{P}}_i\mathbf{X}$ on the ray, **Lx** gives the homogeneous coordinate measuring the 3-D distance from the camera center **C** to the point **X**.

Requiring that the point **u** maps to the line coordinate $[1, 1]$ gives us

$$\begin{bmatrix} s_1 & 0 \\ 0 & s_2 \end{bmatrix} \begin{bmatrix} \mathbf{c} \times \mathbf{n} \\ \mathbf{n} \times \mathbf{d} \end{bmatrix} \mathbf{u} \equiv \begin{bmatrix} 1 \\ 1 \end{bmatrix} \quad \text{or} \quad s_1[\mathbf{cnu}] = s_2[\mathbf{ndu}],$$

which is satisfied by setting $s_1 = [\mathbf{ndu}]$ and $s_2 = [\mathbf{cnu}]$.

Applying this projectivity to points which do not lie strictly on the line introduces errors when taking the resulting line coordinates as the depth values at the given point. The null-space of **L** defines the sets of points in the plane which project to the same line coordinates. For points not on the ray, we take their coordinate to be the same as the coordinate of the perpendicular projection onto the ray. To achieve this, we define the null-space vector to be the point at infinity in the direction perpendicular to the line containing **c** and **d**. This is given by taking the cross product $\mathbf{c} \times \mathbf{d}$, and setting its third coordinate to zero. Thus

$$\mathbf{n} = [c_2 d_3 - c_3 d_2, -c_1 d_3 + c_3 d_1, 0]^\top .$$

Once the distance coordinate along the line is known, it is a simple matter to convert this to a 3-D coordinate. For any distance coordinate λ,

$$\mathbf{X}_\lambda = \begin{bmatrix} \mathbf{C} \\ 1 \end{bmatrix} + \lambda \begin{bmatrix} \mathbf{D} \\ 0 \end{bmatrix}, \tag{5}$$

where again, **D** has been scaled to unity.

3.3. CARVING ALONG A RAY

Ray carving requires projecting a given ray into all the other views. It is more computationally efficient to continue carving down the length of the ray until the visible end of the ray is no longer inconsistent. While updating the visible end of the current ray, moving its front point away from the camera, rays from the other cameras which view this front point are also updated. The carving algorithm proceeds as follows:

1 Determine the 3-D point x which is visible on this ray R as in (5).

2 Project the principal points (**C**,**D**,**U**) of the ray R into the other views i, giving image coordinates $(r, c)_i$ and defining the matrices $\mathbf{L}(R)_i$ as in (4). Recall that **C** is common to all rays from a particular view; its projected coordinate (the epipole) can be saved. Saving other values for the images of the rays is memory intensive.

3 Image coordinates $(r, c)_i$ are used to access predefined rays S_i, the rays which view x in the other cameras.

4 Determine the depth boundaries at which the ray R crosses the edges of the pixels $(r, c)_i$ in each of the views. One of the views, i_{lub} defines the least upper bound on this depth.

5 If the pixels $(r, c)_i$ are inconsistent with the pixel defining the ray R (see below), the portion of the current ray between the visible point and the least upper bound defined above must be removed. The removed region extends onto the second least (unique) depth value found in the previous step.

6 In addition, the ray $S_{i_{lub}}$ defined in the view i_{lub} is also carved, removing from it the region defined by $S_{i_{lub}}$'s intersection with the pixel defining ray R.

7 The position x on ray R is updated, along with the definition of $S_{i_{lub}}$, the ray containing the portion which was carved away. Other rays S_i do not need to be recomputed, or carved, as the point x has moved to a new pixel only in view i_{lub}.

Since visibility information is encoded and updated for each ray, they can be visited in arbitrary order. Our choice is to visit all the rays defined by one image before moving on to the next. Cycling through the images continues until the scene converges and new points are no longer carved away.

4. INTENSITY GRADIENTS AND EDGES IN THREE DIMENSIONS

Typically, voxel carving algorithms have used color consistency as a test function in determining what portions of the scene need to be removed from the object model. Color has several advantages that a simple gray level does not. Color is less sensitive to variation in viewpoint, camera intensity response, and differences in lighting.

Gray-scale images are not without their own properties that can perform equally well. Intensity gradients can perform better than simple intensities, as they are less sensitive to the camera intensity response and differences in lighting. However, intensity gradients are not independent of viewpoint — a simple rotation of the camera in place will induce an opposite rotation of the gradient vectors. Furthermore, gradients which appear at a 3-D point in one image may not be present at all in another image, as at the occluding boundary of a smooth object. As we will see, these viewpoint dependent characteristics can be overcome by computing the 3-D iso-intensity contour.

Intensity gradients arise in images for several reasons. A surface in the scene may reflect or emit different intensities due to texture intrinsic to the surface or due to lighting differences such as shadows. An occluding boundary (discontinuity) in the scene produces a gradient when the occluding and occluded objects are of different colors. Specular reflections and other departures from a Lambertian reflectance model also produce intensity gradients. We do not deal with specularities here, but they could be addressed by including a lighting model of the scene, for example.

The gradient vector $dI/d\mathbf{x} = [I_x, I_y]^\top$ is the intensity change per unit length (usually a single pixel width) in the direction of steepest ascent. The normal to this vector is the direction in which the image intensity remains constant; the iso-intensity contour. Projecting the image intensity values back along their rays into three dimensions, we have a space-filling gradient field, without regard to where the physical surfaces lie. In Euclidean 3-D coordinates $\mathbf{X}$, this field has the brightness gradient

$$\frac{dB}{d\mathbf{X}} = k \begin{bmatrix} \frac{\partial x_1}{\partial X_1} & \frac{\partial x_2}{\partial X_1} \\ \frac{\partial x_1}{\partial X_2} & \frac{\partial x_2}{\partial X_2} \\ \frac{\partial x_1}{\partial X_3} & \frac{\partial x_2}{\partial X_3} \end{bmatrix} \frac{dI}{d\mathbf{x}}, \tag{6}$$

where $k = dB/dI$, i.e. we assume a linear relationship between image intensity and scene brightness.

Using the 3×4 projection matrix $\mathbf{P}$ and homogeneous coordinates $\hat{\mathbf{X}}^\top = \begin{bmatrix} \mathbf{X}^\top & 1 \end{bmatrix}$, we define $\hat{\mathbf{x}} = \mathbf{P}\hat{\mathbf{X}}$. The image of $\mathbf{X}$ is then at the 2-D coordinates

$$x_1 = \frac{\hat{x}_1}{\hat{x}_3}, x_2 = \frac{\hat{x}_2}{\hat{x}_3}. \tag{7}$$

The derivatives of (6) are then given by

$$\begin{aligned} \frac{\partial x_i}{\partial X_j} &= \frac{\partial}{\partial X_j}\left(\frac{\hat{x}_i}{\hat{x}_3}\right) \\ &= \left(\frac{\partial \hat{x}_i}{\partial X_j}\hat{x}_3 - \frac{\partial \hat{x}_3}{\partial X_j}\hat{x}_i\right) / \hat{x}_3^2 \\ &= \left(P_{i,j}\hat{x}_3 - P_{3,j}\hat{x}_i\right) / \hat{x}_3^2. \end{aligned}$$

As in the 2-D case, the gradient vector is normal to the manifold of constant brightness. This is the iso-brightness plane, which must contain the direction of constant brightness lying on the actual surface in the scene.

Each of the views gives a measurement of the image gradient, and therefore a plane on which the iso-brightness direction must lie. With two such planes, a unique line is defined for the edge direction in 3-D. With more than two planes, we can use a fitting technique to find the best direction for the 3-D edge. Furthermore, we can use the quality of this fit to determine whether these image gradients do in fact define a consistent edge in 3-D.

The fitting technique used is a principal component analysis. For N 3-D gradient vectors $\mathbf{g}_i = dB_i/d\mathbf{X}$, what is required is to find the vector $\mathbf{x}$ of unit length which minimizes the sum of projection lengths $\mathbf{x} \cdot \mathbf{g}_i$. This is done by finding the eigenvector for the least eigenvalue of the matrix

$$\mathrm{M} = \sum_{i=1}^{N} (\mathbf{g}_i \mathbf{g}_i^{\top}) \tag{8}$$

where $(\mathbf{g}_i \mathbf{g}_i^{\top})$ is the 3×3 outer product of the vector $\mathbf{g}_i$ with itself.

If the third eigenvalue is not small relative to the first and second, there is no vector which is a satisfactory approximation to the normal of the inputs. In that case, the 3-D location selecting these image measurements must not be a part of a consistent object; we carve the location away.

At surface discontinuities, the image gradient is due to a boundary edge for the object. The 3-D gradient describes the tangent plane passing through the camera center and the limb of the object. The surface at the limb may be a sharp corner, or it the may be a smooth surface. In either case, the tangent plane containing the camera center and the edge will be consistent with any iso-intensity direction on the surface; the 3-D gradient is normal to *all* directions on the surface. If the edge is due to a sharp corner, the same edge may be visible in several views and the iso-intensity contour can be determined precisely. In the case of a smooth surface edge, the iso-intensity direction will have to be determined through texture edges on the surface seen from other viewpoints. A smooth surface with a smooth texture will not have a single iso-intensity direction, but at the limb of the object it can be limited to the tangent plane.

5. THE NORMAL MOTION FIELD IN THREE DIMENSIONS

5.1. NORMAL FLOW

The motion constraint equation is the mathematical formulation of the statement that the brightness of a point in the scene remains constant for small motions. Formally,

$$\frac{\partial I}{\partial x}\frac{dx}{dt} + \frac{\partial I}{\partial y}\frac{dy}{dt} + \frac{\partial I}{\partial t} = 0. \tag{9}$$

This equation relates the component of the optical flow parallel to the image gradient to the time derivative of the intensity. Since this optical flow component is normal to the edges of the image, it is termed *normal flow*.

The tangential component of the optical flow cannot be determined directly without additional assumptions. These extra constraints introduce biases into the computation of flow [5] [6]. Flow smoothness constraints may be marginally acceptable in applications where the camera is moving in a rigid environment. However, with a stationary camera and a non-rigid scene, we expect regions of zero flow to be near regions of quite high flow values. Refusing to compute flow near discontinuities will leave us without the most informative parts of the scene. Rather than accepting additional biases or loss of measurements in order to compute a quantity which is not well-defined in the image, we choose to work with the normal component of the flow.

5.2. THREE DIMENSIONS

Just as in the 2-D case, we start from the premise that motion along the iso-brightness contour cannot be measured locally. This is simply the restatement of the aperture problem in the 3-D framework. The case is not so bad in three dimensions, as we can still determine motion in two out of three principal axes.

The normal motion on an iso-brightness contour is by definition limited to the plane of normals to the contour at a given point. The component of the motion parallel to the contour cannot be measured directly, and doesn't concern us here. Each measurement of normal flow in the image set defines a line in the image, called the normal flow constraint line. Both the optical flow and the projection of the 3-D normal flow must lie along this constraint line. This line, together with the camera center, defines a constraint plane through scene space. The constraint planes from the various views intersect the plane of normals in a set of lines, all of which intersect in the single point defining the 3-D normal flow. If the lines fail to intersect, this indicates that the normal flow measurements in the images are inconsistent.

In practice, there are errors in normal flow measurements, and in gradient measurements. We need to take these errors into account when designing the algorithm which determines the consistency and value of the 3-D normal flow. When more than two normal flow measurements are available, the problem of finding the best intersection point is an optimization problem. The point which minimizes the sum of squared distances from the constraint planes (including the plane of edge normals) is found, while the error measurement determines whether the selected point is sufficiently consistent to use as the 3-D normal flow.

We find the constraint plane for a given image point $\mathbf{x}$, normal flow $[n_1, n_2]$, and the iso-intensity direction defined in the previous section. This plane is defined in homogeneous coordinates by the camera center $\mathbf{C}$, the direction vector $\mathbf{D} = \mathbf{P}^{-1}(x_1 + n_1, x_2 + n_2, 1)^\top$ — as in (2) — and the iso-intensity direction unit vector $\mathbf{W}$. Using homogeneous coordinates for the point $\mathbf{C}$, and representing the vectors $\mathbf{D}$ and $\mathbf{W}$ by the point at infinity in the vector direction, the plane $\mathbf{p}$ containing these (homogeneous) points is given by the determinant

$$\mathbf{p} = \begin{vmatrix} \mathbf{e}_1 & \mathbf{e}_2 & \mathbf{e}_3 & \mathbf{e}_4 \\ C_1 & C_2 & C_3 & 1 \\ D_1 & D_2 & D_3 & 0 \\ W_1 & W_2 & W_3 & 0 \end{vmatrix} \tag{10}$$

$$= [(\mathbf{D} \times \mathbf{W}), -[\mathbf{DWC}]]. \tag{11}$$

Likewise, the plane of normals to $\mathbf{W}$ through $\mathbf{X}$ combines the other two eigenvectors of the matrix $\mathbf{M}$ of (8), $\mathbf{U}$ and $\mathbf{V}$. Noting that $\mathbf{W} = \pm\mathbf{U} \times \mathbf{V}$, the homogeneous coordinate of this plane is

$$\mathbf{q} = [(\mathbf{U} \times \mathbf{V}), -[\mathbf{UVX}]] \tag{12}$$

$$\equiv [\mathbf{W}, -\mathbf{W} \cdot \mathbf{X}]. \tag{13}$$

To find the best candidate for the intersection of these planes, we need to weight the planes equally in Euclidean space. This involves scaling the homogeneous coordinates $\mathbf{p}$ by $1/\parallel [p_1, p_2, p_3] \|_2$. Scaled this way, the homogeneous coordinate can be viewed as a unit vector in the direction normal to the plane, and the negative of the distance from the origin to the plane along this vector. The point $\mathbf{X}'$ is then constrained to have $X_4' = 1$ and is the least squares solution minimizing the error function

$$E = \sum_{i=1}^{i<N} (\mathbf{p}_i \cdot \mathbf{X}')^2. \tag{14}$$

This gives three constraint equations for $k \in \{1, 2, 3\}$ of the form

$$-\sum_{i=1}^{N} p_{i,k} p_{i,4} = \sum_{j=1}^{3} X_j' \sum_{i=1}^{N} p_{i,k} p_{i,j}. \tag{15}$$

The normal motion vector is then $\mathbf{N} = \mathbf{X}' - \mathbf{X}$. In places where the error measure of (14) is excessive, the normal flow values can be deemed inconsistent, and the 3-D point $\mathbf{X}$ can be carved away. Alternately, the reprojection of the vector $\mathbf{N}$ into each of the images can be checked for consistency with the normal flow measurement in that image. The projection of $\mathbf{X}'$ should lie on (near) the motion constraint line.

6. RESULTS

Here we present some results of the algorithm. Input data was obtained from sixteen cameras widely separated around the room, with a person walking through the scene. Cameras were calibrated using images of a known calibration object, and images were corrected for radial distortions. These reconstructions used images of 320×240 pixels. Four of the input images are shown in

Figure 1; Figure 1(a) and (b) are two two raw data images, (c) is an image of the background, and (d) is the foreground silhouette.

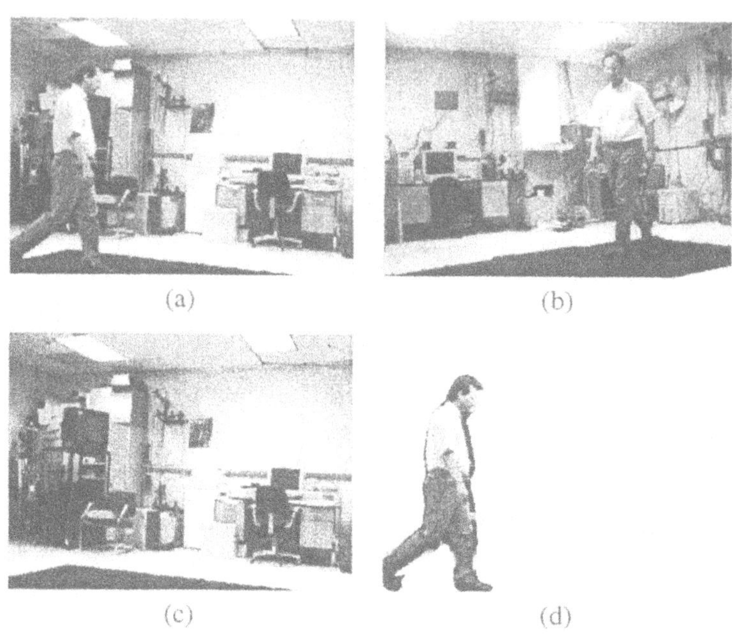

Figure 1 Input Data

In Figure 2, images (a) and (b) show two views of a moving person, after the data structure has been initialized with the silhouette intersection from twenty views. The foreground/background separation procedure purposely favors the foreground, as any missing foreground in a view will generate holes in the initial volume. This also adds a shell around the volume which needs to be carved away, along with any concavities in the moving human. Figures 2(c) and (d) show a depth map of the scene before and after the ray carving. Figures 2(e) and (f) show the agreement in the iso-intensity direction before and after the carving. Light colors represent maximum agreement, darker colors indicate inconsistency. Figures 2(g) through (l) show five views of the scene from viewpoints between the cameras. A virtual floor and shadow are added to the scene, as a simple example of the effects available using full 3-D structure.

7. DISCUSSION AND FUTURE WORK

This paper presents the general framework of ray carving, a method of generating 3-D models by which regions of space with inconsistent images are removed. Previous work in this field has relied on color information as a test of consistency. This paper presents two new criteria for this determination;

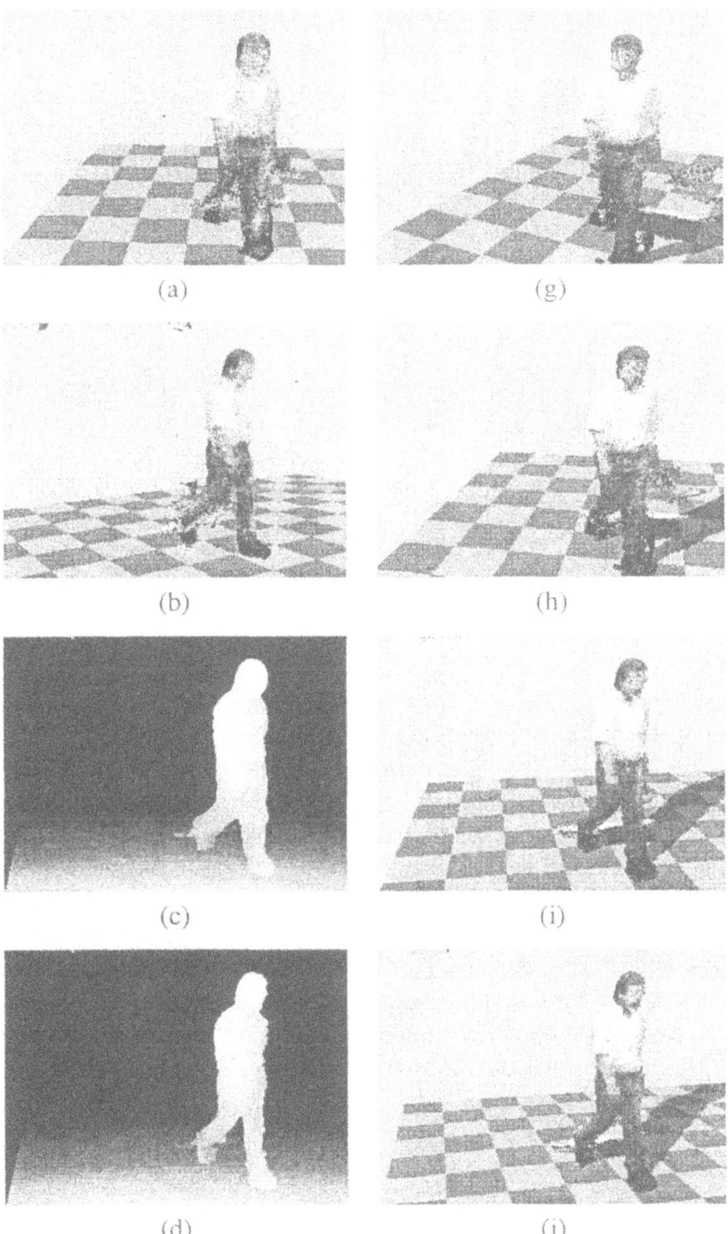

Figure 2 Results

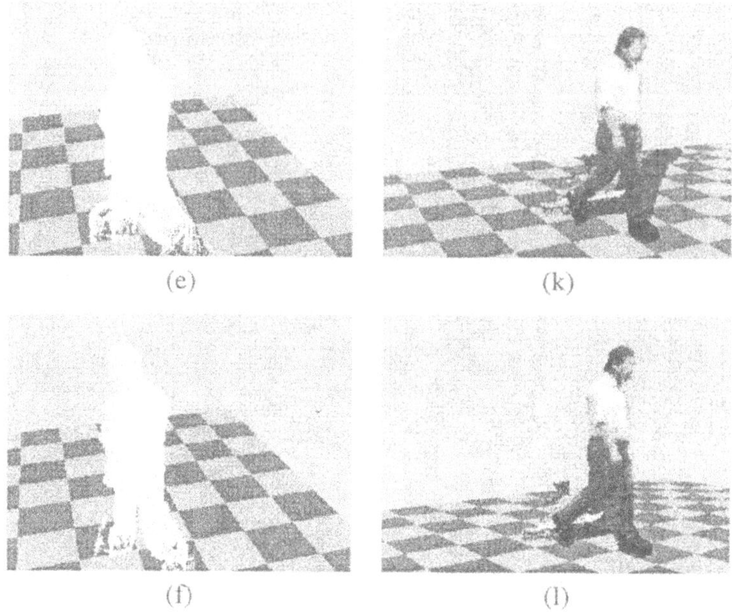

Figure 3 Results (cont.)

consistency of edge gradients in 3-D and normal flow in 3-D. Use of these techniques on sequences of moving people is shown.

This technique is not specific to human motion; it gives the shape and surface motion of general deformable objects. The next step in progressing toward the ultimate motion capture technology for human motion in particular is to use this moving object model to fit trajectories of points in a human model. Simply put, using the recovered models we can create a 3-D motion field sequence representing implicitly the specific animation. Our algorithm implicitly uses this representation during carving. This approach allows motion capture to occur without the need for markers, specialized backgrounds, or sensors on the body. It can capture the complex motions of clothing and nonrigid portions of the body. Ultimately, databases of human activity can be created and used in graphics and recognition systems.

References

[1] P. Baker and Y. Aloimonos. Complete calibration of a multi-camera network. In *Proc. IEEE Workshop on Omnidirectional Vision*, pages 134–141, Hilton Head Island, SC, 2000. IEEE Computer Society.

[2] W. Bruce Culbertson, Thomas Malzbender, and Greg Slabaugh. Generalized voxel coloring. In *Vision Algorithms: Theory and Practice*, Corfu, Greece, 1999. IEEE.

[3] L. Davis, E. Borovikov, R. Cutler, D. Harwood, and T. Horprasert. Multi-perspective analysis of human action. In *Proc. of Third International Workshop on Cooperative Distributed Vision*, Kyoto, Japan, 1999.

[4] O. D. Faugeras. *Three-Dimensional Computer Vision*. MIT Press, Cambridge, MA, 1992.

[5] C. Fermüller, R. Pless, and Y. Aloimonos. Statistical biases in optic flow. In *Proc. IEEE Conference on Computer Vision and Pattern Recognition*, volume 1, pages 561–566, 1999.

[6] C. Fermüller, R. Pless, and Y. Aloimonos. The Ouchi illusion as an artifact of biased flow estimation. *Vision Research*, 40:77–96, 2000.

[7] K. N. Kutulakos and S. M. Seitz. What do N photographs tell us about 3D shape? Computer Science Technical Report 692, University of Rochester, 1998.

[8] P. Narayanan, P. Rander, and T. Kanade. Constructing virtual worlds using dense stereo. In *Proc. International Conference on Computer Vision*, pages 3–10, Bombay, 1998.

[9] H. Saito and T. Kanade. Shape reconstruction in projective grid space from large number of images. In *Proc. IEEE Conference on Computer Vision and Pattern Recognition*, volume 2, pages 49–54, 1999.

[10] S. M. Seitz and C. Dyer. Photorealistic scene reconstruction by voxel coloring. In *Proc. IEEE Conference on Computer Vision and Pattern Recognition*, pages 1067–1073, 1997.

[11] M. E. Spetsakis and J. Aloimonos. A unified theory of structure from motion. In *Proc. DARPA Image Understanding Workshop*, pages 271–283, 1990.

[12] Sundar Vedula, Simon Baker, Peter Rander, Robert collins, and Takeo Kanade. Three-dimensional scene flow. In *Proc. International Conference on Computer Vision*, Corfu, Greece, 1999.

[13] Z. Zhang, O. D. Faugeras, and N. Ayache. Analysis of a sequence of stereo scenes containing multiple moving objects using rigidity constraints. In *Proc. Second International Conference on Computer Vision*, pages 177–186, 1988.

DELAUNAY TRIANGLES MODEL FOR IMAGE-BASED MOTION RETARGETING

Dong Hoon Lee and Soon Ki Jung
Department of Computer Engineering, Kyungpook National University 1370 Sankyuk-dong, Puk-ku, Taegu 702-701, Korea

Key words: vision based motion capture, delaunay triangulation, motion estimation, character animation and image-based modelling and rendering

Abstract: We present an automatic system for retargeting a human body extracted from an image sequence into a new character in a still image. In contrast to analysing the articulated motion of its skeleton in the previous vision-based human body tracking and posture recognition system, we use direct 2-D image warping based on a silhouette. At first, we represent the performer's silhouette with the Delaunay Triangles Model (DTM) of which the boundary points are the critical points of the silhouette. We then use a set of affine transformations of Delaunay triangles for the human body motion, which is applied to a new character for the deformation of the subject's DTM. The final animation of the subject is texture mapped using backward Radial Basis Functions (RBFs). Although our algorithm presented in this paper is not applicable to the human body with self-occluded motion, it allows believable photo-realistic motion retargeting.

1. INTRODUCTION

The pursuit of photo-realism is of major interest in computer graphics and virtual reality. In particular, realistic animations of avatar or an autonomous agent are important essential elements for constructing a virtual environment. Many researchers have studied realistic motion and expression generation and focused on motion control of geometric human body and facial models. Motion capture or motion retargeting is one of these efforts.

In this paper, we will focus on vision-based human body tracking and posture recognition systems.

Systems based on computer vision capture the motion parameters from images. These systems are called kinematics analysis systems [11, 6, 2, 8]. With this approach, the human body model is composed of a number of parts that allows movement among them so that reconstruction of the human body motion should calculate shape and joint angle parameters. The main difficulties are related to modelling humans and to the expensive search procedure for the recovery of shape and motion parameters.

Our method is based on understanding low-level features without an exhaustive search of high-level parameters. Previous similar approaches [1, 13, 7, 3] involve the extraction of the motion flow field and then segmenting it into piecewise smooth surfaces. These surfaces are then grouped and recognized as human parts, maybe using various types of features. Unfortunately, optical flow segmentation methods are rarely sufficiently general, and the recognition process may involve prohibitive search procedures.

Most existing approaches require a skeleton model of human motion. In contrast, we model the human body as a Delaunay Triangles Model (DTM), which has a set of 2-D Delaunay triangles approximating the silhouette of the human body and affine motion for each Delaunay triangle. In order to get a reliable DTM, we perform the following three steps:

First, we extract a set of feature points from the silhouette using the critical point detection (CPD) algorithm described by Zhu and Chirlian [14]. Second, we build a polygon with the set of points. We then tessellate the polygon using Delaunay triangulation [9]. The consistency of Delaunay triangulation between frames is preserved by a model based 2-D tracking of each triangle with piecewise constant affine motion and the adaptation of DTM by managing the critical value of each candidate critical point. Affine motion of each triangle for the subject's DTM is applied to the DTM of the new character for motion retargeting. The motion of the inner part of each triangle is interpolated using backward Radial Basis Functions (RBFs) for image warping of the subject.

We capture the performer's animation footage and the subject's still image (we can also use any picture of famous movie stars) as input data. The subject must have a similar posture to the performer's to ease the correspondence problem. Our algorithm assumes that the person in the image stands facing the fixed camera and does not have self-occluded motion. We assume this because we cannot extract 3-D motion from just one camera. These assumptions show our study is not intended for a challenging case of analysing complicated human motion and animating synthetic modelled character, but rather for rendering a real human appearance.

The overall algorithm is summarized in Figure 1.

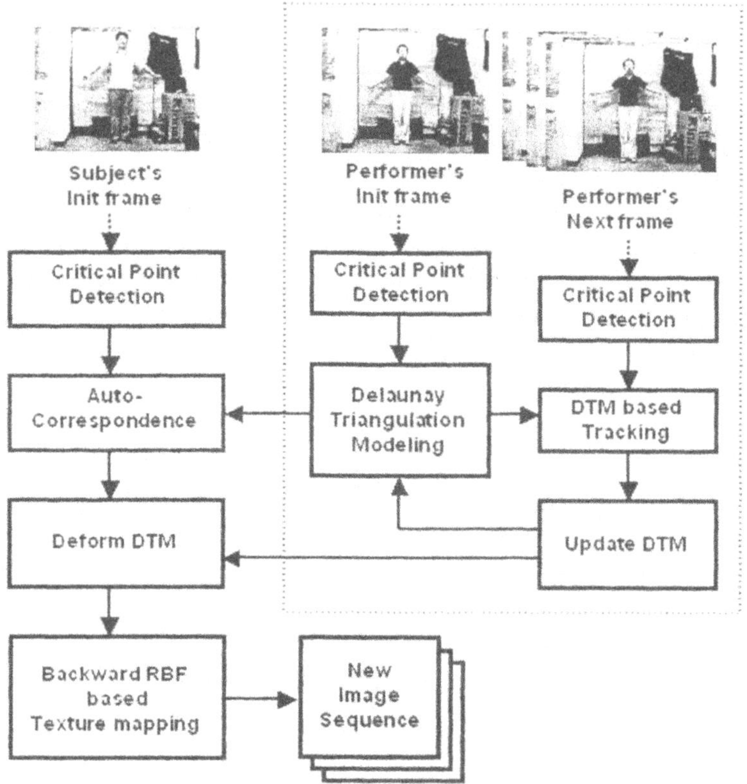

Figure 1. System block diagram.

The rest of this paper is organized as follows. We describe the details of the automatic critical point detection algorithm and the DTM-based tracking of the triangle model in Sections 2 and 3, respectively. Section 4 includes the algorithm of motion retargeting using backward RBFs. We show some results in Section 5. We present conclusions in Section 6.

2. DELAUNAY TRIANGLES MODEL

2.1 Human Body Extraction

To construct a Delaunay Triangles Model (DTM), we first have to extract a human silhouette. Video stream is nearly impossible to get a human silhouette using a manual method because it has a large number of image data, so we design a background modelling strategy for automatic human extraction.

In the first stage, we made a model of a background image with several image frames that do not contain a person. To eliminate the effect of the luminance and shadow, we model each pixel as a mixture of Gaussians in Equation (1). The Gaussian distributions of the adaptive mixture model are then evaluated to determine which are most likely to result from a background process. Based on the persistence and the variance of each of the Gaussians of the mixture, we determine which Gaussians may correspond to background colours. Pixel values that do not fit the background distributions are considered foreground.

$$f(X)=\frac{1}{\sigma\sqrt{2}}e^{-\frac{\|X-u\|^2}{2\sigma^2}} \tag{1}$$

where X is the vector value of each pixel colour element R, G, B, and u is the mean of each pixel about background image.

2.2 Critical Point Detection

The human body is approximately modelled by Delaunay triangles, which consists of triangles connected together by feature points. To generate feature points, we used the critical point detection(CPD) algorithm described by Zhu and Chirlian [14].

2.2.1 Pseudo Critical Points

We assume the human silhouette is a simple closed contour without any interior holes. In a simple closed contour obtained by human body extraction in the previous step and simple border tracing technique, each pixel p_i has two neighbours p_{i-1} and p_{i+1}. We then transfer the contour to polar coordinates because it is easier to handle rotation and scaling changes in polar coordinates than in rectangular coordinates. When the centroid of the shape is used as the origin, the representation of the shape becomes very simple. The 2-D contour can be decomposed into two 1-D curves: $\rho(i)$ and $\theta(i)$, the local maxima and minima (zero crossing points) are more important in describing the curve character than the other points. Therefore, these points are selected as candidate of critical points. We select zero crossing points as pseudo critical points.

2.2.2 Critical Value

The pseudo critical points are just candidates of critical points. Some pseudo critical points must be deleted. The CPD algorithm assigns a critical value to each point on the boundary that is simply the area of the triangle constructed from the given point and its two immediate neighbours. The height of the triangle reflects the information of directional change providing the support region is a constant and the bottom of the triangle reflects the information of feature size. The critical value in each point represents the possibility of becoming a critical point. Thus, a larger critical value has a higher probability to be chosen as a critical point.

An iterative decimation process is used which removes the point with the smallest critical value, recomputes the critical value of the immediate neighbours of the point which has just been deleted and reidentifies the point with the smallest critical value. The process terminates when the remaining smallest critical value is above some threshold set by the user.

2.3 Delaunay Triangles Model (DTM)

The set of feature points from the previous step is tessellated by Delaunay triangulation. The silhouette information is insufficient to model human motion. That is the reason we construct triangle structures for human modelling. Each triangle has the information of a set of feature points with posture data and affine transformation elements. The transformation elements represent a rotation, translation, scale and shear between frames. Each affine motion of Delaunay triangles represents the complicated nonrigid human motion. Figure 2 shows the real human figure and its DTM. The result of tessellation includes the background region, so we should eliminate the triangles outside of human to get the final result.

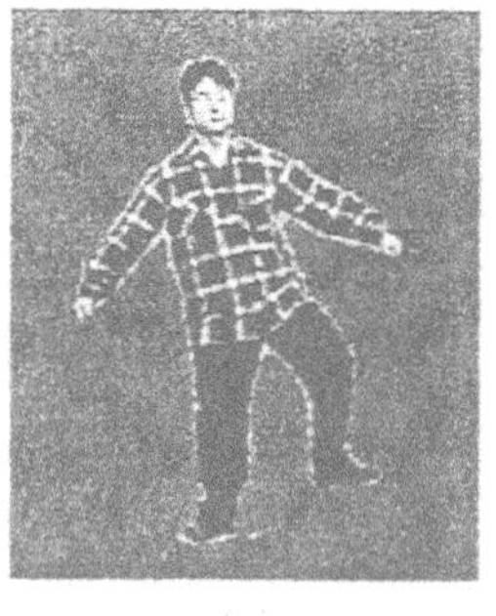

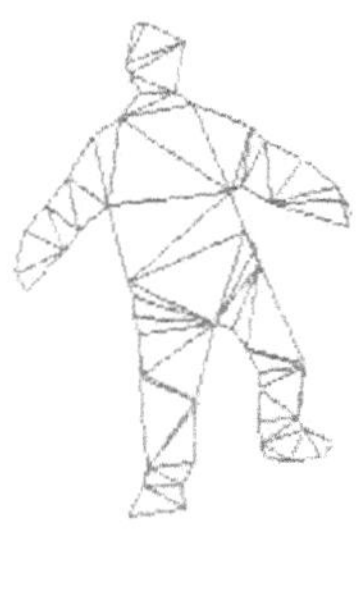

(a) (b)

Figure 2. Delaunay Triangles Model (DTM).

3. DTM-BASED TRACKING

3.1 Tracking

In this section, we describe DTM-based feature tracking using predicted measurements. The human motion is assumed as a 2-D piecewise constant affine motion of each triangle which comprise a DTM. The 2-D motion of a triangle is a general 2-D affine transformation, representing a combination of rotation, translation, scale and shearing.

We predict the posture of each 2-D triangle with affine parameters calculated from a previous triangle and select real measurements from the set of candidate critical points on the silhouette. The candidate critical points are a set of pseudo critical points, not all point on the silhouette because the pseudo critical points have compact features that represent the character of a human silhouette. We can model the error function for selecting real measurements with the weighted nearest neighbour method as below (Equation 2). The critical point with the smallest error value is selected as the real measurement.

$$E(\hat{p}, p_i) = \frac{\lambda \times |\hat{p} - p_i|}{I(p_i)}, \tag{2}$$

where $I(p_i)$ is a critical value of each pseudo critical point, p is a predicted measurement, λ adjusts the weight between the distance and critical value, and the domain of candidate points, p_i, is determined by the user. .

3.2 Update DTM using Critical Value

A DTM constructed from an initial posture does not guarantee to approximate the silhouette after arbitrary human motion such as the bending motion of arms. In this case, some critical points newly appear. The DTM is dynamically updated through missed features, which are not tracked during the tracking step, with a high critical value in the feature extraction step as shown in Figure 3. The update process of the proposed algorithm can be summarized as follows:

1) DTM-based tracking.
2) Calculate the critical value with the tracked real measurement and a critical point with a high critical value.

3) Find the point with the lowest critical value besides the critical value calculated from a triangle that is composed of three real measurements.
4) Compare the lowest critical value with the specified critical value, I. If the lowest critical value is smaller than I, delete the critical point with this critical value, then go to step 2. Otherwise, stop the recursion.
5) Update the DTM.

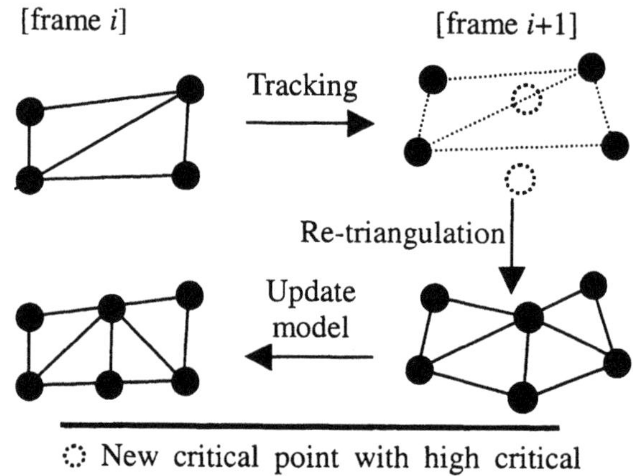

Figure 3. Update object model.

4. MOTION RETARGETING

4.1 DTM-based Motion Retargeting

As mentioned before, we would like to animate the subject from the performer's motion using a set of affine transformations for Delaunay triangles, which compose of the human body. For this purpose, we split the affine motion into several primitive components such as translation, rotation, scale, and shear. First, we extract the stick figure that forms a graph of which the nodes are the center points of triangles and the edges mean the adjacencies between triangles in DTM. We then calculate the translation of the whole body from the translation motion of a specific node, which has the maximum degree of the graph and the maximum area of the triangle. We call the node as the root of the graph. The rotation of each triangle can be extracted by the orientation motion of the corresponding node with respect to the root. The scale factor is calculated from the variation of the distance between the node and the root. Then the remained terms are for the local affine motion of each triangle. The DTM-based motion retargeting is shown in Figure 4.

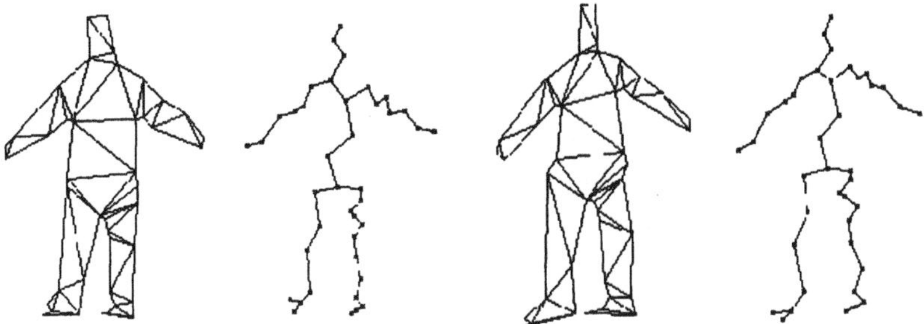

(a) Performer's DTM and graph (b) Subject's retargeted DTM and graph

Figure 4. This figure shows the result of retargeting the performer's DTM into the subject's DTM. The variations of the split affine motion between frames in the performer's graph model are applied to the subject's.

4.2 RBF based Texture Mapping

Classical approximation theory solves the problem of approximating or interpolating a continuous multivariate function by an approximation function with the appropriate choice of a parameter set. Finding a parameter set is often referred to as learning or training in the neural network sense. In the training stage, a goal is to figure out given an approximation function and a set of training examples that will provide the best approximation of F [10]. Radial Basis Functions are often chosen as approximating high dimensional smooth surfaces. Examples of RBFs are Gaussian functions, multi-quadrics and thin plate splines with linear terms added. The RBF training equation is expressed as Equation (3):

$$\Phi \mathrm{w} = \mathrm{d}, \tag{3}$$

where d is defined as the matrix of the coordinate of the performer's feature points, Φ is the matrix of $\{\varphi(\|\mathrm{x} - \mathrm{x}_i\|) \mid i = 1,2,\ldots,N\}$ which is a set of N radial-basis functions which are made with the feature coordinates of the performer's next frame and w is unknown coefficients (weights).

Then, the set of weights, w, is given by

$$\mathrm{w} = \Phi^{-1}\mathrm{d}. \tag{4}$$

The general mapping function can be given in two forms: either relating the output coordinate system to that of the input, or vice versa. These functions are known as forward and inverse mapping. In this paper, we use inverse mapping because it guarantees that all output pixels are computed unlike with the forward mapping scheme.

We already have the spatial transformation parameter, w, from the previous step, so we can get the forward warped image easily by instituting a subject feature in the initial frame into the radial centre. However, we cannot get the initial subject's coordinates for inverse mapping because this information is contained in the radial basis function ϕ.

To operate inverse mapping, we simply obtain the weights of the RBF with the set of subject's feature point in frame i+1 as input x and those in frame i as desired output d in the training step. Then every pixel of subject image in frame i is scanned as input and each output pixel mapped back onto the input via the spatial transformation mapping function.

5. RESULTS AND EXPERIMENTS

The performer's motion is recorded using one video recorder and then captured off-line while playing back frame-by-frame. The system uses a SONY DCR-TRV310 video recorder and we implement the algorithm on a Pentium II PC which has a 350MHz CPU and 128Mbytes memory. The subject must have a similar posture to the performer's to ease the correspondence problem. The person in the experiments stands facing the fixed camera and does not have self-occluded motion. We create a variety of motions of retargeted objects by choosing different motions of source film footage. Figure 5 shows example of results of our proposed scheme.

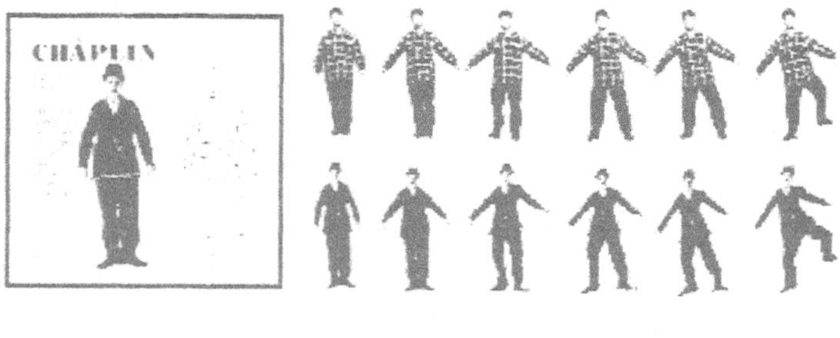

(a) (b)

Figure 5. The example of results of the proposed scheme. The segmentation and feature extraction of subject image is done manually in left image and right image shows its DTM in (a). (b) shows the performer's image sequences (upper) and the result of motion retargeting using Charlie Chaplin still image (below).

6. CONCLUSIONS

In this paper, we have presented an automatic system for retargeting a human body motion extracted from an image sequence into a new character in a still image. In contrast to analysing the articulated motion of its skeleton in the previous vision-based human body tracking and posture recognition system, we have modelled the human body as a Delaunay Triangles Model (DTM), which has a set of 2-D Delaunay triangles approximating the silhouette of the human body and affine motion for each Delaunay triangle. We have used a set of affine transformation of Delaunay triangles for the human body motion that was applied to a new character for the deformation of the subject's DTM. The final animation of the subject was texture mapped using the backward Radial Basis Functions (RBFs).

Our study was not intended to challenge the case of analysing complicated human motion and animating a synthetic modelled character but rather for rendering real human appearance. Therefore, although our algorithm presented in this paper is not applicable to the human body with self-occluded motion, it allows believable photo-realistic motion retargeting. Our system can be utilized in the field of entertainment for the purpose of generation of the motion with old celebrity's image or mimicking the celebrity's motion such as Charlie Chaplin's. Furthermore, this will allow the generation of realistic avatars from widely available video clips.

ACKNOWLEDGEMENT

This work was supported by the Korea Science and Engineering Foundation(KOSEF) through the Virtual Reality Research Center at KAIST and by Korea Research Foundation Grant(KRF-99-041-E00294).

REFERENCES

[1] A. Bottino, A. Laurentini, and P. Zuccone, Toward non-intrusive motion capture, *Computer Vision-ACCV98*, pages 416-423, 1998.

[2] D. M. Gavrila and L. S. Davis, 3-d model-based tracking of humans in action: a multi-view approach, *In IEEE Conf. on CVPR*, pages 73-80, San Francisco, USA, 1996.

[3] I. Haritauglu, D. Harwood, and L. Davis, w^4s: A real-time system for detecting and tracking people in 2½d, *Computer Vision-ECCV98*, pages 877-892, 1998.

[4] Simon Haykin, *Neural networks - A comprehensive foundation*, 2nd Edition, Prentice-Hall, 1999.

[5] Andrew Hill, Chris J. Taylor, and Alan D. Brett, A framework for automatic landmark identification using a new method of nonrigid correspondence, *IEEE Trans. on PAMI*, 22(3), pages 241-251, March 2000.

[6] E. A. Hunter, P. H. Kelly, and R. C. Jain, Estimation of articulated motion using kinematically constrained mixture densities, *In Proceedings of IEEE Non-Rigid and Articulated Motion Workshop*, pages 10-17, Puerto Rico, USA, 1997.

[7] S. Ju, M. Black, and Y. Yacoob, Cardboard People: A parameterized model of articulated image motion. *In 2nd International Conference on Face and Gesture Analysis*, pages 38-44, Vermont, USA, 1996.

[8] I. A. Kakadiaris and D. Metaxas, Model-based estimation of 3d human motion with occlusion based on active multi-viewpoint selection, *In IEEE Conf. on CVPR*, pages 81-87, San Francisco, CA, USA, 1996.

[9] Kazuhiro Nakahashi and Dmitri Sharov, Direct surface triangulation using the advancing front method, *AIAA-95-1686-CP*, pages 442-451, 1995.

[10] Mark J. L. Orr, Introduction to radial basis function networks, technical report, Centre for Cognitive Science, University of Edinburgh, April 1996.

[11] S. Wachter and H. –H. Nagel, Tracking of persons in monocular image sequences, *In Proceedings of IEEE Non-Rigid and Articulated Motion Workshop*, pages 2-9, Puerto Rico, USA, 1997.

[12] George Wolberg, *Digital Image Warping*, IEEE Computer Society Press, 1990.

[13] C. Wren, A. Azarbayejani, T. Darrell, and A. Pentland, Pfinder: Real-time tracking of the human body, *IEEE trans. on PAMI*, 19(7) pages 780-785, July 1997.

[14] Pengfei Zhu and Paul M. Chirlian, On critical point detection of digital shapes, *IEEE trans. on PAMI*, 17(8), pages 737-748, August 1995.

A VECTOR-SPACE REPRESENTATION OF MOTION DATA FOR EXAMPLE-BASED MOTION SYNTHESIS *

Ik Soo Lim† and Daniel Thalmann

Computer Graphics Lab (LIG), Swiss Federal Institute of Technology (EPFL), CH-1015 Lausanne, Switzerland

Keywords: example-based motion synthesis, vector space representation, principal components

Abstract We approach the problem of example-based motion synthesis by transforming motion data into a vector space representation. This allows many techniques successful for stationary object synthesis applicable to that of motion. Especially, by separating generation of motion into a time-consuming preprocess and a fast process, it lets on-the-fly motion synthesis able to use a rich set of examplar motions and handle motion attributes invariant for each individual, both of which are difficult to be addressed by previous approaches based on interpolation.

1. INTRODUCTION

Motion control of articulated figures such as humans has been a challenging task in computer animation [BPW93]. Once an acceptable motion segment has been created, either from key-framing, motion capture or physical simulations, reuse of it is important.

This article describes example-based motion synthesis with parametric manipulation of motion attributes. This is done by transforming motion data into a vector space representation based on a linear combination of prototypical motions in full correspondence/alignment. This representation allows those techniques successful for the synthesis of stationary objects such as 2D images and 3D shapes applicable to motion.

*This work is supported in part by PAVR under the EU Training and Mobility of Researchers program.

†Thanks to Norman Badler for helpful discussions.

By separating motion generation into a time-consuming preprocess and a fast process, it also fits well to real-time animation for applications such as game and virtual reality while taking advantage of a rich set of examplar motions.

In the following sections, we first describe related work of editing and reuse of motion data. A vector-space representation of stationary objects is briefly reviewed. We present its extension to motion data. Taking advantage of the representation, manipulation of motion attributes is introduced. First results of our approach with hand-crafted motion data follow it. We conclude with discussions comparing ours with some of previous works.

2. RELATED WORK

Much of the recent research in computer animation has been directed towards editing and reuse of existing motion data. Stylistic variations are learned from a training set of very long unsegmented motion-capture sequences [BH00]. An interactive multi-resolution motion editing is proposed for fast and fine-scale control of the motion [LS99]. Whereas most of other methods may produce results violating the laws of mechanics [WP95], an editing method maintaining physical validity is suggested [PW99]. Motion editing is also done in frequency-domains [BW95] [UAT95]. Interpolation of existing motion data is employed for the on-the-fly synthesis [RCB98][WH97].

3. LINEAR COMBINATIONS OF STATIONARY OBJECTS

The basic idea of the vector space representation by a linear combination of stationary objects can be described as follows, first proposed by Ulman and Basri [UB91] and followed up for 2D images [BP96][VP97] and 3D geometries [BV99][She00]. It is based on a data set of stationary objects in a same class. All of these exemplar objects are assumed in full correspondence, which can be done using techniques based on optic flow algorithms [BP96][BV99][VP97]. Given a set of m exemplar objects in full correspondence, characterized by feature vectors $\mathbf{X}_1, \ldots, \mathbf{X}_m$ such as pixels for 2D images or vertices for 3D geometries, a linear combination of them produces a new object in the same class:

$$\mathbf{X} = \sum_{i=1}^{m} w_i \mathbf{X}_i$$

This linear combination is meaningful or valid since all the examples are in full correspondence: unless the 2D images align pixel-to-pixel, for example, a simple linear combination of them would look like a transparent superposition of different images rather than a new image in the same class. The vectors $\mathbf{X}_i$ comprise the basis of a linear vector space. The method parametrizes a continuous class of objects and the weight vector $\overrightarrow{w} = (w_1, \ldots, w_m)$ characterizes each object of this class in a compact way. Object transformations, like view point changes in 2D images of an object [UB91] or attribute manipulation in 3D faces [BV99], can be expressed in terms of changes in the weight vector.

4. LINEAR COMBINATIONS OF MOTIONS

Motion can be described by a set of motion curves each giving the value of one of the model's parameters as a function of time, e.g. joint angles over time for articulated objects such as human figures.

For instructional purposes, we start with motion data of just a single curve $\theta(t)$. We represent the motion data with a shape-vector $\mathbf{S} = (\theta_1, \ldots, \theta_n) \in \Re^n$ and a timing-vector $\mathbf{T} = (t_1, \ldots, t_n) \in \Re^n$ where θ_j giving the value of θ at time t_j, i.e. $\theta_j = \theta(t_j)$. Given m exemplar motions, each represented by its shape-vector and timing-vector, an arbitrary motion among them is chosen as a reference motion, $\mathbf{S}_{ref}$ and $\mathbf{T}_{ref}$. Correspondence between all other motions and this reference is computed, which can be done automatically by a time-warp algorithm [BW95]: each shape-vector is warped into the reference $\mathbf{S}_{ref}$ and its corresponding timing-vector is accordingly recomputed. New shapes $\mathbf{S}_{mod}$ and new timings $\mathbf{T}_{mod}$ can be expressed as a linear combination of the shapes and timings of the m exemplar motions in full correspondence:

$$\mathbf{S}_{mod} = \sum_{i=1}^{m} a_i \mathbf{S}_i, \quad \mathbf{T}_{mod} = \sum_{i=1}^{m} b_i \mathbf{T}_i.$$

For motion data consisting of a set of motion curves $\theta^{(1)}(t), \ldots, \theta^{(k)}(t)$ for articulated bodies such as human figures, a shape-vector and a timing-vector can be straightforwardly extended by concatenating those of the single curves such as $\mathbf{S} = \left(\theta_1^{(1)}, \ldots, \theta_n^{(1)}, \ldots, \theta_1^{(k)}, \ldots, \theta_n^{(k)}\right) \in \Re^{nk}$ and $\mathbf{T} = \left(t_1^{(1)}, \ldots, t_n^{(1)}, \ldots, t_1^{(k)}, \ldots, t_n^{(k)}\right) \in \Re^{nk}$. This representation parametrizes a continuous class of motions by the weight vectors $\overrightarrow{a} = (a_1, \ldots, a_m)$ and $\overrightarrow{b} = (b_1, \ldots, b_m)$ in a compact way and motion manipulation / transformation can be expressed in terms of changes in the weight vectors, analogous to that of stationary objects as above.

Principal Component Analysis (PCA) [Jac91] can be employed for a basis transformation to an orthogonal coordinate system with the eigenvectors of the covariance matrices computed over the shape and timing differences with their averages $\overline{\mathbf{S}}$ and $\overline{\mathbf{T}}$, respectively. This will lead to further data compression and level-of-details as explored for stationary objects [AM00][BH00][PW89].

5. MOTION ATTRIBUTES

For the functional relationship between the weight vectors and the continuous parameters of interest, we adopt the technique used for geometric models of 3D faces [BV99]: radial basis functions network [Bis95] [GJP95] are often used for the similar purposes [BP96][She00]. Based on a set of motions $(\mathbf{S}_i, \mathbf{T}_i)$ with labels μ_i describing the markedness of the attribute, we compute the weighted sums

$$\triangle\mathbf{S} = \sum_{i=1}^{m} \mu_i \left(\mathbf{S}_i - \overline{\mathbf{S}}\right), \quad \triangle\mathbf{T} = \sum_{i=1}^{m} \mu_i \left(\mathbf{T}_i - \overline{\mathbf{T}}\right).$$

Multiples of $(\triangle\mathbf{S}, \triangle\mathbf{T})$ can now be added to or subtracted from any individual motion generated by the motion model, which will manipulate a specific attribute while keeping all other attributes as constant as possible. Motion caricature is also possible, analogous to that of a face [Bre85][BV99]. Individual motions are caricatured by increasing their distance from the average motion.

6. RESULTS

We performed experiments with hand-crafted motion data of ten examples similar but distinct (Figure 1). The key-framed data were resampled densely, 64 samplings over 2 seconds or so for each of 75 degree-of-freedom as if simulated/captured data: a vector of 4800 dimension. These examples went through a basis transformation by PCA (Figure 2). To illustrate the manipulation of motion attributes, two attributes vectors were extracted and applied: one for the height of a human figure's right hand, the other for energy (Figure 3). Motion caricatures were also generated with different degree of distinctiveness (Figure 4).

7. DISCUSSIONS AND CONCLUSIONS

A vector space representation of motion data based on a linear combination of prototypes is presented for example-based motion synthesis analogous to that of stationary objects. Due to the representation, many techniques successful for synthesis of stationary objects become applicable to motion synthesis and are done in a compact way with the low dimensional weight vector of the linear combination.

Especially noticeable, among them, is the extraction of motion attribute vectors which, when added to or subtracted from a motion, will manipulate a specific attribute of motion while keeping all other attributes as constant as possible: adopted from a technique to handle attributes such as weight, age, and gender of faces [BV99], the motion attribute vectors can deal with those invariant for each individual. This separates generation of motion into a preprocess that may require complex and time-consuming computations, and a process that is fast and tolerant of various types of complexity: one for the extraction of the motion attribute vectors, the other for the addition/subtraction of them. Even on-the-fly motion synthesis can, hence, take advantage of a rich set of example motions while only a small set of examples are interpolated for the motion synthesis in previous works [RCB98][WH97], hardly handling those attributes invariant for each individual.

The basis transformation to one formed by the eigenvectors of the covariance matrix is often considered for dimension reduction or level-of-details [AM00][BV99][PW89]. Characterizing the variation between the examples, the eigenvector representation also serves well for efficient generation of motion variations which should be especially useful for applications such as crowd motions [MGT99]: altering the weights is more efficient and of better quality than directly perturbing the motion curves in a data-independent way [Per95].

The linear combination of stationary objects is also suggested for computer animation [AM00][BV99][EP00][PW89]. This linear combination in space may be suitable for a single stream of motion data. For a set of motions, however, a linear combination in space-time as done here fits better in terms of computation and storage.

Lately, in computer vision, a similar notion of the vector space representation is proposed for synthesis and analysis of motion patterns [GP00]. Handling video sequences directly without any 3D model, its motion synthesis is limited to, for example, that of similar view angles and the motion correspondence becomes complicated, being a spatio-temporal correspondence problem. In our approach, however, 3D model-based representations such as joint angles are used so that it is suitable for 3D animation and its motion correspondence problem is reduced to that of temporal correspondence for which a time-warp algorithm can be used [BW95].

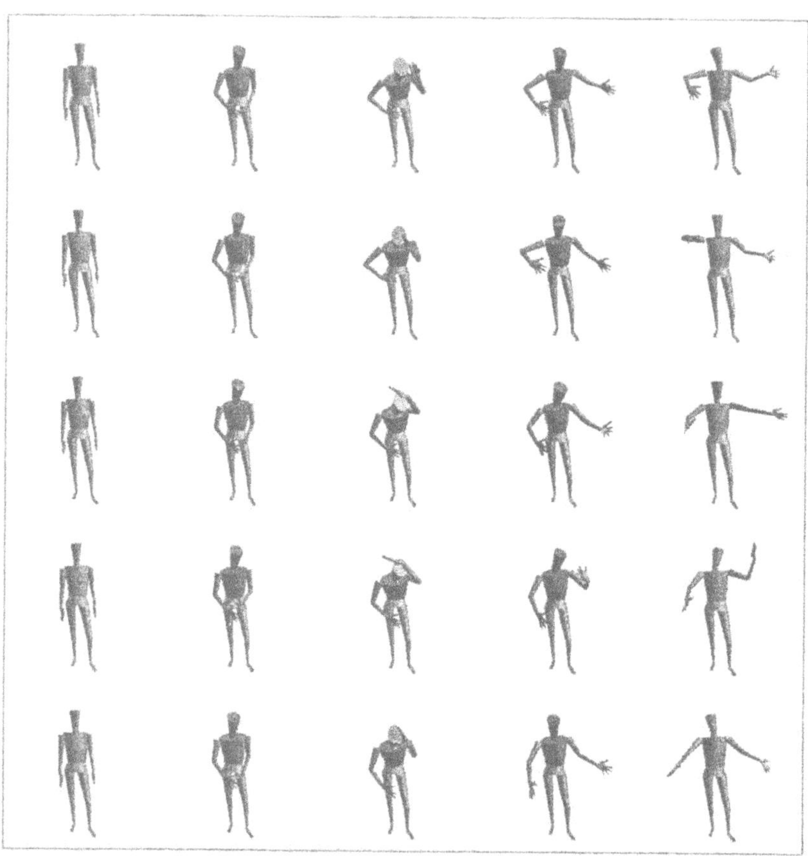

Figure 1 Five of ten similar but distinct example motions used for the motion synthesis.

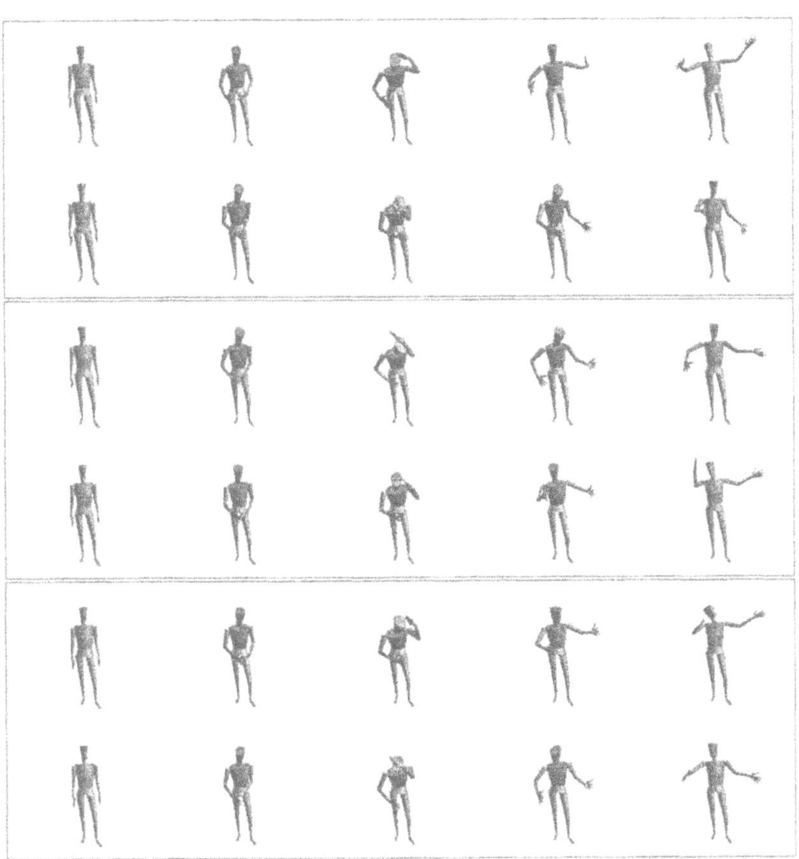

Figure 2 Three of the eigenvectors scaled by ±constants are added to the average motion.

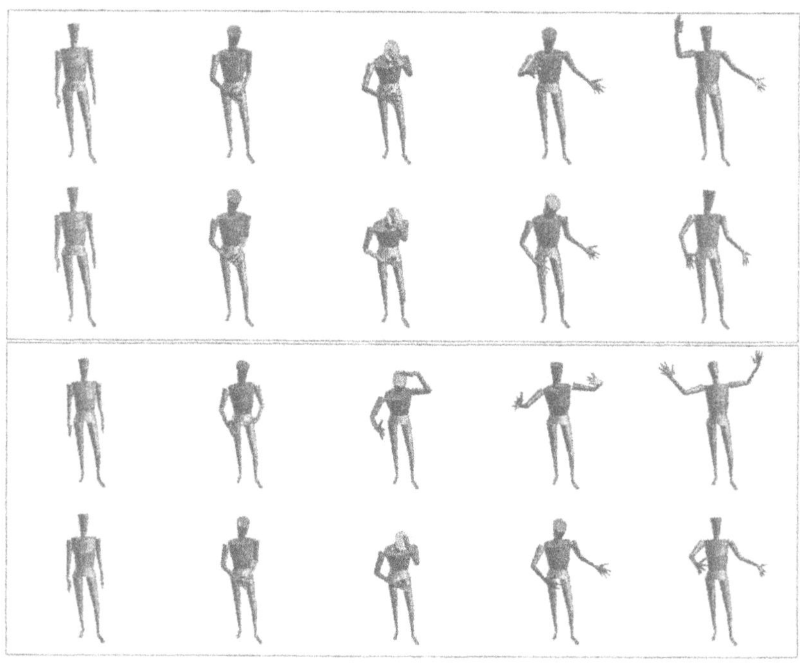

Figure 3 Motion Attributes. (Upper) the height of the human figure's right hand, high/low and (Lower) the energy of the human figure, high/low.

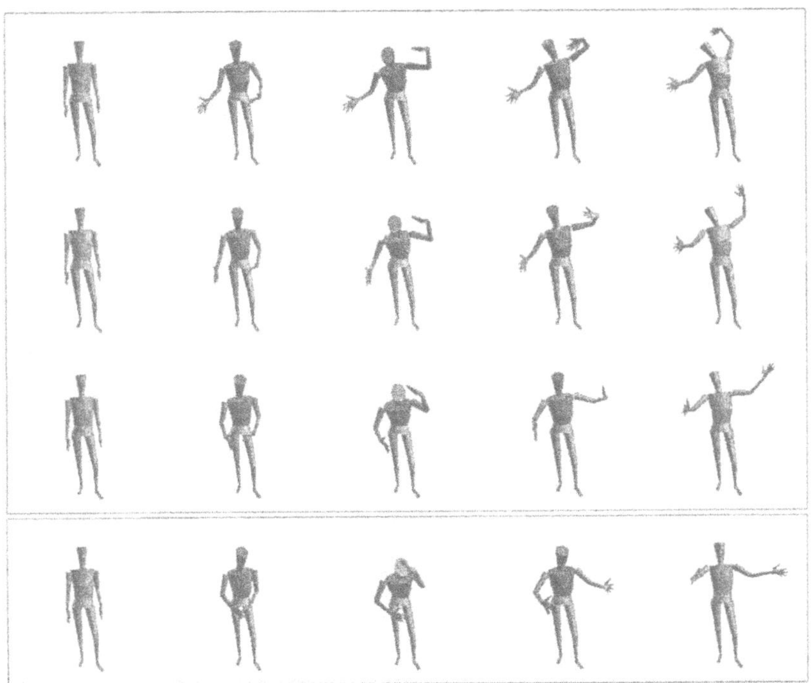

Figure 4 Motion Caricature. (Starting from the bottom) the average motion, the original motion and two of its caricatures with different degrees of distinctiveness.

References

[AM00] M. Alexa and W. Muller. Representing animations by principal components. In *Proceedings of EUROGRAPHICS 2000*, 2000.

[BH00] Matthew Brand and Aaron Hertzmann. Style machines. In *Proceedings of SIGGRAPH 2000*, pages 183 - 192, 2000.

[Bis95] C. M. Bishop. *Neural Networks for Pattern Recognition.* Clarendon Press, Oxford, 1995.

[BP96] D. Beymer and T. Poggio. Image representations for visual learning. *Science*, 272(5270):1905 – 1909, 1996.

[BPW93] N. Badler, C. Phillips, and B. Webber. *Simulating Humans: Computer Graphics, Animation, and Control.* Oxford University Press, 1993.

[Bre85] S. E. Brennan. The caricature generator. *Leonardo*, 18:170 – 178, 1985.

[BV99] V. Blanz and T. Vetter. A morphable model for the synthesis of 3d faces. In *Proceedings of SIGGRAPH 1999*, pages 187 – 194, 1999.

[BW95] A. Bruderlin and L. Williams. Motion signal processing. In *Proceedings of SIGGRAPH '95*, pages 97 - 104, 1995.

[EP00] T. Ezzat and T. Poggio. Visual speech synthesis by morphing visemes. *International Journal of Computer Vision*, 38(1):45 - 57, 2000.

[GJP95] F. Girosi, M. Jones, and T. Poggio. Regularization theory and neural network architechure. *Neural Computation*, 7:219 - 269, 1995.

[GP00] M. Giese and T. Poggio. Morphable models for the analysis and synthesis of complex motion patterns. *International Journal of Computer Vision*, 38(1):59 – 73, 2000.

[Jac91] J. E. Jackson. *A User's Guide to Principal Components.* John Wiley —& Sons, New York, 1991.

[LS99] J. Lee and S. Y. Shin. A hierarchical approach to interactive motion editing for human-like figures. In *Proceedings of SIGGRAPH 1999*, pages 39 - 48, 1999.

[MGT99] S. R. Musse, F. Garat, and D. Thalmann. Guiding and interacting with virtual crowds in real-time. In *Proceedings of Computer Animation and Simulation 1999*, pages 23 - 34, 1999.

[Per95] K. Perlin. Real-time responsive animation with personality. *IEEE Transactions on Visualization and Computer Graphics*, 1(1):5 – 15, 1995.

[PW89] A. P. Pentland and J. Williams. Good vibrations: Modal dynamics for graphics and animation. In *Proceedings of SIGGRAPH '89*, pages 215 – 222, 1989.

[PW99] Z. Popovic and A. Witkin. Physically based motion transformation. In *Proceedings of SIGGRAPH 1999*, pages 11 – 20, 1999.

[RCB98] C. Rose, M. Cohen, and B. Bodenheimer. Verbs and adverbs: Multidimensional motion interpolation. *IEEE Computer Graphics and Applications*, 18(5):32 – 48, September/October 1998.

[She00] C. Shelton. Morphable surface models. *International Journal of Computer Vision*, 38(1):75 – 91, 2000.

[UAT95] M. Unuma, K. Anjyo, and R. Takeuchi. Fourier principles for emotion-based human figure animation. In *Proceedings of SIGGRAPH '95*, pages 91 – 96, 1995.

[UB91] S. Ulman and R. Basri. Recognition by linear combination of models. *IEEE Transactions on Pattern Recognition and Machine Intelligence*, 13:992 – 1006, 1991.

[VP97] T. Vetter and T. Poggio. Linear object classes and image synthesis from a single example image. *IEEE Transactions on Pattern Recognition and Machine Intelligence*, 19(7):733 – 742, 1997.

[WH97] D. Wiley and J. Hahn. Interpolation synthesis of articulated figure motion. *IEEE Computer Graphics and Applications*, 17(6):39 – 45, November/December 1997.

[WP95] A. Witkin and Z. Popovic. Motion warping. In *Proceedings of SIGGRAPH '95*, pages 105 – 108, 1995.

PARAMETRIZATION AND RANGE OF MOTION OF THE BALL-AND-SOCKET JOINT

Paolo Baerlocher and Ronan Boulic
Computer Graphics Lab (LIG), Swiss Federal Institute of Technology (EPFL), 1015 Lausanne Switzerland

Key words: Ball-and-socket joint, joint limits

Abstract: The ball-and-socket joint model is used to represent articulations with three rotational degrees of freedom (DOF), such as the human shoulder and the hip. The goal of this paper is to discuss two related problems: the parametrization and the definition of realistic joint boundaries for ball-and-socket joints. Doing this accurately is difficult, yet important for motion generators (such as inverse kinematics and dynamics engines) and for motion manipulators (such as motion retargeting), since the resulting motions should satisfy the anatomic constraints. The difficulty mainly comes from the complex nature of 3D orientations and of human articulations. The underlying question of parametrization must be addressed before realistic and meaningful boundaries can be defined over the set of 3D orientations. In this paper, we review and compare several known methods, and advocate the use of the swing-and-twist parametrization, that partitions an arbitrary orientation into two meaningful components. Finally, we review two joint boundaries representations based on this decomposition, and show an example.

1. INTRODUCTION

In fields such as robotics [8] and biomechanics, and in Computer Animation as well [11], hierarchical structures are used to model articulated bodies like (real or imaginary) robots, humans and other creatures. An articulated body is made of a set of segments, connected by *joints*. The essential feature of a joint is that it permits some degree of relative motion between the two segments it connects. Ideal kinematic joint models are defined in order to formalize this permitted relative motion, called *range of motion*, characterized by the number of parameters that describe the motion space, and constrained by joint limits. Modeling real joints can be very complex, since the range of motion depends on many factors, especially in the articulations of living organisms and the human in particular [2]. Moreover, joints may be dependent on each other. In this paper, the coupling between joints is ignored.

The simplest example of joint model is the *revolute joint* that allows a rotation about an axis fixed in both segments it connects, usually within some angular limits. This joint is said to have one degree of freedom (DOF) and, because of its simplicity, is by far the most used joint in robotics. In human modeling, it is a convenient model of the interphalangeal joints of the hands and feet, for example. For more complex articulations such as the shoulder and hip, joint models allowing more degrees of freedom are required. The kinematic modelling of such articulations is a difficult task. First, a clear mathematical description of the allowed relative motion must be given by a proper parametrization: because of the complex non-Euclidean nature of rotations, this must be done carefully, because of the problem of singularities. Second, the range of motion must be constrained to restrict the parameter space to a more realistic subset. The problem is complex for ball-and-socket joints, because the boundaries on the three independent parameters are generally coupled.

In Computer Animation, these topics have already been addressed by Badler [1, 2], Korein [5], Wang [9, 10], Grassia [4] and Maurel [7]. In this paper, we summarize and compare their results, and try to provide some more insight on the topics.

1.1 Notation and conventions

Vectors are denoted by small boldface letters such as $\boldsymbol{v}$. The three basis vectors of a coordinate frame are noted $\boldsymbol{x}$, $\boldsymbol{y}$ and $\boldsymbol{z}$. Matrices are denoted by capital letters such as M.

The rotation by an angle θ about an axis passing through the origin and whose direction is given by vector $\boldsymbol{a}$, is noted $R_{a}(\theta)$.

Given two unit vectors $\boldsymbol{a}$ and $\boldsymbol{b}$, we define $R_D(\boldsymbol{a},\boldsymbol{b}) := R_{\boldsymbol{a}\times\boldsymbol{b}}(acos(\boldsymbol{a}^T\boldsymbol{b}))$ as the *direct rotation* that transforms $\boldsymbol{a}$ into $\boldsymbol{b}$, with the minimum angle of rotation. If $\boldsymbol{b}+\boldsymbol{a}=0$, $R_D(\boldsymbol{a},\boldsymbol{b})$ is undefined.

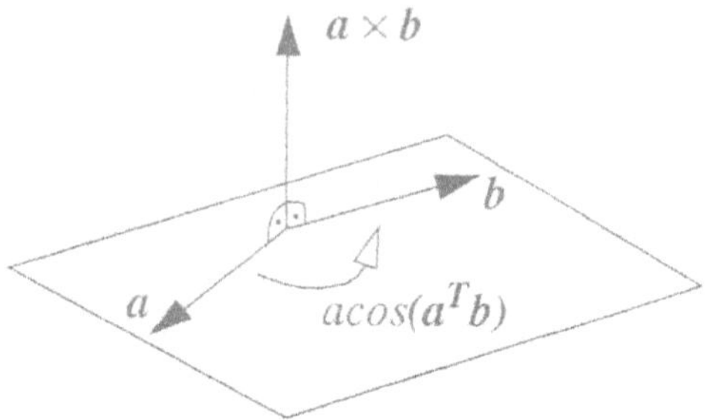

Figure 1. A direct rotation transforms a unit vector $\boldsymbol{a}$ into a unit vector $\boldsymbol{b}$.

2. PARAMETRIZATION OF A BALL JOINT

A ball-and-socket joint possesses three rotational degrees of freedom. Hence, it is the most mobile of the purely rotational joints. It allows an axial motion (or *twist*) of the segment (one DOF), as well as a *spherical* motion (or *swing*) that determines its direction (two DOFs). Ball-and-socket joints are used to model articulations such as the human shoulder and hip. By convention, the moving segment is aligned with the z axis of the local joint frame (see Fig. 2).

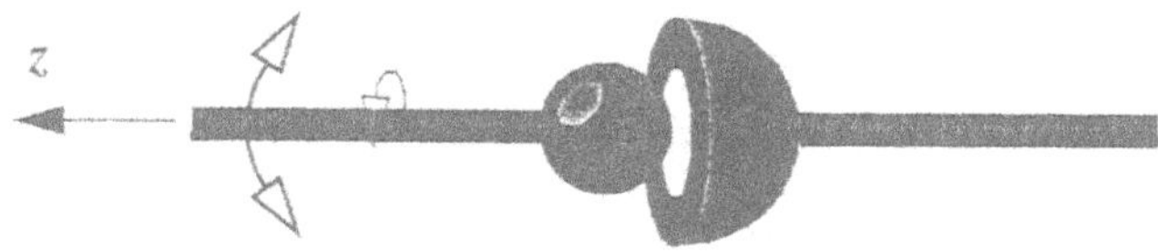

Figure 2. Mechanical illustration of a ball-and-socket joint.

2.1 Parametrization of rotations

The motion space of a ball-and-socket joint is the set of 3D rotations. There are many well-known parametrizations of rotations, such as: the *Euler angles* (the angles of three successive rotations about main axes), the *unit quaternion* (also known as the *Euler parameters*), the *axis-angle* vector (also known as the *exponential map*).

Good comparisons of such parametrizations for the purposes of animation of articulated bodies can be found in [4] and [11]. As noted by [4], no single parametrization of rotations is best. Each one possesses its advantages and drawbacks, with respect to the intended application. Hence, it is likely that several parametrizations be used simultaneously, with conversions between them. For example, the unit quaternion is ideally suited for interpolation [11], while the axis-angle vector is more appropriate for differential control with inverse kinematics [4]. Euler angles would not be a good choice in both applications. Instead, they are a more intuitive set of parameters to manipulate a ball-and-socket joint in a graphical user interface.

An important point to consider when comparing two parametrizations is the presence of singularities. Singularities are locations in the parameter space that result in the same orientation of the joint. Sometimes these singularities are purely mathematical and only result from the choice of parametrization, but they may also reflect a physical reality. In that case, we encounter the problem known as gimbal lock [11, 4]. Because of the problems induced by the singularities not only at the singular point but also in their neighborhood, the configuration of a joint should always be kept as far as possible from these points.

It is well-known that any three-dimensional parametrization of rotations presents at least one singularity [8]. Those of the Euler angles are discussed in [4], and will be recalled later. The unit quaternion parametrization is singularity-free, but at the cost of requiring four parameters instead of three, and a quadratic constraint (unit norm) must then be ensured [4].

2.2 Parametrization for range of motion definition

For the purpose of defining a range of motion, an appropriate parametrization is needed. Certainly, one can impose limits on any parametrization. For example, it is possible to impose limits on Euler angles or on quaternion parameters. For example, Lee [6] describes simple analytical constraints (such as axial, spherical or conical constraints) enforced directly in quaternion space. More complex constraints can then be defined by combining the simple ones with boolean operators. While simple and elegant, this method is not precise enough for an accurate modelling of the limits of complex joints such as the shoulder, and placing more complex meaningful limits on quaternions is difficult.

To simplify the problem, the joint limits may be decoupled. For example, independent limits may be specified on each Euler angle, or on each element of the axis-angle. However, the resulting range of motion can hardly match real motion ranges with sufficient precision [7].

For the purpose of defining a range of motion, neither the axis-angle nor the unit quaternion reflect the intuitive decomposition of the rotation into a swing and a twist component. Euler angles do, since the third angle may be used to perform the twisting motion. However, in the following sections we see that the first two Euler angles can be replaced by an axis-angle vector with zero component along the z axis: this alleviates the problem of singularities that affects the Euler angles.

2.3 The swing and twist decomposition of an orientation

Intuitively, the orientation R of a ball-and-socket joint can be thought as being composed of a swing component, that controls the direction of the limb directly attached to it, and a twist component that lets the limb rotate about itself [5, 4]. This may be written as: $R=R^{twist}R^{swing}$

The twist component is easily parametrized by a single angle of rotation, noted τ: hence, $R^{twist}=R_z(\tau)$. However, this rotation must be done with respect to a well-defined orientation, here called the *zero twist reference orientation*. In fact, this reference orientation merely results from the swing rotation, and is not necessarily a good reference. Hence a relative twist, τ_{offset}, as a function of the swing parameters, can be added. An example of such an offset function is given by Badler [1].

The purpose of the swing motion is to orientate the outgoing limb in a prescribed direction given by a unit vector $\boldsymbol{d}$. To transform the $\mathbf{z}$ vector into the $\boldsymbol{d}$ vector, a rotation matrix R^{swing} must be defined. We consider two solutions.

The first is to perform two successive rotations, for instance one about the $\boldsymbol{x}$ axis and then a second one about the rotated $\boldsymbol{y}$ axis: $R^{swing}=R_y(\beta)R_x(\alpha)$. This is equivalent to the first two rotations of the ZYX Euler angles sequence [8] (Fig. 3).

The second is to perform a single, direct rotation: $R^{swing}=R_D(z,\boldsymbol{d})$ (Fig. 3). Note that the axis of rotation always lies in the $\boldsymbol{x}$-$\boldsymbol{y}$ plane. This solution has been used by Korein [5] and Grassia [4].

As already noted by Korein [5], the difference between the two solutions lies in the final twist about the $\boldsymbol{d}$ axis, which is given by the different orientations of the rotated $\boldsymbol{x}$ and $\boldsymbol{y}$ vectors. Table 1 shows a sampling of the zero twist on the sphere for the two parametrizations: the outgoing arrow at each point on the sphere indicates the direction of the rotated $\boldsymbol{x}$ axis, which is taken as a reference to indicate the twist.

As said before, the singularities of a parametrization must also be considered, because the presence of singularities may be problematic for several applications. For the purpose of defining a range of motion, the twist component is affected by a singularity of the swing component: for example, no zero twist may be defined at a singularity, since an infinity of twists are possible. An arbitrary twist may be assigned to this point, but there is still a discontinuity with respect to its neighborhood. Table 1 compares the position of the singularities on the sphere, and the next two sections discuss and compare these singularities.

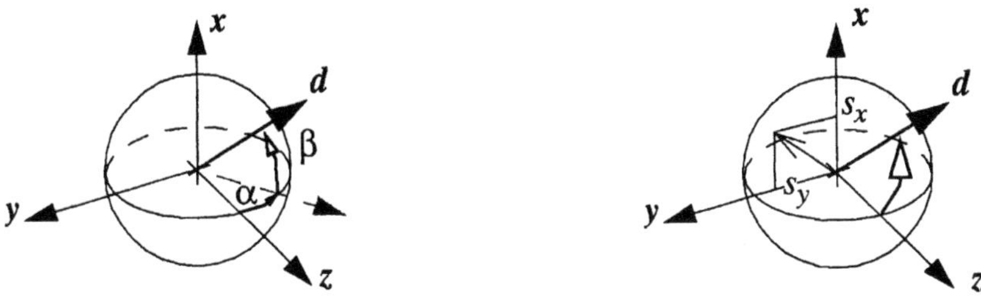

Figure 3. Euler angles parametrization (left) and axis-angle (right) of the swing motion.

2.4 Singularities of the XY Euler angles parametrization

This parametrization possesses two singularities: one at $\beta=\pi/2$ and another at $\beta=-\pi/2$. In Cartesian space, these singularities correspond to directions $d_1=[1\ 0\ 0]^T$ and $d_2=[-1\ 0\ 0]^T$ respectively, and any twist is possible there. Furthermore, moving close to these directions results in wild variations of twist. For example, moving along a closed path close to, and around the singularity, results in a complete rotation of the segment about itself (i.e. a twist of 2π radians).

To understand the meaning of the singularities, consider a universal joint, made as a sequence of two revolute joints whose axes of rotation are orthogonal, as shown in Fig. 4. A rotation about the $\boldsymbol{x}$ axis or the $\boldsymbol{y}$ axis changes the direction of the outgoing segment, and apparently no twisting is performed. However, this is not always true. When $\beta=\pm\pi/2$, which is the angle of rotation about the $\boldsymbol{y}$ axis, the outgoing segment becomes aligned with the $\boldsymbol{x}$ axis (Fig. 5): as a consequence, a change in α does not change its direction anymore, but its twist. Actually, any twist is possible in this direction, but the segment cannot move up and down anymore. This phenomenon is known as *gimbal lock*, and is a well-known flaw of Euler angles [11]. Also note how the vertical swing component (along the $\boldsymbol{x}$ axis) gradually transforms into a twist of the outgoing limb, as the singular configuration is approached. This shows that the problem not only exists at the singularity, but also in its vicinity.

Table 1. Comparison of "zero" twist and singularities (**O**) for two parametrizations of swing.

View (axes)	Axis-angle parametrization of swing (one singularity)	Euler angles parametrization of swing (two singularities)
Front (x/y)	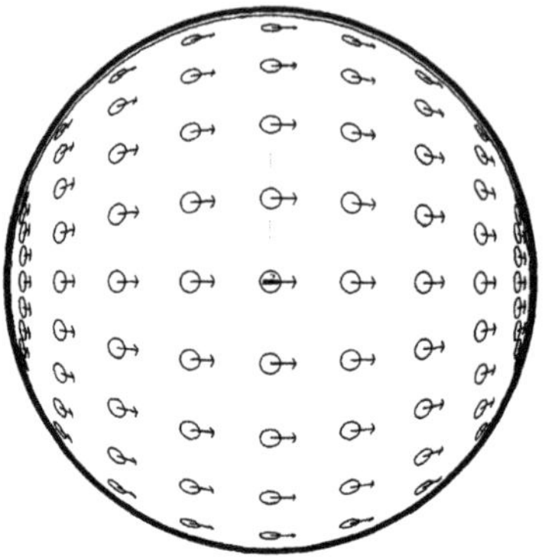	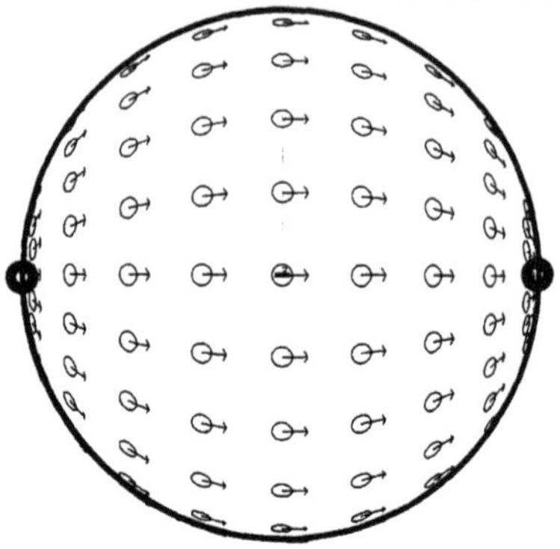
Side (z/y)	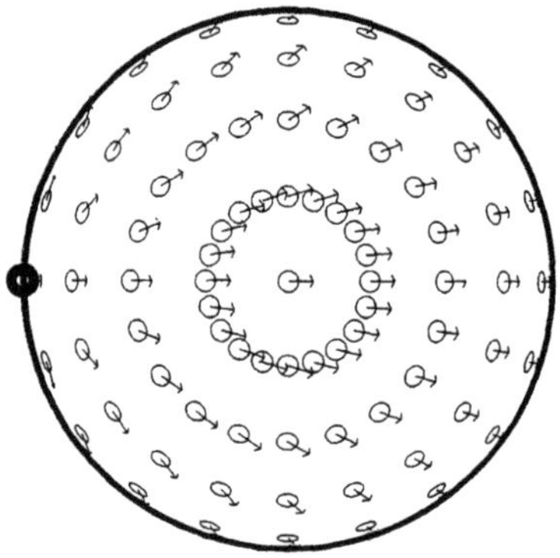	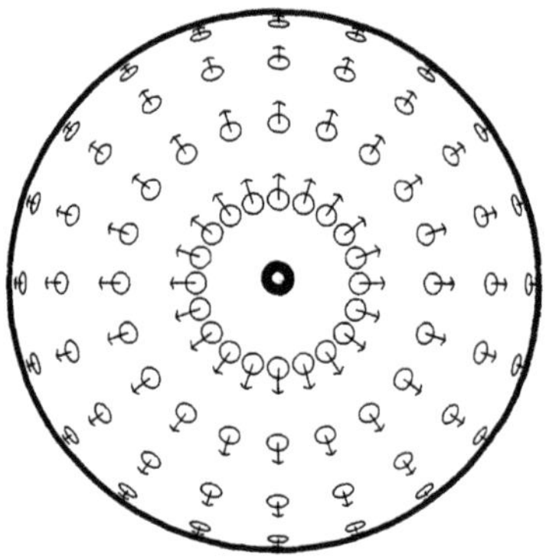
Rear ($-x/y$)	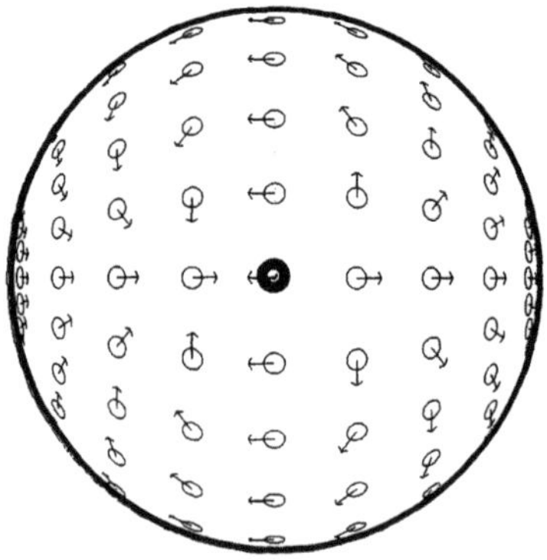	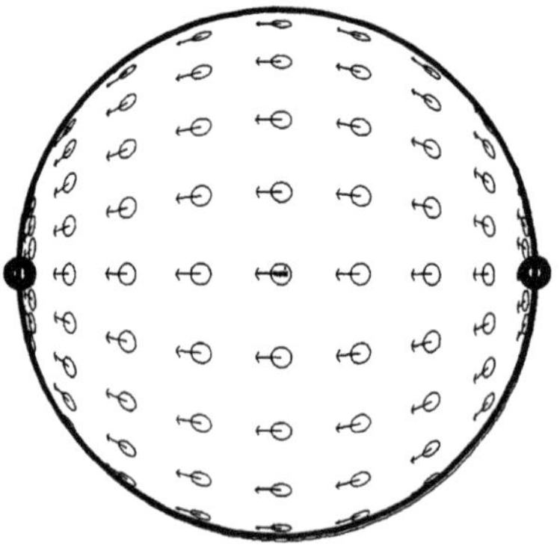

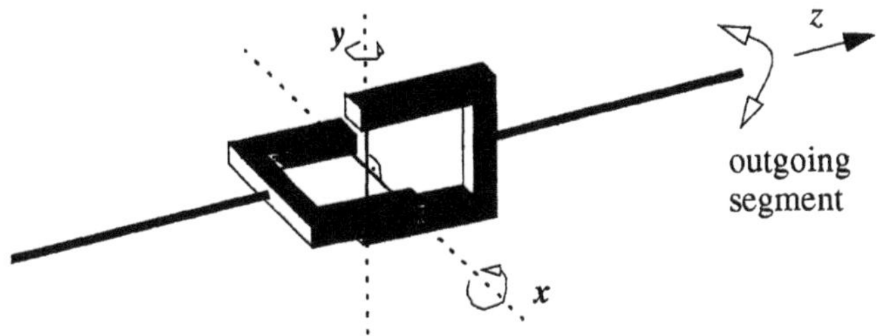

Figure 4. Illustration of the universal joint, with two orthogonal rotation axes.

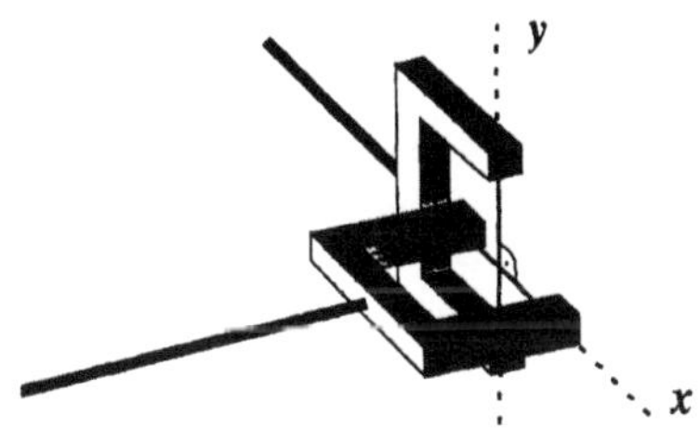

Figure 5. The universal joint in a singular configuration (β=π/2).

2.5 Singularity of the axis-angle swing paramatrization

The axis-angle possesses only one singularity on direction $\boldsymbol{d}=[0\ 0\ -1]^T$, where $s_x^2+s_y^2=\pi^2$. Again, any twist is possible there. However, this singularity is more "severe" since a closed path close to, and around the singularity, performs two complete rotations of the segment (i.e. a twist of 4π radians).

To summarize, the axis-angle parametrization is preferable to the Euler angles parametrization, since it is easier to avoid one single singular point than two antipodal singular points on the sphere. To stay as far as possible from the singularity, the motion range should be centered about the z axis in its "zero" configuration, or at least the singular point should not be part of the motion range.

3. THE DEFINITION OF JOINT LIMITS

Based on the swing and twist decomposition, independent limits can be imposed on both components. The limits of the swing component are best visualized as a curve on a sphere centered at the joint center. This curve delineates the valid region for the limb, and can be seen as the directrix of a general conical surface whose vertex is the center of the joint. In the following two sub-sections, we review two possible methods for defining this curve. The third section discusses the limits of the twist component.

3.1 Swing function : the spherical ellipse

An analytical method is to use a function $f(s_x,s_y)$ which is negative only for valid swings $[s_x\ s_y]^T$. A simple example given in [4] is an ellipse with semi-axes r_x and r_y, that describe the maximum angle of rotation around the x axis and the y axis respectively: in this case, the function is given by $f(s_x,s_y)=(s_x/r_x)^2+(s_y/r_y)^2-1$, with $r_x<\pi$ and $r_y<\pi$. This results in a "spherical" ellipse in the Cartesian space (see Fig. 6).

The advantage of the spherical ellipse is that, with a minimum of parameters, a meaningful boundary can be defined for the swing component.

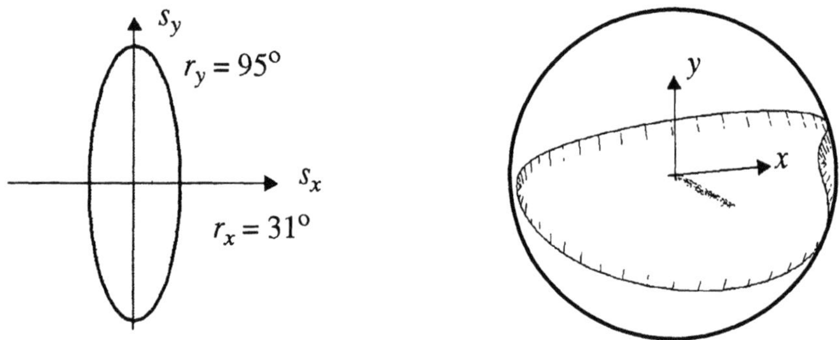

Figure 6. An example of spherical ellipse (the ticks indicate the inside region).

3.2 Spherical polygons

In his excellent book, Korein [5] uses a spherical polygon as directrix for the limiting cone. The edges of the spherical polygon are great arcs connecting its vertices lying on a unit sphere, and specified by three Cartesian coordinates. A great arc is the shortest path that binds two points on a sphere (it is a *geodesic*). The order of the vertices defines an inside region: inverting this order swaps the inside and outside regions of the polygon. Korein described an algorithm to test the inclusion of a point lying on the sphere within an arbitrary (possibly concave) spherical polygon.

Of course, spherical polygons are more general than spherical ellipses. They are also more complex to deal with. A similar method has been used by Maurel [7], but with planar polygons. As a consequence, the possible motion ranges are less general than those obtained with spherical polygons.

However they may suffice for the human joints, and the *point-in-planar-polygon* test algorithm is much simpler than its spherical counterpart.

3.3 Twist limits

The twist motion possesses a single degree of freedom, parametrized by the angle of rotation τ about the outgoing segment. The important point is that that limits are relative to the zero twist resulting from the swing motion.

In the following globographic representations, the twist range of motion is visualized as a circular arc: it indicates the orientations that can take the reference vector (which is the $\boldsymbol{x}$ basis vector of the joint frame).

4. AN EXAMPLE OF SHOULDER BOUNDARY WITH SWING AND TWIST COMPONENTS

Fig. 7 shows two boundaries for the shoulder complex, based on a spherical ellipse on the left and on a spherical polygon on the right. The distal segment (the arm) is shown in its default position. The twist limits are constant over the range of swing motion (the twist motion range is about 105°). However, in reality the twist limits depend on the position of the arm, and the range can vary between 104° and 160° on average [10]. The data for the spherical polygon, are obtained from the results of Engin [3].

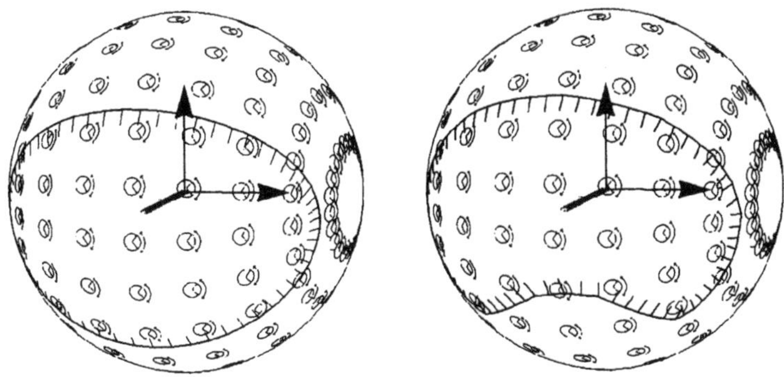

Figure 7. Shoulder motion range: spherical ellipse (left) and spherical polygon (right).

5. CONCLUSION

The swing-and-twist parametrization is a good basis for the definition of simple yet meaningful joint limits for ball-and-socket joints. This decomposition has been previously discussed by Korein and Grassia. In this paper, we have emphasized and illustrated the difference between the well-known Euler angles parametrization and the swing-and-twist parametrization.

We have reviewed and illustrated two methods to set joint limits on the swing and twist components. The spherical ellipse proposed by Grassia is a good compromise between simplicity and accuracy, while spherical polygons are more complex but can better match real limits.

ACKNOWLEDGEMENTS

Research supported by the Swiss National Foundation for Scientific Research, grant 20-53809.98.

REFERENCES

[1] N. Badler, J. O'Rourke and B. Kaufman, "*Special problems in human movement simulation*", Computer Graphics (SIGGRAPH 80), 14(3), pp. 189 - 197, 1980.

[2] N. Badler, C. Phillips, B. Webber, *Simulating Humans, Computer Graphics Animation and Control*, New York, Oxford University Press, 1993.

[3] A.E. Engin, S.T. Tuemer, "*Three-dimensional kinematic modelling of human shoulder complex - Part I: Physical model and determination of joint sinus cones*", Journal of Biomechanical Engineering, 111, pp. 107 - 112 , 1989.

[4] F.S. Grassia, "*Practical Parameterization of Rotations using the Exponential Map*", Journal of Graphics Tools, 3(3), pp. 29 - 48, 1998.

[5] J.U. Korein, "*A Geometric Investigation of Reach*", The MIT Press, Cambridge, 1985.

[6] J. Lee, *A Hierarchical Approach to Motion Analysis and Synthesis for Articulated Figures*, Ph.D. thesis, Department of Computer Science, KAIST, 2000.

[7] W. Maurel and D. Thalmann, "*Human Upper Limb Modeling including Scapulo-Thoracic Constraint and Joint Sinus Cones*", Computers & Graphics, 24(2), pp. 203 - 218 , 2000.

[8] R. Murray, Z. Li, S. Sastry, *A mathematical introduction to robotic manipulation*, CRC Press, 1994.

[9] X. Wang and J.-P. Verriest, "*A geometric algorithm to predict the arm reach posture for computer-aided ergonomic evaluation*", Journal of Visualization & Computer Animation, 9, pp. 33 - 47, 1998.

[10] X.G. Wang, F. Mazet, N. Maia, K. Voinot, J.P. Verriest and M. Fayet, "*Three-dimensional modelling of the motion range of axial rotation of the upper arm*", Journal of biomechanics, 31(10), pp. 899 - 908, 1998.

[11] A. Watt, M. Watt, *Advanced Animation and Rendering Techniques*, Addison-Wesley, ACM Press, 1992.

TOWARDS BEHAVIORAL CONSISTENCY IN ANIMATED AGENTS

Jan M. Allbeck and Norman I. Badler
University of Pennsylvania

Key words: animated agents, believability, communication, consistency

Abstract: We are seeking to outline a framework to create embodied agents with consistency both in terms of human actions and communications in general and individual humans in particular. Our goal is to drive this consistent behavior from internal or cognitive models of the agents.

1. INTRODUCTION

Consciously or not, people spend their entire lives observing other people. We have unconscious and cultural norms of human behavior and are more likely to notice the unexpected rather than the natural or expected. In the *embodied agent* research community, agent behaviors created with an attempt to conform to our nominal expectations are termed *believable*. Unfortunately, this term is awkward to define. *Believable* means "to accept as real." But *real* is itself a loaded term, as there are numerous aspects of real people that embodied agents do not or cannot portray. Usually, it is the character's *actions* and *communications* that ought to appear similar enough to those of real people that we accept the animation as having believable thoughts or emotions. If these conditions are satisfied we are capable of ignoring significant non-human variants in form, appearance, or structure. One only need look at the wide range of animated cartoon characters that communicate their presumed thoughts and feelings to see that reality in expression is the stronger determiner of believability (Thomas and Johnson 1981).

If actions and communications are the triggers for our understanding of animated characters, then these must be manifest on the character in human-like ways. For example, mechanical speech may destroy the believability of an otherwise accurately rendered character (unless we need to believe that it is a robot!); an awkward mechanical walk can distract us from seeing well-executed and subtle facial expressions. Herein lies the first major goal of this study. What we are seeking is an animated embodied agent with *consistency* both in terms of our expectations of human actions and communications in general and our expectations of individual humans in particular. The agent's behaviour must be consistent from moment to moment and from situation to situation. There should be no wild mood swings or complete loss of focus. Departures from consistency might be interpreted as dramatic effects or, more likely, as internal conflicts within the agent's own cognitive state. Normally, we should expect the cognitive state of the agent to be consistent with every level of its behavior: the expression on its face, the affect of its movements, the actions it performs, and the goals which it pursues. Also, cognitive state (and thus actions) must be consistent with the context or situation in which the agent finds itself.

Inconsistencies at any level can cause mixed messages and miscommunication. As Burgoon et al (1989) indicates, "When enacting multi-channel nonverbal presentations, common sense says that one should coordinate the channels to produce a consistent message." Sometimes mixed messages are deliberate as in the case of jokes and sarcasm. Other times, mixed messages are indicative of internal confusion (Burgoon et al 1989). There may, of course, be times when internal confusion is our intent, but it seems more prudent to first model unconfused internal states and demonstrate consistent communication. If the theory works, we should be able to portray inconsistent behaviours and have observers infer conflicted or unbelievable states within the agent.

Our second major goal is to drive this consistent behavior from internal or cognitive models of the agent. It is somewhat surprising that agent modellers have been so heavily influenced by Ekman and Friesen (1977) that they concentrate only on the basic facial expressions of happy, sad, anger, fear, and disgust and do not include internal reflective states such as determination, confusion, vacillation, and anxiety. Similarly, human gesture performance appears to reflect internal agent state in subtle but observable ways(Chi et al 2000). Only by representing the agent's internal cognitive state and thus the information, beliefs, desires, and intentions that motivate it, can we achieve consistent externalised actions.

In this paper, we will concentrate on nonverbal communication and the cognitive states or parameters that effect it. We will propose a parameterized agent model that creates consistent behaviors and allows controllability at different levels. We will describe the importance and interaction of the components and their manifestation in the channels of nonverbal communication.

2. MANIFESTATIONS OF NONVERBAL COMMUNICATION

Though verbal communication is the standard channel of communication used by people, nonverbal communication also contains valuable information. In fact, the information contained in nonverbal communication may be more valuable in some situations. In *Snow Crash* (Stephenson 1992), Neal Stephenson describes an international business meeting taking place in a virtual world:

> They come here [The Black Sun] to talk turkey with suits from around the world, and they consider it just as good as a face-to-face. They more or less ignore what is being said--a lot gets lost in the translation, after all. They pay attention to the facial expressions and body language of the people they are talking to. And that's how they know what's going on inside a person's head--by condensing fact from the vapor of nuance.

The internal or cognitive state of a person can manifest itself in all of the channels of nonverbal communication. According to (Lewis 1998) the channels of nonverbal communication are:

- facial expressions (smiles, nods)
- gestures (especially hand and arm movements)
- body movements
- posture
- visual orientation (especially eye contact)
- physical contacts (handshakes, patting)
- spatial behaviour (proximity, distance, positions)
- appearance (including clothes)

- non-verbal vocalizations

We will briefly describe each of these channels and some of the research that has been done in the embodied agents community.

2.1 Facial Expressions

Facial expressions are known to express emotion (Ekman and Friesen 1997), but facial expression can indicate what a person is thinking as well as feeling. The face reflects interpersonal attitudes, provides nonverbal feedback on the comments of others, opens and closes channels of communication, complements or qualifies verbal responses, and replaces speech (Knapp and Hall 1992).

Both Brand (1999) and Poggi and Pelachaud (2000) have researched ways of generating facial expressions for speech. Brand generates facial animation from information in an audio track. Poggi and Pelachaud concentrate on the visual display of intentions through facial animation based on semantic data. They model performatives, which are the type of action a sentence performs, such as requesting or informing. They also discuss how the degree of certainty, the power relationship, the type of social encounter, and the affective state effect the facial animation.

Cassell, Bickmore, Campbell, Vilhjalmsson, and Yan (2000) present a system which automatically generates and animates conversations between multiple agents. A dialogue planner creates the conversation and generates and synchronizes appropriate facial expressions, intonation, eye gaze, head motion, and arm gestures.

2.2 Gestures and Body Movements

Gestures are voluntary or involuntary movements that are intended to communicate. They may involve any part of the body. They are used to emphasize, clarify, or amplify a verbal message. They can also regulate or control a human interaction, or display affect (Lewis 1998).

By contrast body movements are not intended to convey information. Body movements include, walking, reaching, turning, bending, etc. The manner in which these actions are done can help convey the cognitive state of the performer. People can walk in dramatically different ways: fast, slow, straight, swerved, proudly, sadly, joyfully, etc.(Rose et. al 1998).

Gestural communication and body language have been studied by several groups, e.g., Morawetz and Calvert (1990), Kurlander, Skelly, and Salesin(1996). The EMOTE tool of Chi, Costa, Zhao, and Badler (2000) controls the expressive shape and effort characteristics of gestures. Amaya, Bruderlin, and Calvert (1996) studied the expression of emotion on the body.

2.3 Postures

Posture is an indicator of the degree of involvement, the degree of status relative to the other participants, or the degree of liking for the other interactants. A forward leaning posture, for example, can indicate higher involvement, more liking, and lower status in situations where the participants do not know each other very well. Posture is also a key indicator of the intensity of some emotional states. A drooping posture is associated with sadness and a rigid, tense posture is associated with anger. The extend to which the communicators reflect each other's posture may also be an indication of rapport or an attempt to build rapport (Knapp and Hall 1992).

Becheiraz and Thalmann (1996) present a model of nonverbal communication where agents react to one another in a virtual environment based on their postures. Relationships between the agents evolve based on the perceptions of postures.

2.4 Visual Orientation

What a person pays attention to and how much attention they pay is another channel of communication. A person's gaze and even the dilation and constriction or their pupils can be an indicator of interest, attention, or involvement (Knapp and Hall 1992).

Johnson and Rickel (1997) present an animated pedagogical agent, which uses both gestures and attention to aid in the instruction of manual tasks. Vilhjalmsson and Cassell (1998) created an interface for chat room avatars that allows the user to give conversational cues through attention control. If a user sees an agent that he is talking to begin to look away from his avatar more and more, then this is probably an indication that the agent no longer wants to participate in the conversation.

2.5 Physical Contacts and Spatial Behaviour

Physical contacts may be self-focused or other-focused. Self-focused touching may reflect a person's cognitive state or a habit and include nervous mannerisms. There are many kinds of other-focused touching, including, irritating, condescending, comforting, and electric. The meaning of a touch behavior is often derived more from its context and manner than from its configuration.

Spatial behaviour refers to social and personal space. Spatial behaviour can vary based on many aspects of individuals including, age, gender, status, roles, culture, personality and context. Studies show that conversational distance is related to general comfort level (Sommer 1961).

Physical contacts and spatial behaviors are types of behaviors that animation artists do well, but embodied agents researchers do not focus on. In order to create consistent communication these two channels of communication will have to be coordinated with the other channels.

2.6 Appearance

Among other things, appearance can provide information about, behaviour, values and attitudes, and occupation. An immaculate appearance can indicate that a person pays attention to details. Wearing hiking boots can indicate that the person likes the outdoors. An old-fashioned appearance sometimes indicates old-fashioned values, and excessive jewellery can indicate materialism. Wearing attire that is functional and protective can indicate a blue collar job, whereas white collar workers wear more formal clothing (Lewis 1998).

There are many companies and research laboratories, including Blaxxun Interactive and MIRALab, working on modelling virtual human bodies, skin, hair, and clothing.

2.7 Nonverbal vocalizations

Nonverbal vocalizations are vocal sounds other than words. This includes tone of voice which is known to convey emotional information (Argyle

1992). For example, depressed people speak in a low, slow voice, with falling pitch.

The Sims is a good example of the use of nonverbal vocalizations in embodied agents. In this game, the characters live their daily lives including, participating in polite conversations and angry discussions, but the characters have no discernible spoken language. The game's characters communicate through gestures, thought-bubbles, and nonverbal vocalizations. In the game, it is easy to distinguish a polite conversation from an heated argument by the volume and frequency of the nonverbal vocalizations.

3. AGENT COGNITIVE MODEL

In order to create an agent whose cognitive state is reflected in these channels of communication and therefore create consistent communication and behavior, we need to examine what cognitive processes effect the channels of communication. Books concerning nonverbal communication(Knapp and Hall 1992, Lewis 1998, and Burgoon et al 1989) often talk about the effects of the following cognitive processes on communication: age, status, gender, culture, role, context, emotion, mood, and personality.

3.1 Age and Status

In any interpersonal situation, one person's status is always at least a little above or below the other person's (Johnstone 1979), and age is often a component of status. Age and status are reflected in many different communication channels. In order to present consistent agent behavior, these channels should all indicate the same age and status cognitive states.

For example, gestures change and become more subtle with age(Lewis 1998). Young children immediately cover their mouths when lying to an elder. Teenagers also bring a hand to their mouth, but they do so more slowly and just rub the fingers around the mouth. Adults telling spontaneously lies sometimes also bring their hand toward the mouth, but often then rub their nose instead. Status tends to effect the frequency of gesturing. People of higher status seem to gesture less frequently (Lewis 1998).

Interpersonal distance also changes with age. Distance seems to increase with age, but is always closer with peers than with those that are younger or older (Burgess 1983). Physical contacts change with age and status. For example, older people are more likely to touch younger people than vice versa (Henley 1973). This is probably a factor of both status and age.

Status effects visual orientation. People of more dominance are more likely to engage in unwavering, direct looks and to break eye contact last. Looking away, however, increases your status, but only if you do not look back right away. In other words, ignoring someone can increase your status. People tend to lower their eyes to show deference to authority figures, and submission is often marked by raised eyebrows, which connote deference and possibly appeasement (Burgoon et al 1989).

Postures, spatial behavior, and body movements are also effected by status. Proper posture signals dominance. High status people are more confident and therefore comfortable in their space. They will allow their space to flow into other people's. Low status people will adjust their posture or position to avoid the flow. Minimal head movement signals dominance, as does smooth movements. Nonverbal vocalizations are also effected by status. A short "er" at the beginning of a sentence is weak, but a long "er" is strong (Knapp and Hall 1992).

The agents research community has, to some extend, modeled status. Hayes-Roth, van Gant, and Huber (1996) have explored the use of status with embodied agents in the form of a master-slave relationship. They illustrate how the postures and actions of the characters change as the servant becomes the dominant character in the environment and then returns to his submissive role. Poggi and Pelachaud (2000) model status through facial expressions called performatives, which are facial expressions that accompany and add interpersonal relationship information to speech. Musse and Thalmann (1997) included dominance in their crowd simulations.

3.2 Gender

Physical appearance is an obvious channel to communicate gender, but gender should also be consistent with the other channels of communications. For instance, pairs of women tend to engage in more eye contact than pairs of men (Exline 1963). Burgoon et al (1989) discusses many gender differences that effect the channels of nonverbal communication, including: postures in which males tend have more dominant, less affiliative, and less intimate postures than woman, and spatial behavior in which in small groups and interpersonal interactions, women require less personal space than men.

Though both men and women have been modeled in virtual environments, we currently know of no implementation that models gender as a component of the cognitive state of the agents.

3.3 Culture

It is said that cultural information is a minimum prerequisite for human interaction--in the absence of such information communication becomes a trial and error process (Knapp and Hall 1992). Cultural differences in communication can be extensive and do not only include the language spoken. First, different cultures have different distances for interacting. In some cultures standing close and directly in front of a person while speaking is considered either an intimate or a hostile act. In other cultures, not standing close and directly facing a person would be considered rude. There are also different touching behaviors, gestures, and eye gaze patterns (Knapp and Hall 1992).

It is also well known that there are some similarities across cultures. Studies have shown that the six basic facial expressions can be distinguished across cultures (Ekman et al 1969). Also, some behaviours have cross-cultural similarities, e.g. coyness, flirting, embarrassment, open-handed greetings, and a lowered posture for showing submission (Eibl-Eibesfeldt 1972).

While culture is a very important component of human behavior and communication, it has been neglected as a focus for the embodied agents research community, perhaps due to its complexity.

3.4 Role

Every character in a virtual environment should have a role that it is playing, whether it is a professor of astrophysics, a tour guide, or just a man walking down the street. Roles involve expectations, both from the individual playing the role and from those interacting with the individual playing the role. In order for a character in a virtual environment to be consistent, it must meet the expectations of the role it is playing.

Roles are learned, generalized guidelines for behavior. Among other things, a role can stem from an individual's occupation, kinship, age, sex, prestige, wealth, or associational grouping. In a situation, one participant normally establishes his or her role and the other participant(s) must either go along or counter with a different role definition. There must be an agreement on the roles in order to effectively interact. Otherwise, communication will break down (Danziger 1976).

Roles influences many of the channels of nonverbal communication. Take for example the roles of doctor and mechanic. We have certain expectations about these roles. The appearance of a doctor is expected be clean and neat, while a mechanic may be very messy. We would also expect the interpersonal distance with a doctor to be smaller and the physical contacts more frequent (when comforting as well as examining). Confusion and alarm might result from a mechanic standing too close or touching too often (even if try to comfort someone after showing them the bill).

Isbister and Hayes-Roth (1998) have explored roles in relation to intelligent interface agents. They found that making the role of an interface agent clear helps to constrain the actions users will take in their corresponding roles.

3.5 Context

People all perceive situations differently, and form different mental representations of the environment, people, and actions of a situation. This implies that their behavior is predicated on their knowledge and understanding of the situation. An embodied agent's behaviour should be consistent with the current context (or its perception of it). We would not expect the same behavior in an opera-house as a football stadium.

The problem is that context is a difficult thing to represent. Not only must we take into account all of the people and objects in the environment, and the embodied agent's feelings about them, and all of the action taking place in the environment, and the feelings about the actions, and feelings about past events, and the overall feeling of the environment, but we must then decide what the significance of all of these factors are.

Although context is an important feature for agents in virtual environments, it has not been heavily researched by the community. It requires attention, synthetic vision, a representation of the situation, and a way to determine what is important in the situation based on the agent's current cognitive state.

Once the environment has been perceived and the situation represented, the context can be used to create behaviour which is contextually consistent.

3.6 Emotion and Mood

Emotions and mood effect many of the channels of nonverbal communication. The effect of emotions on facial expressions is well-known and well-studied (Ekman and Friesen 1977), but other channels are effected as well. Lewis (1998) indicates that tense moods cause postures that are rigid and upright, or slightly leaning forward. Extreme inhibition tends to cause withdrawal movements and general motor unrest. When depressed, movements are slower, fewer, and hesitating. By contrast, elation causes fast, expansive, emphatic, spontaneous movements.

The embodied agents research community has studied emotion and mood more than any of the other cognitive processes (EBAA 1999, Cassell et al 2000).

3.7 Personality

Personality is a pattern of behavioral, temperamental, emotional, and mental traits for an individual. There is still a lot of controversy in personality research over how many personality traits there are, but the OCEAN model by is popular(Wiggins 1996). See Table1.

Table 1. OCEAN Model of Personality

	High Score Traits	**Low Score Traits**
Openness	Creative, Curious, Complex	Conventional, Narrow interests, Uncreative
Conscientiousness	Reliable, Well-organized, Self-disciplined, Careful	Disorganized, Undependable, Negligent
Extraversion	Sociable, Friendly, Fun-loving, Talkative	Introverted, Reserved, Inhibited, Quiet
Agreeableness	Good-natured, Sympathetic, Forgiving, Courteous	Critical, Rude, Harsh, Callous
Neuroticism	Nervous, High-strung, Insecure, Worrying	Calm, Relaxed, Secure, Hardy

Like the other cognitive processes described, the modeling of personality may lead to more consistent communication, and because personality is a pattern of behavior (longer temporal extent) it should lead to more consistent behaviour from situation to situation. This may aid in observers of the character developing a sense of *knowing* the character. It may become an individual instead of just another computer character.

In spatial relations, introverts generally prefer greater interpersonal distances. Aggressive and violence-proned (not agreeable) individuals tend to need even greater interpersonal distances in order to feel comfortable. Introverts also tend to resist visual interaction. People who are more neurotic and introverted have more restrained and rigid behavior, and display more uncoordinated, random movements (Burgoon et al 1989).

Though often personality traits are confused with emotions in embodied agents research, there has been research done in embodied agents with personality (Trappl and Petta 1997).

3.8 Interaction of Cognitive Processes

These cognitive processes can influence and even conflict with one another. An extremely introverted person, for example, is unlikely to express anger in the same way as an extroverted person. An agreeable person is less likely to feel anger or to feel it as intensely as a disagreeable person. Perhaps personality also influences the types of roles a person performs. Would we want an unconscientious, neurotic person as a doctor? An introverted person who is forced into a public role would feel uncomfortable. Only by representing the agent's internal cognitive state, can we hope to depict such interactions and contradictions that result in anxiety, vacillation, or confusion.

3.9 Individuals

What is important to people, what they value, and what they desire are important aspects of their individuality. at any moment a person's actions are motivated by their goals and the interactions and conflicts of their goals. In order to achieve consistent external actions for embodied agents, we also need to model their goals and the processes involved in planning for goals and resolving conflicts between goals. AI research has studied many aspects of planning and conflict resolution in planning (Russell and Norvig 1995), but what is move important for consistent communication is the manifestation of these processes in the channels of nonverbal communication. Imagine a young child whose mother asks if he pulled up all of her newly-planted flowers. The child values being honest with his mother, but he also values the dessert which will be taken away as punishment. He will express confusion and anxiety as he decides what to do. The manifestations of his cognitive processes will communicate valuable information to his mother.

A person's goals and their other cognitive processes are related. Age influences an individual's perceptions, actions, decisions. Dominant individuals tend to claim scarce and desirable resources. In our society, males are traditionally thought of as more task oriented, while females are considered more interpersonal oriented. Culture helps in determining the importance and immediacy of the activities of life. Roles can be defined by what goals are valued while the person is performing the roles, and personality can be defined by what goals are valued and how those goals are achieved through time.

4. CONCLUSION

We are seeking an animated embodied agent with consistency both in terms of our expectations of human actions and communications in general and our expectations of individual humans in particular. We believe that modelling the cognitive processes of embodied agents is a step in this direction, and will facilitate the communication of internal reflective states such as determination, confusion, and anxiety.

We have discussed the type of cognitive processes an embodied agent should have in order to create consistent communication. We must also address how to create and control these cognitive processes. Ideally our model will provide varying levels of control. There are times when a virtual environment create wants to specify every detail of the characters behavior, and there are other times when he or she wants autonomous characters. We envision a system where a user sets only the parameters that they are interested in, and the system sets the rest. For example, if a user only desires to create a character who is close-minded, unconscientious, extroverted, disagreeable, and neurotic, then the system would set the other parameters based on these personality traits. This character, for example, might tend toward anger. If the roles in the system included nun and boxer, boxer would probably be chosen. The user could always go back and fix settings that were undesirable.

This paper has focused on nonverbal communication, but these channels of communication would have to be coordinated with verbal communication including vocabulary, tone of voice, and intonation.

5. REFERENCES

Amaya, K., A. Bruderlin and T. Calvert. Emotion from Motion. *Proceedings of Graphics Interface '96*, pages 222-229.

Argyle, M. *The Social Psychology of Everyday Life*, London: Routledge, 1992.

Badler, N. and M. Costa and L. Zhao and D. Chi. To gesture or not to gesture: What is the question? *Proceedings of Computer Graphics International*; 2000, pages 3-9.

Becheiraz, P. and D. Thalmann. A Model of Nonverbal Communication and Interpersonal Relationship Between Virtual Actors. *Proceedings of Computer Animation '96*, pages 58-67.

Blaxxun Interactive, http://www.blaxxun.com/.

Brand, M. Voice puppetry. *Proceedings of SIGGRAPH '99*, pages 21-28.

Burgess, J.W. Developmental trends in proxemic spacing behavior between surrounding companions and strangers in casual groups. *Journal of Nonverbal Behavior*, 7: 158-169, 1983.

Burgoon, J.K., D.B. Buller and W.G. Woodall. *Nonverbal Communication, the unspoken dialogue*. New York: Harper and Row, 1989.

Cassell, J., T. Bickmore, L. Campbell, H. Vilhjalmsson and H. Yan. "Human Conversation as a system Framework: Designing Embodied Conversational Agents," In *Embodied Conversational Agents*. Cambridge, MA: The MIT Press, 2000.

Cassell, J., J. Sullivan, S. Prevost, and E. Churchill. *Embodied Conversational Agents*. Cambridge, MA: The MIT Press, 2000.

Chi, D., M. Costa, L. Zhao, and N. Badler. The EMOTE model for Effort and Shape. *Proceedings of SIGGRAPH '00.*

Danziger, K. *Interpersonal communication*. New York: Pergamon, 1976.

EBAA, Emotion-Based Agent Architectures Workshop of the Third International Conference on Autonomous Agent. May 1999. http://www.ai.mit.edu/people/jvelas/ebaa.html.

Eibl-Eibesfeldt, I. "Similarities and differences between cultures in expressive movements," In *Non-verbal communication*. Cambridge University Press, 1972.

Ekman, P. and W.V. Friesen. *Manual for the Facial Action Coding System*. Palo Alto: Consulting Psychologists Press, 1977.

Ekman, P., E. R. Sorenson, and W. V. Friesen. Pan-cultural elements in facial displays of emotions. *Science*, 164: 86-88, 1969.

Exline, R. V. Explorations in the process of person perception: Visual interaction in relation to competition, sex, and the need for affliation. *Journal of Personality*, 31: 1-20, 1963.

Hayes-Roth, B., R. Van Gent and D. Huber. *Acting in Character*. Technical Report KSL-96-13, Knowledge Systems Laboratory, Stanford University, Stanford, CA, 1996.

Henley, N.M. Status and sex: Some Touching Observations. *Bulletin of the Psychonomic Society*, 2: 91-93, 1973.Johnson, W.L and J. Rickel. An animated pedagogical agent for procedural training in virtual environments. *ACM SIGART Bulletin*, 8(1-4): 16-21, 1997.

Isbister, K. and B. Hayes-Roth. Social Implications of Using Synthetic Characters: An Examination of a Role-Specific Intelligent Agent. Technical Report KSL-98-01, Knowledge Systems Laboratory, Stanford University, Stanford, CA, 1998.

Johnstone, K. Status: *Impro: Improvisation and the Theatre*. New York, NY: Theatre Arts, 1979.

Knapp, M.L. and J.A. Hall. *Nonverbal Communication in Human Interaction.* Fort Worth, TX: Harcourt Brace Jovanovich College Publisher, 1992.

Kurlander, D., T. Skelly and D. Salesin. Comic chat. *Proceedings of SIGGRAPH '96*, pages 225-236.

Lewis, H. *Body Language, a guide for professionals.* New Delhi, India: Response Books, 1998.

MIRALab, http://miralabwww.unige.ch/.

Morawetz, C.L. and T. W. Calvert. Goal-Directed Human Animation of Multiple Movements. *Proceedings of Graphics Interface '90*, pages 60-67.

Musse, S.R. and D. Thalmann. A Model of Human Crowd Behavior: Group Inter-Relationship and Collision Detection Analysis. *Proceedings of Workshop of Computer Animation and Simulation of Eurographics '97.*

Poggi, I. and C. Pelachaud. "Performative facial expressions in animated faces." In *Embodied Conversational Agents.* Cambridge, MA: The MIT Press, 2000.

Rose, C., M. F. Cohen, and B. Bodenheimer. = Verbs and Adverbs: multidimensional motion interpolation using radial basis functions. IEEE Computer Graphics and Applications, 18(5): 32-40, 1998.

Russell, S. and P. Norvig. Artificial Intelligence: A Modern Approach. Englewood Cliffs, NJ: Prentice Hall, 1995.

Sommer, R. Leadership and group geography. *Sociometry*, 28: 99-110, 1961.

Stephenson, N. *Snow Crash.* New York: Bantam Books, 1992.

The Sims, http://www.thesims.com/.

Thomas, F. and O. Johnson. *The Illusion of Life.* New York: Abbeville Press, 1981

Trappl, R. and P. Petta. *Creating personalities for synthetic actors: Towards autonomous personality agents.* Berlin, Germany: Springer Verlag, 1997.

Vilhjalmsson, H.H. and Cassell, J. BodyChat: Autonomous Communicative Behaviors in Avatars. *Proceedings of Autonomous Agents '98*, pages 269-276.

Wiggins, J.S. *The Five-Factor Model of Personality: Theoretical Perspectives.* New York: The Guilford Press, 1996.

PECS
A Reference Model for Human-Like Agents

Christoph Urban
University of Passau
Chair for Operations Research and System Theory
94032 Passau, Germany
email: urban@fmi.uni-passau.de

Key words: autonomous human-like agents, agent architectures, agent-based simulation

Abstract: In recent years autonomous agents have significantly gained in importance for the modelling of human behaviour. With this development a need for adequate design methodologies for complex agents emerges which are capable of modelling essential characteristics of human beings in connection with their decision making and behaviour control. In this article the *PECS* reference model for the construction of human-like agents is introduced which enables an integrative modelling of physical, emotional, cognitive and social influences within a component-oriented agent architecture. Furthermore the case study *Adam* is introduced which demonstrates the practical application of the design methodology. Also a perspective should be drawn on how the reference model could be used for the control of virtual humans.

1. INTRODUCTION

In recent years agents play a vital role for modelling and simulation in empirical sciences. Parts of real systems or systems as a whole are modelled on the basis of autonomous agents. Agents are especially useful as a modelling paradigm when creatures or even human beings are part of the system to be examined. Agents act as virtual representatives of real world entities here. A very prominent example in which agents are used to construct an artificial social system is given by the *Sugarscape* experiments conducted by Epstein and Axtell (1996). Further examples for the application of agent technology in the social sciences, psychology, economics, ecology or other related areas can easily and numerously be found in literature (see e.g. Sichman, Conte & Gilbert, 1998; Urban, 2000a; Suleiman, Troitzsch & Gilbert, 2000).

In contrast to the application of agent technology to technical domains the structure, the properties and the behaviour of agents must not be selected freely when they are used in the context of modelling. In fact it is a basic requirement for good models to display structural and behavioural similarity with the original system. For the design of agents this means, that they have to be constructed in a way, which makes them quite similar to their real counterparts with respect to their structure and behaviour. When an agent is used for modelling a human being for example, the agent has to be equipped with all properties and behavioural patterns of the real human which are of relevance in the given scenario.

Looking at agent-based models of social systems in the literature one can find that human behaviour is often reduced to cognitive abilities and cognitively controlled actions. Human beings are often seen as pure rational decision makers. But recently these "classical" approaches which are often based on BDI architectures (Rao & Georgeff, 1995) are criticised more and more. The view of human beings as rational decision makers who are perfectly informed and maximise an exogenously given utility function seems to be too restrictive. At the same time in psychology more complex theories about human behaviour come into the foreground. Such theories, as e. g. introduced by Dörner (1999), are not restricted to cognitive aspects, but also take physical or emotional influences as well as interactions with the social environment into account.

With the increasing complexity of models for human beings the demands made on the design methodology for agent-based simulation models rise, too. There is a need for agents which are capable of modelling quite complex internal states as well as interactions between physical and psychical processes. The *PECS* (Physis, Emotion, Cognition, Social Status) reference model which will be introduced in the following chapters provides concepts for the construction of such human-like agents. In the second part of this paper a case study is described which shows the practical application of the reference model in the context of a psychological problem.

2. THE *PECS* REFERENCE MODEL

The *PECS* reference model is intended to support the design process of agent-based simulation models in which individual human behaviour and decision making, interactions between individuals as well as interactions of individuals with their environment are in the centre of interest. Therefore the reference model provides a concept for the construction of agents, a communication infrastructure and an environment component. The reference model provides a domain independent model architecture. It proposes a general, methodologically founded construction scheme which can be applied to various application areas and therefore must be filled with specific attributes and dynamic behaviour.

In the following sections the basic ideas of the reference model and the agent architecture will be discussed in further detail.

2.1 Basic Ideas of the *PECS* Reference Model

In order to reach a high degree of comfort in model description and a clear structure of resulting models, *PECS* is designed according to two major design principles.

The first principle relates to the structuring of models and is called *component-oriented, hierarchical modelling* (Urban, 2000b). According to this principle it is possible to functionally decompose complex models into a set of smaller model components. Each model component is responsible for modelling a special part of the required functionality and may be connected to other model components. By connecting components to each other it is possible to generate more complex components on a higher level of abstraction. Following this principle leads to clearly structured and well understandable models.

The second principle concerns the description of attributes and model behaviour. *PECS* follows a *system-theoretic approach* (Urban, 2000b) here. Every component is characterised by an internal state *Z* which is defined by the current values for the given set of model quantities at each calculated point in time. This internal state may be influenced by a time-dependent input and also an output may be produced according to the given dynamic behaviour. For the dynamic behaviour of a model component time-continuous as well as time-discrete state transitions may be specified. This system-theoretic approach leads to a comfortable handling of complex internal states and state transitions and is therefore especially useful for the description of agents which are strongly influenced by complex internal processes.

2.2 The *PECS* Agent Architecture

The *PECS* agent architecture grounds on the opinion that an agent must be capable of integrating physical, emotional, cognitive and social attributes and processes in order to provide an adequate means for modelling human behaviour. For that reason the *PECS* agent architecture is structured as shown in Fig. 1.

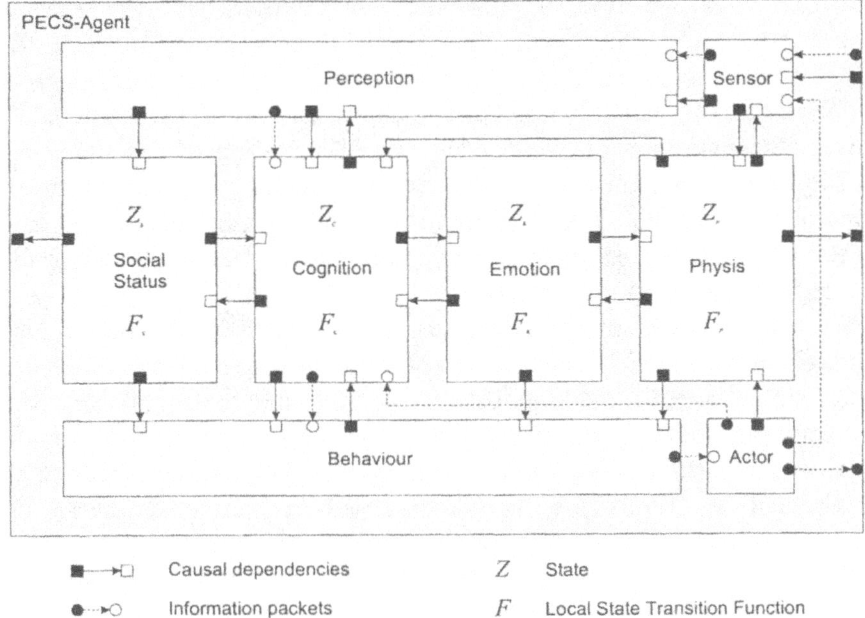

Figure 1: Basic Architecture of *PECS* Agents

The architecture may be divided up into three different horizontal layers. The input layer consists of the components *Sensor* and *Perception* and is responsible for the processing of input data coming from the environment of the agent. The internal layer is composed by the components *Physis*, *Emotion*, *Cognition* and *Social Status*. This group of components models the internal state of the agent. And finally in the output layer, covering the components *Behaviour* and *Actor*, the behaviour of the agent is calculated and the actions are executed.

The *Sensor* component receives sensory input from the environment of the agent. The incoming information may be divided into visual information and audible information. The visual information is about current processes going on in the environment of the agent and the audible information packets cover messages produced by other agents or also by the environment.

The sensory input received in the *Sensor* component is forwarded to the *Perception* component for further processing. In the *Perception* component for example information filtering mechanisms or other perceptional processes my be realised. In general percepts are generated in this component which contain information about the external world of the agent. In subsequent stages of information processing these percepts may be used for updating the mental model of the agent about its environment or for learning purposes.

The internal state of the agent may in general be composed of physical, emotional, cognitive and social attributes and processes. In order to achieve a clear structure of the agent architecture, these different attributes and processes are distributed to the four components *Physis*, *Emotion*, *Cognition* and *Social Status*. Nevertheless there could be various kinds of interactions between these components which can be modelled by causal dependencies.

The *Physis* component is responsible for modelling physical or material properties of agents. These properties could be influenced either by vegetative processes like ageing or by actions performed by the agent itself or even by the actions of other agents.

As emotions are considered as strongly relevant for the behaviour of human beings the *PECS* agent architecture provides a component *Emotion* which is able to model emotional states and processes of agents. Concerning the triggering of emotions we currently prefer cognitively oriented emotion theories (see e.g. Plutchik, 1993) which assume that emotions emerge as a consequence of information processing and cognitive appraisal. The consequences of emotions may be observed via the behaviour of an agent. Emotions can on the one hand modulate the behaviour of an agent and on the other hand even determine its behaviour.

The *Cognition* component models the knowledge base of the agent and related operations. In the centre of this component is a kind of memory which stores a mental representation of the agent's environment and of its own state. By incoming percepts this model may be extended and updated. Furthermore the mental representation provides information for the agent's decision making and planning. Deliberative agents are for example able to construct plans for their future behaviour based on their knowledge. Also learning processes may be modelled within this component which enable the agent to improve or adapt its behaviour in different situations. But not only the extension and elaboration of the knowledge base can be taken into consideration here. Also existing deficiencies like loss of information by forgetting may be modelled in the *Cognition* component.

An agent is in many cases embedded in a society and therefore a social entity. For that reason agents often have to be equipped with a set of attributes which describe their social properties. Such properties can for example be a social role of an agent in a given situation, the social status of an agent within a group or even social needs which direct the agent's behaviour. All these attributes and phenomena can be modelled within the *Social Status* component.

The repertoire of possible actions and the action selection processes are modelled in the components *Behaviour* and *Actor*. *PECS*-agents are able to display simple reactive behaviour which can be described by condition-state-action rules. But agents can also be equipped with more complex deliberative behaviour which includes planning processes and is based on goals the agent has in mind. Depending on a given goal which can be described by a certain state to be reached, a planning process is triggered. As a result of the planning process a plan is generated. Such a plan determines in an abstract way which activities have to be undertaken in order to reach the given goal. The *Behaviour* component selects the individual actions or even sequences of actions that are connected with the currently triggered activity. An action instruction is generated by the *Behaviour* component and handed over to the *Actor* component where finally the execution of the action is triggered. The *Actor* component accordingly stores the set of actions the agent is able to perform and realises the output interface of the agent.

As can be seen from the previous paragraphs, with the *PECS* reference model we intend to provide a model architecture which enables an integrative modelling of the various aspects and processes that essentially influence human decision making and behaviour.

3. THE CASE STUDY *ADAM*

In the following chapter the model *Adam* (see also Schmidt, 2000) will be introduced. This model is strongly influenced by Dörner's ? (1999). But in contrast to Dörner's approach which is intended to model psychological reality, the major goal of *Adam* is to demonstrate as simply as possible, how various control mechanisms for human behaviour can be integrated within the *PECS* architecture.

The chosen scenario is quite simple. We start with only one agent called *Adam*. Adam may be thought of as a prehistoric man at a very early stage of development – perhaps a member of the early *homo habilis* species which inhabited the savannah.

3.1 Adam's World

Adam lives and moves in a world consisting of a matrix with 12×12 fields. There are danger points, food sources and other fields with no special meaning in this world. Fig. 2 shows one possible configuration for Adam's world as an example.

A danger point is marked by a dark square. When Adam steps onto such a field, he gets into danger, looses a lot of energy and time, and becomes fearful for a certain period of time.

Adam's world also contains bright squares which provide the food that he needs to satisfy his energy requirements. As soon as Adam is hungry and reaches a food source, he will eat the food he finds there. Fortunately for Adam, the food grows again. The food regeneration is modelled by a logistical growth curve.

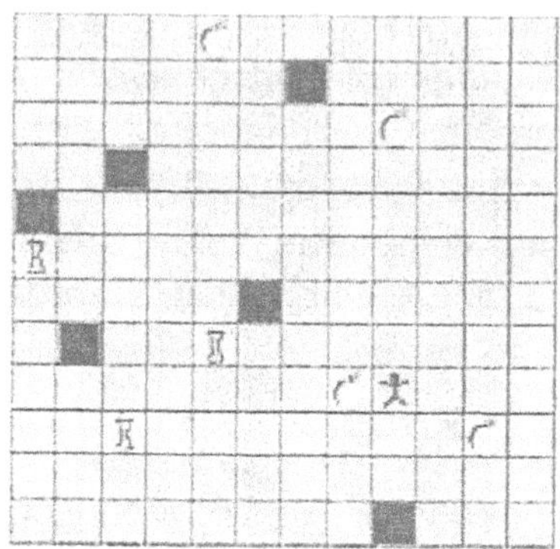

Figure 2: Adam's World

3.2 Adam's Internal State

Adam's internal state spans over physical, emotional and cognitive variables. Social attributes are not necessary as Adam lives alone in his world.

Adam's physical state is determined by his energy level. The state variable *energy* indicates how much energy Adam possesses and therefore how vital he still is. When Adam's energy has been used up, his life ends. Every action that Adam performs consumes a certain amount of energy. In order to replace lost energy, Adam must keep visiting food sources and intake food provided there.

The range of emotions accessible to Adam is for simplicity reasons very limited. His emotional state is described solely by the state variable *fear*. It will suddenly and abruptly reach a high level when Adam comes across a danger point. When Adam is in a fearful state, he will examine every new field for danger points before entering it.

The knowledge that Adam possesses of his environment and of himself is represented in the cognition component. For the description of this mental representation, state variables are used. There are two basic processes that influence the mental model essentially: *learning* and *forgetting*. By a learning process Adam gets more detailed knowledge about the growing behaviour of food sources. Forgetting reduces the knowledge of Adam, i. e.

he forgets information about fields he has not visited for a long period of time.

Independently of the mental representation two further variables *competence* and *level_of_knowledge* exist. *Level_of_knowledge* denotes the number of fields that Adam knows as opposed to the total number of fields in the environment. The *level_of_knowledge* variable triggers a knowledge acquisition motive. The state variable *competence* is intended to describe in the simplest possible form an element of self-awareness. In the present model, when Adam displays high competence he will choose riskier strategies in cases of uncertainty.

3.3 Adam's Repertoire of Actions

Adam is able to perform internal and external actions. Internal actions trigger processes that modify attributes and structures within the agent itself. They are delegated from the *Actor* component to another internal component of the *PECS* agent architecture. External actions are actions which are directed at the external world of the agent and produce changes in the environment.

The set of internal actions consists of the actions *planning*, *examination* and *exploration*.

Planning is an action that is delegated from the *Actor* component to the *Cognition* component. As the consequence of a *planning* action Adam devises a plan according to a given goal. The plan consists of partial goals which must be achieved one after another in order to achieve the final goal.

Examination is an action which activates the *Sensor* component and is related to a field that is part of Adam's environment but where Adam is not at present located. By means of examination Adam wishes to find out whether an adjacent field is a danger point to be avoided or whether he can enter it unimpeded. Adam examines only if he is in a state of fear.

The *Exploration* action also activates the *Sensor* component. Via this action Adam examines the field on which he is currently located.

The set of external actions consists of the actions *walking*, *food_intake* and *escaping*. All external actions are passed on by the *Actor* component to the *Environment* component where the resulting state transitions are executed.

The action *walking* enables Adam to move from one field to a neighbouring field in the environment. Using the action *food_intake* Adam is able to eat the food he finds on a food source in his environment. After Adam entered a danger point in his environment as a consequence of incautious behaviour he can use the action *escaping* for climbing out of the trap and freeing himself.

3.4 From States to Actions – Basic Principles of Adam's Behaviour Control

Looking at a scenario in which our agent Adam gets hungry and therefore has to seek for food, the basic elements of the behaviour control used in this case study should be illustrated in this section.

The entire behaviour of Adam is guided by *motives*. In general motives are activated in connection with certain *needs* and needs are immediately connected to *state variables*.

In our example the whole process starts with the internal state variable *energy* which is calculated in the *Physis* component. Depending on the actions Adam performs, his energy level goes up and down over time. The energy level is directly connected with a variable describing Adam's *need for food*. From his need for food a motive called *hunger* results. The intensity of the motive depends on the strength of the need. For modelling this relation, a logarithmic function as shown in Fig. 3 is assumed.

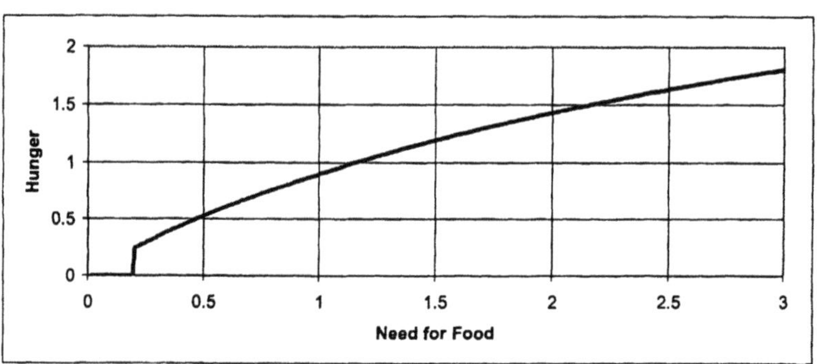

Figure 3: Intensity of the Motive *Hunger* in Relation to the *Need for Food*

On the next stage of behaviour control all existing motives struggle for the right to determine the actions of the agent and become so-called *action-guiding motives*. In our example besides the motive *hunger* there is a second motive called *knowledge acquisition*. It is derived from the wish and the conscious effort to discover more about the environment. For choosing an action-guiding motive the motive intensities are decisive. The motive with the highest intensity will be action-guiding. Fig. 4 shows the intensities of both given motives over time. One can see that Adam's behaviour will alternately be dominated by his need for food and by his thirst for knowledge.

For continuing this example let us assume that the motive *hunger* has been selected as the action-guiding one. In order to satisfy his need for food, Adam has to start a food search now. Let us further assume that Adam has information about the location of food sources stored in his mental representation (in any other case there is no other chance for Adam than starting a trial and error search in his environment). Then Adam locates the place on his mental map which is closest to his current position and provides some food. This place is declared as the goal of a sequence of actions that is to be planned now.

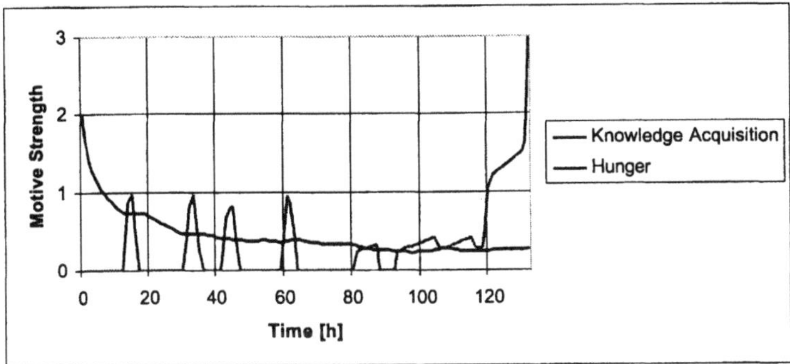

Figure 4: Temporal Sequence of Motive Intensities

An action plan is strategic in nature and consists of partial goals which have to be reached one after another in order to reach the superordinated goal. In the case of our example within the planning process a sequence of fields is calculated which leads our agent from his current position to the intended food location.

As soon as the action plan has been finished the first partial goal is released for execution. Therefore first of all the *Behaviour* component is activated. Within the *Behaviour* component a sequence of elemental actions is determined which depends on the overall internal state of the agent and which should lead to the fulfilment of the given partial goal. In case of a situation where Adam is very fearful such an action sequence could have the form *(examination – walking – exploration)*. In another case Adam may leave out the *examination* action and simply decide for *walking* and *exploration*.

As soon as the action sequence is fixed the first action is handed over to the *Actor* component which immediately starts with its execution. When the execution of this action is finished the subsequent action will be performed etc. In this way all actions of an action sequence must be executed successfully before the next partial goal of the action plan can be activated. This cyclic process ends when the last partial goal which equals the superordinated goal of the action plan has been reached. In this case a new plan must be conducted or a new motive may be selected as the guiding one and thus the whole process starts over again.

4. SUMMARY AND OUTLOOK

The *PECS* reference model provides an architectural pattern which can be used to construct agent-based simulation models in which human behaviour is of particular interest. Up to now, the reference model was exclusively used for modelling purposes. But looking at virtual human-like agents or avatars and new approaches in the context of human-computer interaction it seems to be worth spending some effort on the question if *PECS* could also be used as a basic architecture for designing control systems for virtual human-like agents.

One of many examples one could think of here could be found in the context of distance learning systems. Approaches in this area introduce so-called tutor agents for example which take over the role of human teachers. In order to make these agents more believable to the human user it could be useful to equip them with a control system that enables such agents to display human-like behaviour.

In this context the *PECS* agent architecture seems to provide a useful starting point for designing control systems of autonomous human-like agents and avatars. This question has to be discussed in further detail in the near future.

5. REFERENCES

Dörner, D. (1999). *Bauplan für eine Seele*. Reinbek bei Hamburg: Rowohlt.

Epstein, J. M., Axtell, R. (1996). *Growing Artificial Societies: Social Science from the Bottom Up*. Washington, DC: Brookings Institution Press.

Plutchik, R. (1993). Emotions and their vicissitudes: Emotions and their psychopathology. in: Lewis, M. & Haviland, J. M. (Eds.). *Handbook of Emotions*. New York: Guilford Press. 53-66.

Rao, A. S., Georgeff, M. P. (1995). BDI Agents: From Theory to Practice. in: *Proceedings of the First International Conference of Multi-Agent Systems (ICMAS)*, San Francisco.

Schmidt, B. (2000). *The Modelling of Human Behaviour*. Ghent: SCS European Publishing House.

Sichman, J., Conte, R. & Gilbert, N. (Eds.). (1998). *Multi-Agent Systems and Agent-Based Simulation*. Lecture Notes in Artificial Intelligence 1534. Berlin: Springer.

Suleiman, R., Troitzsch, K. G. & Gilbert, N. (2000). *Tools and Techniques for Social Science Simulation*. Heidelberg, New York: Physica-Verlag.

Urban, C. (Ed.) (2000a). *Workshop 2000 – Agent-Based Simulation*. Ghent: SCS European Publishing House.

Urban, C. (2000b). PECS - A Reference Model for the Simulation of Multi-Agent Systems. in: Suleiman, R., Troitzsch, K. G., Gilbert, G. N. (Eds.): *Tools and Techniques for Social Science Simulation*. Heidelberg, New York: Physica-Verlag. 83-114.

COMMUNICATIVE AUTONOMOUS AGENTS

Angela Caicedo, Jean-Sébastien Monzani and Daniel Thalmann
Computer Graphics Lab, Swiss Federal Institute of Technolog y (EPFL), CH 1015 Lausanne, Switzerland

Key words: Agent control, communicative virtual humans, trust.

Abstract: We present a way to mix the lower control of agents with the high level specifications of their goals. This paper addresses various topics required to animate virtual humans in a distributed way such as combining primary actions into tasks, using verbal communication between virtual humans and directing them with high level orders. Our models have been tested into a multi-languages / multi-modules application as described below.

1. INTRODUCTION

During the last years, the entertainment industry have produced a lot of exciting movies, games or TV shows involving realistic virtual humans. However, most of the work is hardly designed by artists and these impressing animations still require huge efforts. Furthermore, since movies are now integrating more and more virtual humans, there is a need for authoring tools specifically decicated to *autonomous* agents animation. This has been clearly demonstrated by the famous Improv system [17] or similar commercial tools, such as Motion Factory's Motivate [15] or Virtools' NeMo [19]. Efforts are continuously spent in order to obtain more and more realism: the use of speech, better animation, improved autonomy contribute to go toward life-like characters. Target applications do not only include the entertainment industry, but any inhabited virtual world might benefit from this kind of work. For example, we are now working on a simulator into which policemen have to deal with panic situations, with virtual humans running all around: this kind of training into a virtual environment is a good test for realistic autonomous agents.

Unfortunately, the animation of a virtual human is not an easy process: it actually involves various topics such as: motion control, action selection and verbal communication. Consequently, the *integration* of these domains altogether is a motivating technical challenge. The work presented by Bindiganavale *et al.* [2] is a good illustration of this goal. Our research is focusing on the same topic, that is the animation of autonomous virtual humans which are able to communicate verbally as we do. We are now going to briefly summarise the contributions and previous research for these domains.

From the animator's point of view, it is difficult for one agent to handle concurrent motions at the same time: how can one walk while carrying a box and looking around? If we are able to do this everyday, the simulation of simultaneous gestures and motions is a particular research subject. Models have been proposed to deal with that, such as Granieri's Parallel Transition Networks [10]. For the specific case of gestures involved in virtual humans conversation, Cassel *et al* [8] studied an automatic generation of movements and facial expressions (during conversation), based on the content of the dialog itself.

Regarding realistic verbal communication, we also need some sound propagation models. While Funkhouser, Min and Carlbom [9] introduced interesting algorithms for fast rendering of sound occlusion and diffraction effects, we think that simpler models simulating sound within a room and taking almost no CPU time have many useful applications in social simulations. A good example would be the simulation of a party, with many people speaking at the same time, and background music disturbing them. Our model is able to simulate such situations, without high computational cost.

Finally, an autonomous agent has to select its actions by itself. Research has been driven by people from different areas: ethologists such as Tinbergen [20], and computer scientists such as Brooks [6], Maes [13] and Minsky [14] who lead the school of Behaviour-Based Artificial Intelligence (BBAI). Our model, as proposed in the BBAI, does not attempt to build models of the world, and the agent has to reevaluate its course of action on every slot of time. Some points are not directly addressed by the BBAI such as the interplay between internal factors (emotional levels) and external factors (common world situations). Other authors such as Travers [21] have modelled a behavioural system where the agents are described in terms of *if-then* rules. However, we show in this paper that a simple predicate approach is not sufficient for modelling complex human behaviours based on different levels of emotions.

We are now going to present briefly our system and the various components embedded into it. We will continue with in section 3 with the *agent's brain*. Finally we describe in section 4 the agent's brain implementation in LISP, before concluding.

2. AGENT COMMON ENVIRONMENT

We have developed a system called: the *Agent Common Environment* (ACE) which animates virtual humans able to perceive their shared environment, perform different motions and have facial expressions. It also provides an easy way to plug-ins different behavioural modules.

ACE understands a set of different commands to be able to control the simulations: (i) Creation and location of 3D objects, virtual humans, and smart objects [12], (ii) Performance of different motion motors and facial expression: playing key-frames animation, using inverse kinematics [1], walking actions, etc. (iii) Virtual human interactions with smart objects. And (iv) Query of perception pipelines for a given virtual human [4].

All these commands are easily accessible from Python scripts, where different behavioural libraries can be created and plugged into ACE. Those scripts are basically ensuring the low level 3D animation of the virtual humans, while the high level decisions and behaviours are selected by the external Intelligent Virtual Agent behavioural module (see section 5). Thanks to the available packages coming with Python, one can manage easily concurrent processes with threads (such as, walking while looking at something), while a TCP/IP connection is maintained between the scripts and the Intelligent Virtual Agent. We are now going to describe the Agent Common Environment in details.

2.1 Agent design philosophy

The behaviour of agents is decomposed into two modules: the low-level animation and the high-level decisions taking. As many 3D environments, ACE is mainly coded in C++ to ensure high performances. For convenient user-interaction, it also provides the **Python layer** which interprets on the fly commands and animates the virtual humans. Python is an all-purposes scripting langage that we have extended to fit our needs. More precisely, when the application is launched, a simple environment is created and displayed in a window, and a command shell is prompted, ready for entering commands in Python. ACE provides the basic commands for loading, moving, animating humans and objects, giving a powerful set of functionalities straight from the scripting language. It is very convenient indeed to reuse a language and extend it to match our purposes, rather than developing a new syntax from scratch: this saves time and gives the opportunity to reuse third-party modules, which have been already implemented and tested by others. On the other hand, the **Intelligent Virtual Agent** (IVA) is in charge of making decisions, e.g. choosing the next action to take place, deciding what are the new goals of the agent, managing the dynamics of the agent's emotions during the simulation, and so on. Information is stored here in an abstract way, leaving the high to low level binding to the Python layer. For instance, to indicate a specific furniture in an office, we will specify it as *the chair next to the window* rather than x, y and z coordinates: this mapping is handled directly in Python. To conclude, the IVA can be consider as the agent's *brain*.

2.2 Multiple inheritance architecture

Running into ACE, the script for each agent should handle various capabilities, such as: perception, verbal communication, performing actions and connecting to the IVA behavioural module. Thus, we split each capability into one class and merged all of them into the definition of what an agent should be able to do. Using UML [3], we present in *Figure 1* the definition of the **Agent** class, as implemented in Python.

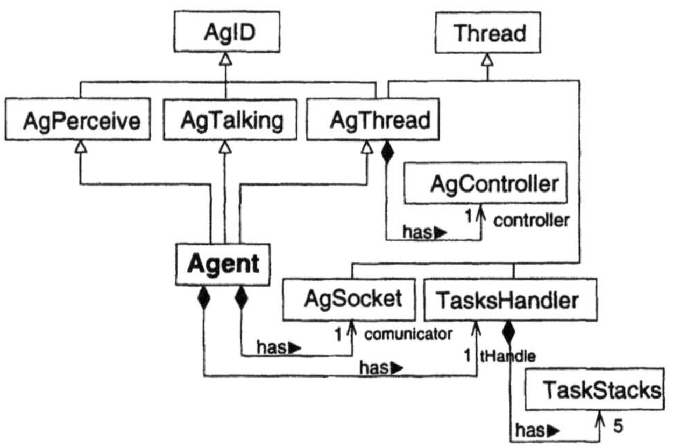

Figure 1. Multiple inheritance architecture defining one agent

Since each agent has a unique ID, we start by defining the AgID class as a super class, sharing the ID among the inherited classes. From this, we derive three basic classes, for the various capabilities, as pointed out before: the **AgPerceive** class encapsulates all the methods that allow the agent to visually perceive objects and remembers when objects get on/out of focus.

AgTalking lets the agent communicate by speaking to and hearing other agents. **AgThread** is the basic class for running one thread per agent, which means that each agent is running its own code in its thread (these functionalities are provided by the standard Thread class). Each thread is registered into an AgController which is then in charge of monitoring them. It also provides a shared space for exchanging information between the threads.

The final **Agent** class inherits from these three basic classes, which of course means that our **Agent** is able to speak to someone, hear when someone speaks and perceive the objects in the environment. But the **Agent** still needs to use some other modules: the **TasksHandler** which is in charge of handling parallel tasks like walking, looking, playing keyframes, applying facial expressions or interacting with objects and the **AgSocket**: each agent should be connected in some way to its IVA behavioural module and this is achieved by this class. The AgSocket class is able to decode orders coming for the IVA or send stimuli like visual perception back to the it. By using sockets and TCP/IP connection, the system can run in a distributed way, reducing the CPU cost on the machine which is responsible of the 3D environment display. The communication between the **Agent** object and the corresponding IVA is summarised in *Figure 2.*

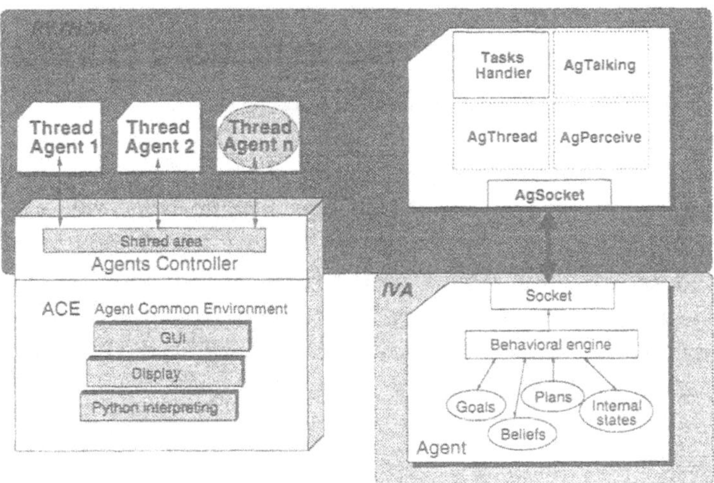

Figure 2. ACE system and connections to the Intelligent Virtual Agent (IVA)

2.3 The use of threads

One major improvement in adding the Python interpreter is the easy way of creating threads within it. Threads all run in parallel and efficient synchronisation primitives are available, such as events. This is a very convenient way to perform actions in parallel. Blocking actions such as waiting for data or event (for instance, a task to finish) could easily be handled by such threads. While it is very tempting to use threads to mimic human capabilities of performing various actions at the same time, one should take care of not creating too many threads (let's say, one per action), since it might take too much CPU time. That is why we are concerned in the next sections by simulating parallel behaviours within non-concurrent instructions too.

Our **Agent** has mainly three threads: the **Agent itself**, the **Tasks Handler**, and **the Agent Socket**. The main task of the **Agent** is to be alert of what he sees, or hears, and to give the appropriate response when one of these events happens. Even if the agent is managing socket connections and parallel tasks, it has not to worry about this matters, because this is continuously handled by separated threads. The **Tasks Handler** is a thread that is managing the stacked tasks performed or to be performed by the **Agent**. This thread is in charge of choosing the tasks that will be triggered in the next time slot. The **Agent Socket** monitors the activity of the socket, this means, is in charge of reading from the socket the incoming data, and writing the outgoing data or feedback data to the **IVA brain**.

3. INTERCONNECTING THE ANIMATION AND BEHAVIOURAL MODULES

As we have already mentioned earlier, the agent's animation in handled by Python scripts (and by the **Agent** class) while behaviour selection and decisions are chosen into the Intelligent Virtual Agent. Both are connected through sockets, and the **Agent Socket** (defined in Python)n is in charge of interconnecting the high level orders coming from the IVA with orders understandable by the **Agent** defined in Python, and vice-versa. We can basically distinguish three kinds of communications:

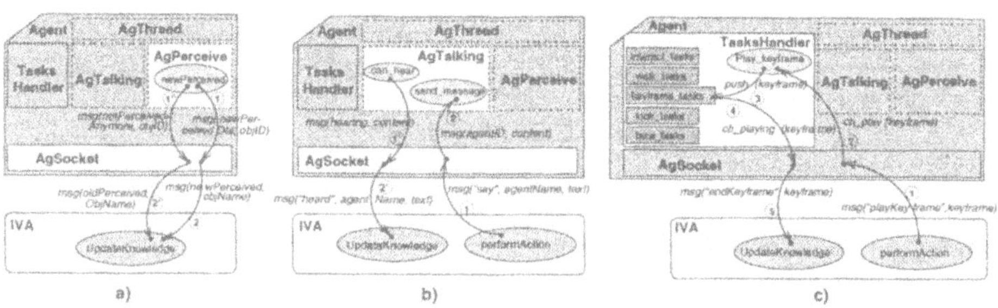

Figure 3. Communication between the Agent Python class and the IVA

1. **Perceiving an object or another agent**: whenever any new object is perceived, the method *newPerceived* inherited from AgPerceive returns *true*, and a message is created for the AgSocket (see *Figure 3a*). This message consists of a short description of what happened, and the ID of the perceived object. The AgSocket receives this message and translates it for the IVA brain, which finaly maps the ID to the corresponding object name. Similarly, the method *newPerceived* is also used to update the objects that are not visible anymore.
2. **Speaking to and hearing another agent**: when someone starts to speak, the method *can-hear* inherited from AgTalking returns *true*, and the **Agent** receives the incoming message. The *is-speaking* and the *end-of-message* messages are ignored, because these ones are just used for synchronisation purposes. The AgSocket again is in charge of extracting the relevant information for the IVA brain, and creates a new message that contains the name of the agent who spoke, and the utterance. The speaking process is a little bit different, because it is the IVA this time which starts the conversation, as presented in *Figure 3b*. The message consists of the action that will take place (in that case, the action *say*), the agent receiver's name, and the text that the agent wants to say. The AgSocket receives this message and generates three new *SpokenMessages*: *is-speaking*, *message-interchange* (which carries the semantic) and *end-of-message* to finish the communication [16].
3. **Walking, looking, playing keyframes or applying face actions**: these tasks are treated in the same way by the **Agent** in Python, specifically by the **Agent's Tasks Handler**. Again, the IVA brain triggers the need of performing one of these tasks, sending a message to the AgSocket, which then activates the corresponding **task callback** associated with the task and push it into its **Tasks Stack**. The **Tasks Handler** keeps checking for the termination callback of all the tasks inside the **Tasks Handler**, and when the termination callback is triggered, a new message is sent to **AgSocket** to reflect the changes into the **Agent's** brain (see *Figure 3c*).

4. THE IVA BRAIN: INTELLIGENT VIRTUAL AGENT

The Intelligent Virtual Agent is based on a BDI architecture (Beliefs, desires and intentions), widely described by Georgeff [18]. This architecture is promising but needs some extensions for achieving our goal: giving to the virtual human the ability to act by itself in a dynamic environment relying on its beliefs, internal states, current state of the surrounded world and assumptions about other agents. It should also allow us to control it in real time [7].

4.1 IVA's components

An IVA has all its knowledge organised into sets, which are distributed according to their functionality (*Figure 4*): the set of *Beliefs*, the set of *Goals*, the set of *Competing Plans*, the set of *Internal states*, the set of *Beliefs About Others*. Based on all its knowledge, the IVA is able to select the correct action to perform, in order to achieve its goal. This process is done by the *Behavioural Engine* which will be explained later in this paper.

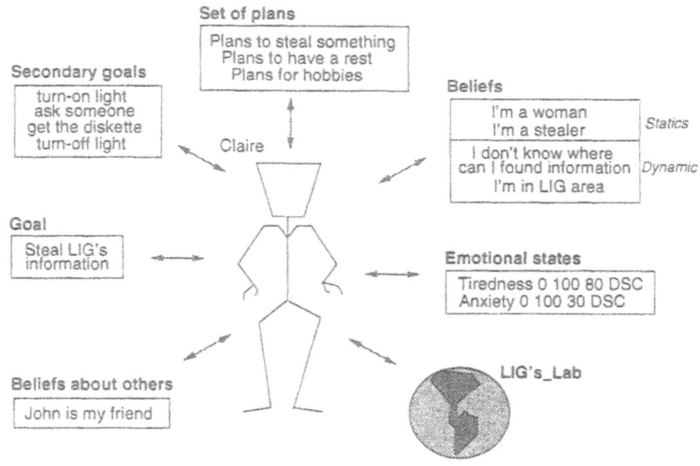

Figure 4. The Intelligent Virtual Agent (IVA)

1. **Beliefs** are a set of statements that the IVA believes to be true. The agent's beliefs are organised to let us simulate *short term memory* by the **Short term beliefs (STB)**, and *everlasting memory* by the **Long term beliefs (LTB)**.
2. IVAs have one main **Goal** and one or several **Subgoals**. The main goal is the objective that the IVA is trying to achieve at a certain moment. During this process, an IVA has to deal with smaller subgoals on which the outcome of the larger one relies on.
3. Internal states: The agent stores a set of internal states representing physiological or psychological variables of the virtual human. Internal state act as stimulus for the agent, i.e. *a high hunger level will stimulate the agent to eat*. An internal state is_i is described as a tuple: (n_i, min_i, max_i,c_i, cat_i), where for any given internal state *i*: n_i is its name, min_i is its minimum accepted value, max_i , the maximum accepted value, c_i

the current value, and cat_i is its category. Internal states are constantly being adjusted, as the simulation evolves and plans are adopted. Changes in the internal state are consequences of: the **autonomous growth or damping** associated with the internal state and the **side-effects** of an active behaviour. We categorise the internal states as ascendant (the higher the level the better), descendants and not categorised.

4. **Competing plans:** An IVA uses a set of competing plans that specified a sequence of actions required to reach its main goal. A competing plan P_i is described as: $P_i = (is_i, pc_i, ef_i)$, where: is_i is a list of internal states to be checked before the plan can be executed. Each of the internal states has an associated valid value or range. pc_i is a list of preconditions which have to be true before the competing plan can be triggered. The preconditions belong either to the agent's beliefs or to the general knowledge stored in the world. ef_i is a list which contains the effects of a plan execution. When a plan is selected, changes at agent or world level will occur (new knowledge will be added and old one will bc deleted). These changes are consequences of the plan's effects.
5. **Beliefs about others:** In our model each IVA is autonomous, and can accept or reject an order coming from the user or from another agent. Each IVA includes a set of Beliefs about others into which it stores the trust levels associated with them. An IVA sees the user as another agent, and depending on the user's category it will accept an order or not. The levels of trust will evolve during the simulation [7], following the Hinde statement: *"Trust, once established in some degree, is often self-reinforcing because individuals have stronger tendencies to confirm their prior beliefs than to disprove them."* [11]. All IVAS contain the name of the other agents and the level of trust associated to them. The value of acceptance for any order coming from a user is handled so that the higher/lower the trust level, the higher/lower the possibility of accepting the order.

4.2 The Behavioural Engine (BE)

The behavioural engine is in charge of updating the internal states of the IVA and selecting its next action. It is composed of some controllers as shown in *Figure 5*. First the *Event Controller* checks in the pending events list for those events that trigger in a specific time slot to be integrated in the IVA's knowledge. Then the *Plan Seeker* sequentially passes the plans to the *Plan Controller* which verifies if the plan will be trigger or not. A plan to be triggered needs to have the suitable internal states levels and to full-fill all the preconditions. The *State Controller* checks the internal states levels and if all of them have the appropriate values it will give the control to the

Precondition Controller, otherwise the *Plan Seeker* will search for the next plan to evaluate. The *Precondition Controller* searches if all the preconditions are full-filled from its local knowledge, or from the external knowledge (*World Agent*). If the *Precondition Controller* agrees with all the preconditions the *Effects Performer* will be called, in order to perform all the necessaries updates inside the IVA or in the *World Agent*, and send the selected action (if there is one) to the *Virtual Human*.

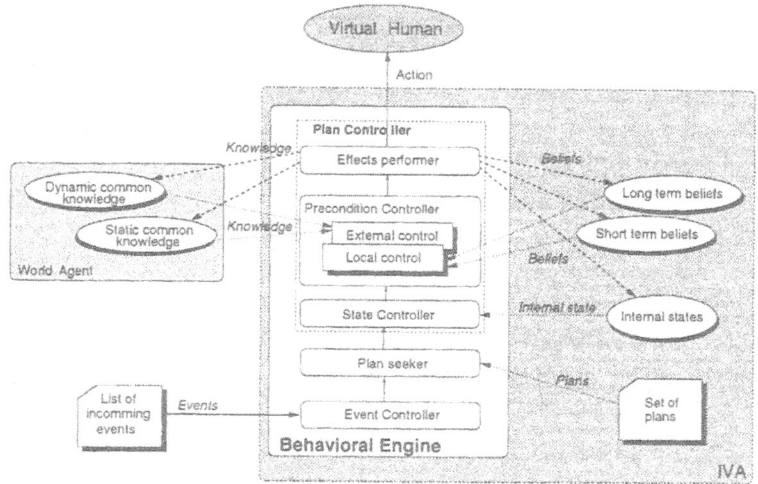

Figure 5. Behavioural Engine

5. CONCLUSION

We have presented in this paper various requirements to go toward life-like agents: our system has a multi-layered and distributed multi-languages architecture. We used **Tasks** to combine primary actions altogether, and we have presented a model for simulating verbal communication. The high level IVA brain, independent of graphics specification, is able to intelligently interact with a lower level module to create one single unit: the *Agent*.

REFERENCE

[1] P. Baerlocher and R. Boulic. Task priority formulations for the kinematic control of highly redundant articulated structures. In *IEEE IROS' 98*, pages 323–329, 1998.

[2] R. Bindiganavale, W. Schuler, Allbeck J., Badler N., Joshi A., and M. Palmer. Dynamically altering agent behaviors using natural language instructions. In *Autonomous Agents 2000 Proceedings*, 2000.

[3] Grady Booch, Ivar Jacobson, James Rumbaugh, and Jim Rumbaugh. *The Unified Modeling Language User Guide.* Addison-Wesley, 1998.

[4] C. Bordeux R. Boulic and D. Thalmann. An efficient and flexible perception pipeline for autonomous agents. In *Proceedings of Eurographics' 99,*.

[5] R. Boulic, P. Becheiraz, L. Emering, and D. Thalmann. Integration of motion control techniques for virtual human and avatar real-time animation. *ACM Symposium on Virtual Reality Software and Technology*, September 1997.

[6] R. Brooks. A robust layered control system for a modbile robot. *IEEE Journal of Robotics and Automation RA-2*, 1986.

[7] A. Caicedo and D. Thalmann. Virtual humanoids: let them be autonomous without losing control. In *The Fourth International Conference on Computer Graphics and Artificial Intelligence*, 2000.

[8] J. Cassell, C. Pelachaud, N. Badler, M. Steedman, B. Achorn, T. Bechet, B. Douville, S. Prevost, and M. Stone. Animated conversation: Rule-based generation of facial expression gesture and spoken intonation for multiple.*Proceedings of SIGGRAPH 94*

[9] Thomas A. Funkhouser, Patrick Min, and Ingrid Carlbom. Real-time acoustic modeling for distributed virtual environments. *Proceedings of SIGGRAPH 99*

[10] J. P. Granieri, W. Becket, B. D. Reich, J. Crabtree, and N. L. Badler. Behavioral control for real-time simulated human agents. *1995 Symposium on Interactive 3D Graphics*

[11] Robert Hinde and Jo Groebel. Cooperation and prosocial behaviour. Cambridge University Press, 1991.

[12] M. Kallmann and D. Thalmann. A behavioral interface to simulate agent-object interactions in real-time. In IEEE Computer Society Press, editor, *Proceedings of Computer Animation 99*, pages 138–146, 1999.

[13] P. Maes. How to do the right thing. *Connection Science Journal*, 1:291–323, Dec 1989.

[14] M. Minsky. *The society of mind.* Simon and Schuster, 1988.

[15] Karen Moltenbrey. All the right moves. *Computer Graphics Word*, 22, October 1999.

[16] J.-S. Monzani and D. Thalmann. Verbal communication: Using approximate sound propagation. In *Autonomous Agents'2000 Conference Proceedings*, 2000.

[17] Ken Perlin and Athomas Goldberg. Improv: A system for scripting interactive actors in virtual worlds. *Proceedings of SIGGRAPH 96*, pages 205–216, August 1996.

[18] A. S. Rao and M. P. Georgeff. Modeling rational agents withing a bdi-architecture. *Proceedings of the Third International Conference on Principles of Knowledge Representation and Reasoning.* Morgan Kaufmann, 1991.

[19] Dan Teven. Virtools' NeMo. *Game Developer Magazine*, September 1999.

[20] N. Tinbergen. *The study of Instinc.* Oxford University Press, 1951.

[21] M. Travers. *Agar: An animal construction kit.* PhD thesis, The Media Lab, MIT, 1988.

DESIGN ISSUES FOR CONVERSATIONAL USER INTERFACES: ANIMATING AND CONTROLLING 3D FACES

W. Müller[1], U. Spierling[2], M. Alexa[1], I. Iurgel[2]
[1] *Technische Universität Darmstadt, Interactive Graphics Systems Group, Darmstadt, Germany*
[2] *ZGDV Computer Graphics Center, Darmstadt, Germany*

Keywords: Avatars, anthropomorphic conversational interfaces, facial animation, behavioral animation.

Abstract: Software agents and assistants, together with their adequate visual representations, lead to so-called social user interfaces, incorporating natural language interaction, context awareness and anthropomorphic avatars. Today's challenge is to build a suitable visualization architecture for anthropomorphic conversational user interfaces, and to design believable and appropriate face-to-face interactions, including human attributes, such as emotions. An integrated approach to these tasks is presented.

1. INTRODUCTION

With the end of the 20th century, the vision of a new human-computer interaction paradigm of "assistance" seemed destined to overtake the as yet still valid paradigm of the "computer as a tool" (Maes 94). However, recent discussions in research and development for human-computer interaction have lead to the following agreements:

1. The introduction of task delegation to software assistants will not replace, but complement, the direct manipulation of software tools. (Maes et. al. 97)

2. The delegation of tasks to an assistance software and their monitoring claims for special and social interfaces, which resemble a human-human relationship rather than tool usage. (Nass et. al. 94)
3. Consequently, so-called conversational interfaces evolve, not only relying on natural speech interaction, but also on non-verbal behavior, such as facial expressions and gestures. (Cassell et. al. 00)

Especially in the home area, a convergence between TV, VCR, and household appliances with desktop computer and web interfaces is apparent. In this context, a unique approach is undertaken to suggest and evaluate prototypes and solutions for face-to-face interaction with virtual characters (here called “user interface agents” or "avatars") integrated in traditional interaction concepts. This approach is interdisciplinary and addresses the following challenges:

1. Human factors research towards an academic basis for non-verbal communication: Evaluation of human-human interaction as a starting point for the design and generation of human-computer interaction.
2. Technological platform for animated behavior: A lean behavior animation platform with emphasis on real-time interaction and flexibility.
3. Design for appropriate usage and acceptance: Integrated design of face-to-face scenarios regarding human and technical requirements, as well as context of interfaces and contents.

In this contribution, we present current results of our ongoing projects with respect to the last two points, technology and design.

2. STATE OF THE ART

In the area of facial animation, the first synthetic faces based on a parametric model were created by Parke in 1972 (Parke 72). Psychological studies from Ekman and Friesen (Ekman and Friesen 69) built the bases for most of today's approaches, allowing for a control on a higher level of abstraction. Their Facial Action Coding System (FACS) describes the facial muscle activities based on 58 action units. A current adaptation of this work can be found in Facial Animation Parameters (FAPs) in MPEG-4 (Ostermann 98). A good overview of FACS and FACS-based approaches can be found in (Parke 98). Though MPEG-4 also targets small and medium platforms, FAPs implementations are usually relatively complex and real-time performance can hardly be achieved. An alternative approach based on a modification of standard morph targets has currently been introduced by Alexa et al (Alexa et. al. 00), providing good performance, scalability, and better control during authoring.

There have been several approaches to control the emotional appearance of a synthetic character. Bates (Bates 94) introduced virtual characters with their own personalities based on individual goals and emotions. Similarly, Perlin and Goldberg (Perlin and Goldberg 96) developed an interactive animation system with hierarchical goal descriptions and artificial personalities for automated choreography. André et al (André et. al. 98) worked on a virtual presenter with internal models of emotion. However, all these approaches target the control of a virtual character's general behavior and have not yet proven to provide sufficient modeling for believable, complex facial expressions. Rule-based models have been introduced for this purpose by Cassell and Pelachaud (Cassell et. al. 94). Another example in this context is the work of Beskow (Beskow 95). Our work described in this paper borrows from Cassell and Pelachaud. However, we are using greatly simplified models due to a different application context. Here, a sound and believable appearance on small systems is a sufficient criterion for success.

3. AVATAR ANIMATION PLATFORM

We target at a UI control module appropriate for rendering animated characters with speech output and lip sync on standard PC platforms while communicating over low bandwidth connections. These technological constraints, as well as considerations for the future design of successful conversations, have been considered for the realization of a new and flexible Avatar Platform (see Figure 1):

The overall human-machine dialogue is controlled by a preceding dialogue manager, which manages all user-interface components and modalities. It also decides on explicit sentences to be spoken.

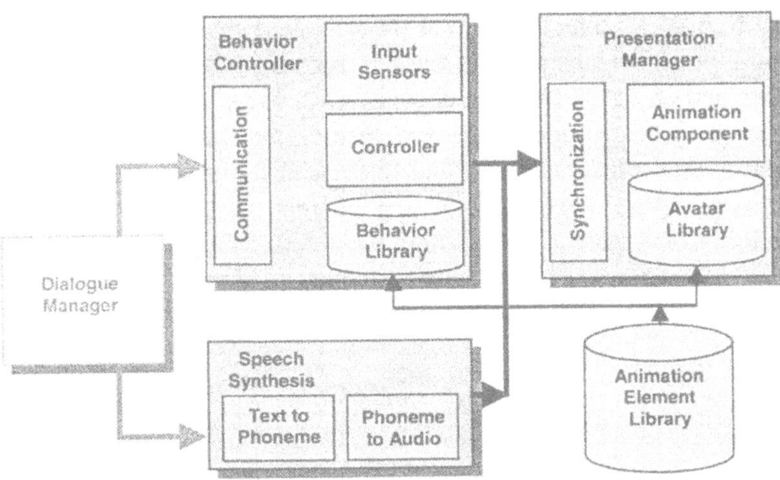

Figure 1: *Architecture of the Avatar Animation Platform (with preceding Dialogue Manager)*

3.1 PRESENTATION MANAGER

This module provides the functionality to present animated artificial characters, to perform facial animations, and to achieve lip sync. Animated characters are represented in a structure conforming to H-ANIM (H-ANIM 99). H-ANIM joints are augmented by a facial structure based on Morph Targets (see Figure 2) and efficiently realized as a Morph Node (Alexa et. al. 00). Hereby, a much broader range of facial expressions can be provided than in known real-time systems, while the parametrization of the face is kept simple.

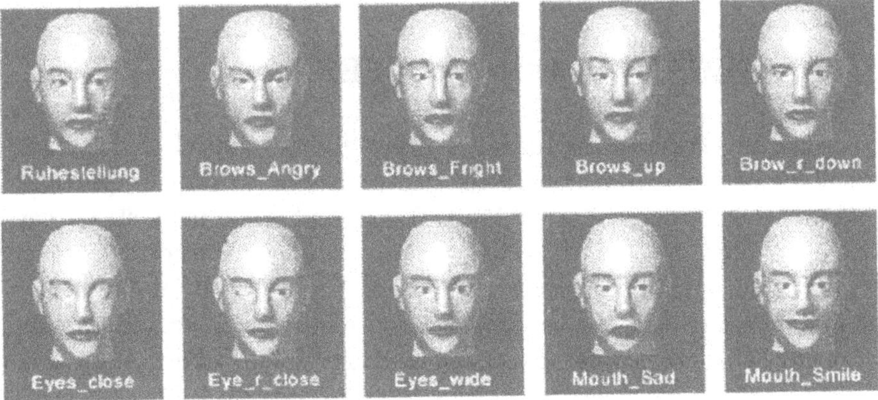

Figure 2: *Example set for basic morph targets*

Key-frames defining the state of the animated character consist of only a small number of values and playback is possible even over low-bandwidth networks and on small, portable devices. Moreover, facial animations can be easily mapped to different even very cartoon-like faces. Figure 3 depicts a different avatar representation, able to present the same behaviors, though partly with different expressions (e.g., using ear movements to express certain emotional states). Even within the same topology of a generic avatar face the expression range could be extended to morph targets that lead to different character representations (see Figure 4).

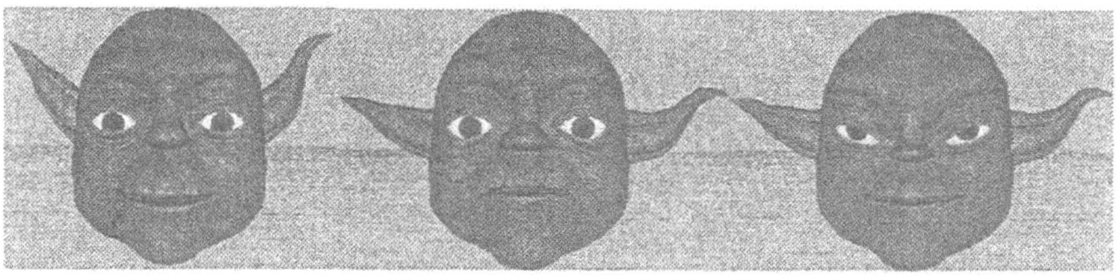

Figure 3: *Alternative avatar representation based on a Yoda geometry (Platinum 2000)*

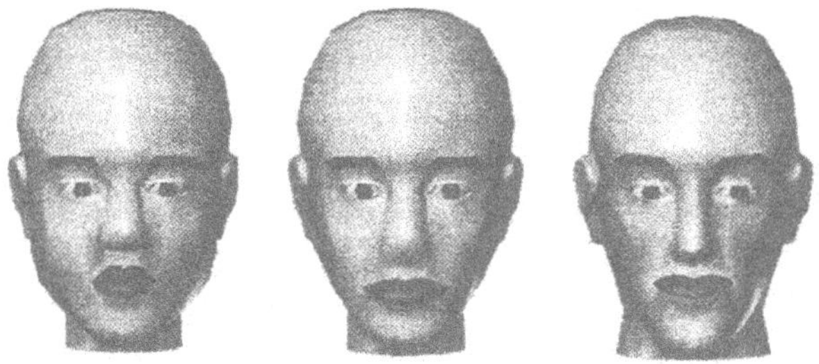

Figure 4: *Alternative character representations (baby, young, elder) within consistent topology*

3.2 BEHAVIOR CONTROLLER

While the Presentation Manager allows for the control of the avatar on the fundamental geometric levels, the Behavior Controller provides an interface on a more abstract level. Tasks and even motivations can be specified and the corresponding actions are performed automatically. Examples of such actions are gestures and movements of the avatar. In addition, behavior patterns for specific motivations or moods can be activated. This corresponds to a rule-based (possibly stochastic) activation of behavior elements. Applications for this are simple Avatar actions (e.g. accidental looking around or smiling) to avoid repetitive behavior. Another possible application is to provide emotional expressions to emphasize system states, such as a puzzled look in case of an unexpected user input.

As base behaviors, we provide emotional states corresponding to the human universal prototype emotions, which are: fear, happiness, sadness, surprise, anger, disgust (Ekman and Friesen 69), and embarrassment (Castelfranchi and Poggi 90). Typically, the first four of these emotions are more relevant for our application field, since user interface agents tend to be polite.

The Avatar Platform is controlled by the dialogue manager, which is responsible for managing the multimodal and multimedia dialogue with the user. The application context is provided by the assistance functionality behind the dialogue manager.

3.3 SPEECH SYNTHESIS

In order to achieve a realistic appearance, an important requirement for the Avatar is a realistic synchronization of speech output with lip sync motions, facial expressions, gestures, and head movements. Since the dialogue with the user is not known in advance, prerecorded animation sequences with lip and facial animation cannot serve as a solution. Instead, text segments provided by the dialogue manager have to be converted automatically by a text-to-speech (TTS) engine. The speech synthesis system used is expected to generate phoneme information with appropriate timing information, which will be mapped to corresponding visemes and facial animation. This concept offers several advantages:

- Lip sync is realized automatically assuming that speech synthesis works in real time.
- Interactive applications with speech generation during and based on the interaction are possible.
- It is easy to implement a transparent system providing speech synthesis for different languages.
- New developments in the area of speech synthesis systems are readily usable. Even new features of such systems appear to be easy to include.

Our concept is based on a Hadifix-based text-to-phoneme conversion (Portele 97, Portele 96) and MBROLA (MBROLA 99). Here, phonemes are communicated using the international standard SAMPA. The mapping to visemes or sequences of visemes is based on timing and frequency information available in SAMPA.

In addition, heuristics are used to generate non-verbal facial expressions from phoneme information. Similar to (Poggi and Pelachaud 2000), we animated the eyebrows, eyelids, eye movement, and head movement based on typical structures in the phoneme stream. The rules applied include:

- Tone pitch attendance: In human communication, a tone pitch increase is usually connected with a raising of the eyebrows. The eyebrows are raised if the tone pitch exceeds a specified level by an amount dependent on the tone pitch.
- Semantic accentuation: When the tone pitch increases over a longer time frame, we assume an accentuation in the spoken sentence. The animation is accentuated by an raising of the eyebrows and a nod with the head. In addition, we direct the gaze of the avatar towards the user.
- Pause attendance: A longer pause between some words or sentences is accompanied by the avatar closing its eyes.
- Speech Rhythm attendance: We achieved good results by not blinking completely at random, but in coordination with the duration of a long vowel and of the following phoneme. This seems to support accordance to speech rhythm.
- Turn signal support: After finishing a speech act, we automatically supply some non-verbal behavior to signal a switch in the speaker role, that is, the user may interact with the system now. Here, we again supply a nod of the head. As a default, we accompany this nodding with a smile.

3.4 PSYCHOLOGICAL COHERENCE

An additional module ensures that the facial display will always appear to be psychologically coherent, giving the impression of the avatar undergoing psychological processes. The coherence module is derived from psychological literature, but all dependencies are simplified and adapted to the avatar's function of assistance (e.g. Smith and Lazarus 90, Ekman and Friesen 69, Kemper 84). The avatar is not an agent that makes choices on its own, but it does show considerable autonomy in the ways commands are displayed (comparable to IMPROV, Perlin and Goldberg 96). Arousal and mood are two important parameters governing the display of emotions.

Our goal is a fully parametrizable set of rules, supplemented by databases of idiosyncratic facial expressions, so that many different "actors" can easily be defined, each one interpreting the same directions according to its "personality". For example, an avatar that reads news would show almost no arousal or mood changes, while an assistant that is part of the extended family should show deep concern for problems. An assistant for the elderly will always be serene, while another for children will never show aggression.

3.5 IMPLEMENTATION

The implementation has to fulfill the following requirements:

- **Short response time.** The delay between request and display of the processed animation of a single sentence should be less than a second.
- **Expressive dynamics.** Mainly for movements of the head, varieties of acceleration are important for an appealing impression.
- **Resolution of conflicts in rules.** Conflicts between rules are common, e.g. between a rule to blink and a rule to open the eyes widely.
- **Continuous behavior.** Even if the avatar is not displaying commands of the dialogue manager, it should continuously show some simple behavior patterns – yawning, for instance.

We met these requirements by decomposing the module that determines morph weights and transformations. The resulting bundle of concurrent animations is coordinated by a blackboard and a multiplexer. Figure 5 depicts the architecture.

We use two distinct types of animations to set weights and positions:

- Computing a key frame sequence in advance. For example, expensive prosody-dependent animation parts are all preprocessed and stored as key frames.
- A real time animation, which does only a minimum of preprocessing and relies on a finite state machine to determine in real time weights or transforms. Eye blinks, for example, are produced this way.

Thus, the first three requirements mentioned above are met. Continuous behavior is assured by the generation of specific animations in the background.

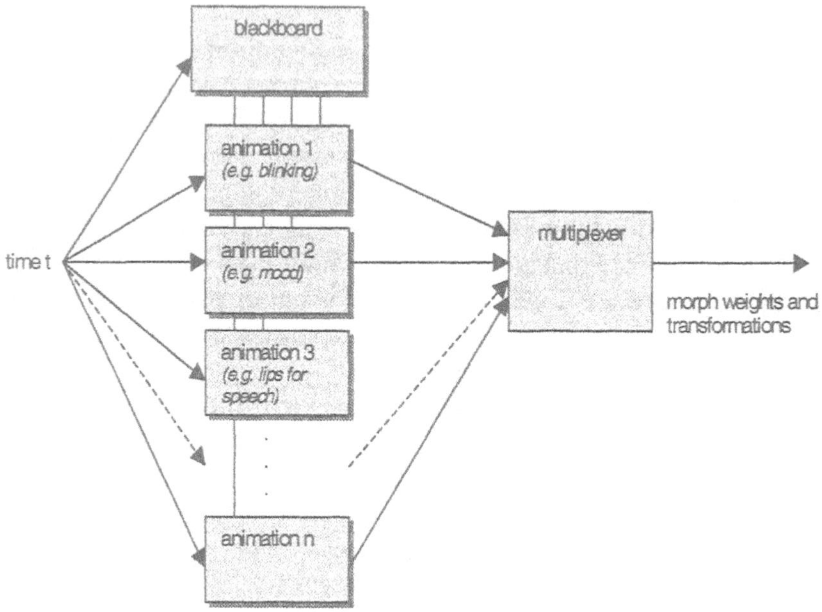

Figure 5: *Determination of morph weights and transforms by a coordinated bundle of animations*

4. FACIAL EXPRESSIONS FOR CONVERSATIONAL INTERFACES

The avatar platform is conceived as part of the rendering pipeline in the multimodal system and covers several anthropomorphic output modalities. User interface designers of the future must utilize these possibilities in an integrated way along with traditional output media such as graphics (Spierling 2000).

Up to now, there have been no known user interface design tools or common methods that allow the integrated design of anthropomorphic interfaces, but input can be taken from several existing concepts, such as UI design, character design, 3D animation, TV show design, and film grammar. The key aspects are:

- Believable animation of the user interface agent, making use of an autonomous behavior engine: creating a character, assigning characterized behavior and a role of assistance, animation and dialogue design.

- Integration of the avatar into context with other interface elements: giving stage directions for screen layout, and synchronizing camera and screen elements in time.

It is to be expected that with regard to converging systems, not only rules of building interfaces, but also influences from the realms of entertainment and storytelling will shape the future platform. The challenge is to provide authoring possibilities on top of the rather autonomously working user interface agent software. The separation of the geometry database and the behavioral animation library is the key concept for our solution.

One goal, for example, is to allow an intuitive scripting of avatar behavior by interface designers, comparable to stage directions. Stage directions tell an actor what to do, but give certain degrees of freedom to the performer. This can be done on various levels of abstraction, from a precise instruction up to a more improvising level. In our system, this is reflected by four hierarchical layers (direct, feature, task, motivation), that can be employed for different scenarios.

Facial expressions and the expression of emotions, as well as distinct character, are important aspects along with believable storytelling. Measurement of effectiveness and efficiency of conversational user interfaces has to be expanded to include a measurement of acceptance. The function and semantics of single features in facial expressions have not yet been analyzed or evaluated by human factors research and the effort is expected to be enormous. At this point, a potential risk of non-acceptance is obvious, just as with every other media that includes emotional attributes.

Our proposed solution is to give responsibility not exclusively to the engine, but to writers and storytellers, by opening the system for entertainment designers. Instead of completely building upon research results, designers can make suggestions based on intuition, or on experience in traditional animation (Thomas and Johnson 81) and experimental problem solving strategies. Figure 6 shows an environment for experiments.

5. APPLICATION EXAMPLE

We used the system in various test scenarios. One application of the Avatar Platform is a Virtual News Reader. Here, a web-based news service is polled and new messages are presented by the Avatar. In addition, the Avatar's emotional behavior is based on the content of the news message. For this, the news text is scanned for keywords stored in a database, and corresponding emotional expressions are automatically selected.

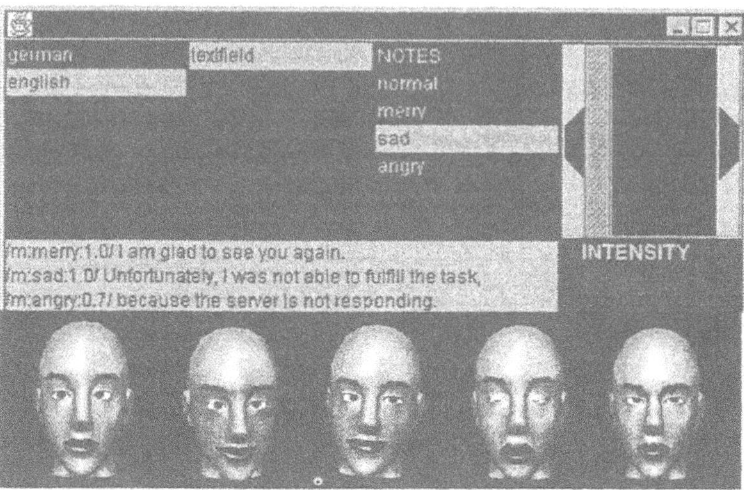

Figure 6: *Animation sequence automatically produced based on speech information*

6. CONCLUSIONS

In this paper, we presented the conception and realization of a presentation engine for conversational user interface agents. This software engine distinguishes itself from other solutions in using a novel approach for the representation and animation of facial expressions, enabling real-time lip-sync animations even on small machines. Furthermore, the system allows for an easy exchange of the animated face during runtime.

Based on a behavior controller and a library with animation elements and animation rules, the Avatar can be easily controlled at a task level and by making use of the motivation layer. Very complex animations can already be achieved automatically just from the phonetic information of speech output employing psychological rules of communication.

The Avatar Platform has been applied successfully to realize a Virtual News Reader. For broader application in more complex scenarios, however, usability studies and a better understanding of human communication rules and the use of non-verbal cues are needed.

7. ACKNOWLEDGEMENTS

This work has been partially funded by the German "Bundesministerium für Bildung und Forschung," BMB+F through the Focus Project EMBASSI (BMB+F-No. FKZ 01 IL 904 U8) [http://www.embassi.de]).

8. REFERENCES

Alexa, M., Behr, J., and Müller, W.: The Morph Node. In: Proc. Web3d/VRML 2000, Monterey, CA., 2000, pp. 29-34.

André, E., Rist, T., and Müller, J.: Integrating Reactive and Scripted Behaviours in a Life-Like Presentation Agent. Proc. 2nd Int. Conf. on Autonomous Agents '98, 1998, pp. 261-268.

Bates, J.: The Role of Emotion in Believable Agents. Communication of the ACM, Vol. 37, No. 7, 1994, pp. 122-125.

Beskow, J.: Rule-based Visual Speech Synthesis. in: Proc. of Eurospeech '95, Madrid, 1995

Castelfranchi, C. and Poggi, I.: Blushing as a discourse: Was Darwin wrong? in: Crozier, R. (ed.), Shyness and Embarrassment: Perspectives from Social Psychology, 1990, pp. 230-251, Cambridge Univ. Press, Cambridge, MA.

Cassell, J., Pelachaud, C., Badler, N.I., Steedman, M., Achorn, B., Beckett, T., Douville, B., Prevost, S., and Stone, M.: Animated conversation: rule-based generation of facial display, gesture and spoken intonation for multiple conversational agents. Computer Graphics (Proc. SIGGRAPH '94), 28 (4), 1994, pp. 413-420.

Cassell, J., Sullivan, J., Prevost, S., and Churchill, E. (eds.): Embodied Conversational Agents. MIT Press, Cambridge, MA, 2000.

Ekman, P. and Friesen, W.: The repertoire of nonverbal behavior: Categories, origins, usage, and coding. Semiotica 1, 1969.

Humanoid Animation Working Group (H-ANIM): http:// ece.uwaterloo.ca:80/~h-anim/ 1999.

Kemper, T. D.: Power, Status, and Emotions: A Sociological Contribution to a Psychophysiological Domain. in: K. Sherer and P. Ekman (eds.), Approaches to Emotion, Hillsdale 1984, pp. 369-383.

Maes, Pattie: Agents that Reduce Work and Information Overload. Communications of the ACM Vol.7/7, July 1994.

Maes, Pattie, Shneiderman, Ben, and Miller, Jim (Mod.): Intelligent Software Agents vs. User-Controlled Direct Manipulation: A Debate. Panel Description, ACM CHI '97, 1997

The MBROLA Project: Towards a Freely Available Multilingual Synthesizer. http://tcts.fpms.ac.be/synthesis/mbrola.html, 1999

Nass C., Steuer J., and Tauber, E.: Computers are Social Actors. Proceedings of ACM CHI '94, Boston. MA, 1994.

Ostermann, J.: Animation of Synthetic Faces in MPEG-4. Computer Animation, Philadelphia, Pennsylvania, June 1998, pp. 49-51.

Parke, Frederic I., and Waters, Keith: Computer Facial Animation. 1998.

Perlin, Ken and Goldberg, Athomas: Improv: A system for scripting interactive actors in virtual worlds. Proc. SIGGRAPH '96, 1996, pp. 205-216, http://www.mrl.nyu.edu/improv/

Platinum Multimedia Pictures Inc.: 3dCafe, http://www.3dcafe.com/asp/anatomy.asp, 2000

Poggi, Isabella and Pelachaud, Catherine: Performative Facial Expressions in Animated Faces. in: Cassell et al (ed.): Embodied Conversational Agents, MIT Press, Cambridge, 2000.

Portele, Thomas: Hadifix. http://www.ikp.uni-bonn.de/~tpo/Hadifix.html, 1996.

Portele, Thomas: Txt2pho - German TTS front end for the MBROLA synthesizer. http://tcts.fpms.ac.be/synthesis/, 1997.

Smith, C.A., & Lazarus, R.S.: Emotion and Adaptation. In: Pervin (ed.), Handbook of Personality: theory & research, Guilford Press, NY, 1990, pp. 609-637.

Spierling, U.: Conversational Integration of Multimedia and Multimodal Interaction. Development Consortium "Beyond the Desktop", Ext. Abst. of ACM CHI 2000, Den Haag.

Thomas, F. and Johnson, O.: The Illusion of Life. New York Abbeville Press, 1981.

CONSTRUCTING VIRTUAL HUMAN LIFE SIMULATIONS

Marcelo Kallmann, Etienne de Sevin and Daniel Thalmann
Swiss Federal Institute of Technology (EPFL), Computer Graphics Lab (LIG), CH-1015 Lausanne, Switzerland.

Keywords Artificial Life, Agents, Virtual Humans, Virtual Environments, Behavioral Animation, Object Interaction, Python.

Abstract This paper describes an approach to construct interactive virtual environments, which are suitable for the development of artificial virtual human life simulations. Our main goal is to have virtual human actors living and working autonomously in virtual environments. In our approach, virtual actors have their own motivations and needs, and by sensing and exploring their environment, an action selection mechanism is able to determine the suitable actions to take. Such actions often involve interaction with the environment and thus a specific technique to define actor-object interactions is used, where pre-defined interaction plans are put inside interactive objects, and just selected during the simulation. We explain in this paper the steps taken in order to construct and animate such environments, and we also present a test simulation example.

1. INTRODUCTION

Virtual human simulations are becoming each time more popular. Many systems are available targeting several domains, as: autonomous agents, human factors analysis, training, education, virtual prototyping, simulation-based design, and entertainment. As an example, an application to train equipment usage using virtual humans is presented by Johnson et al [1].

Simulations with autonomous virtual humans, or *actors*, may use different techniques for their behavioral programming. Common approaches are based on scripts [2] and hierarchical finite state machines [3].

Such techniques are powerful and may serve to define a large range of behaviors. However, achieving complex and emergent autonomous behaviors will always be a difficult and challenging task.

We show in this paper how we construct interactive virtual environments, which are suitable for autonomous actors simulations. Our main goal is to have actors living and working autonomously in virtual environments, according to their own motivations and needs.

We focus on common-life situations, where the actor senses and explores his environment, and following an action selection mechanism, determines the suitable actions to take. Actions often involve object interaction, and so a specific technique to model actor-object interactions is used, following the *smart object* approach [4]. Smart objects contain interactivity information based on pre-defined interaction plans, which are defined during modeling phase.

We construct our interactive virtual environment using the *Agents Common Environment* (ACE) system [13], which provides the basic requirements for the implementation of autonomous actors simulations:

- Load and position different actors and smart objects.

- Apply an action to an actor, as: walking [7], inverse kinematics [10], facial expressions, etc. Actions can be triggered in parallel and are correctly blended, according to given priorities, by a specific internal synchronization module [8].

- Trigger a smart object interaction with an actor. Each smart object keeps a list of its available interactions, which depends on the object internal state. Each interaction is described by simple plans that are pre-defined with the use of a specific graphical user interface application called *somod*. These plans describe the correct sequence of actions and objects movements required to accomplish an interaction.

- Query *pipelines of perception* [9] for a given virtual human. Such pipelines can be configured in order to simulate, for example, a synthetic vision. In this case, the perception query will return a list with all objects perceived inside the specified range and field of view. As an example, figure 1 shows a map constructed from the results of the perception information received by an agent.

We have thus implemented in Python a motivational action selection model [11], which permits to use internal actor motivations and environment information in order to select which actions and object interactions to take.

Following this architecture, the action selection algorithm works on a very high level layer, and ACE guarantees the smooth control of low-level motions, as walking and interacting with objects.

In the following sections we show how we have built smart objects with coherent behavioral information, and how they are coherently linked to our action selection model.

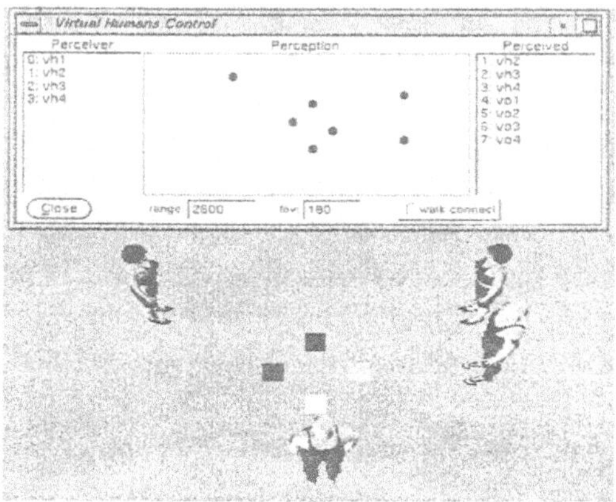

Figure 1. Perception map of the lowest agent in the image. In this example, a range of 2.6 meters and a field of view of 180 is used. The darker points in the map represent the positions of each perceived agent and object.

2. THE ACTION SELECTION MODEL

We have implemented in Python a motivational model for the action selection problem specifically for virtual human actors. This model is composed of a free flow hierarchy [11], associated to a hierarchical classifier system [12]. Such a model permits to take into account different types of motivations and also information coming from the environment perception. During the propagation of the activity in the hierarchy, no choices are made before the lowest level in the hierarchy represented by the actions.

Motivations correspond to a "subjective evaluation" of internal variables. When such variables pass over a threshold, the motivation becomes stronger. This generates a higher activity being propagated through the hierarchy, and the actions having more influence to reduce the motivation have more chance to be chosen. The system chooses always the most activated action at each iteration.

In another words, the main role of the action selection mechanism is to maintain the internal variables under the thresholds by choosing the correct actions. Actions involving interactions with smarts objects are preferably chosen because they are defined to be directly beneficial for the virtual human. Otherwise, the virtual human is instructed to reach the place where the motivation can be satisfied.

Take as an example the eat motivation depicted in figure 2. The behaviors "go to known location" or "go to a visible food" control the actor displacement to a specific direction, using the low level action of walking. Note also that distinct motivations can control the same action, and in this case their influences are added.

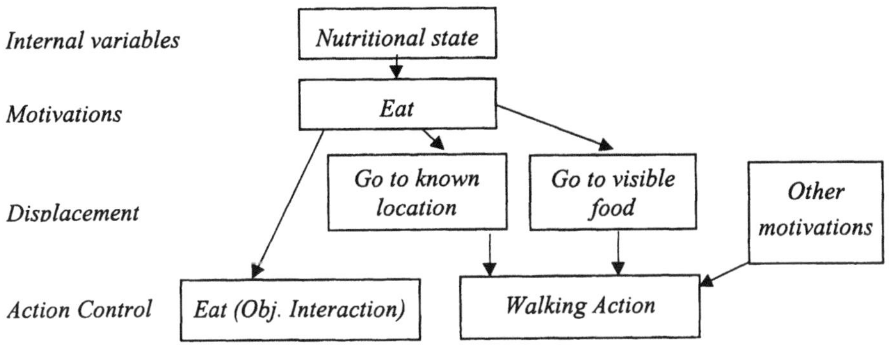

Figure 2. A part of the hierarchical decision graph for the eat motivation, which is evaluated on each iteration.

The simulation being presented in this paper uses five main motivation types: eat, drink, rest, work, and go to the toilet. The action selection mechanism is then fed with the parameters describing the current state of the actor concerning each of these motivations and by flowing inside the hierarchical structure, will correctly trigger the concerned actions.

After an action is selected as a response to satisfy one of the actor's motivations, the state parameter of the motivation is adapted accordingly. For example, after the action of eating is completed, the "hungry" parameter will decrease. In this way, each action needs to be associated to a motivation, closing the loop: motivation parameter evaluation, action selection, action animation, and motivation parameter adjustment.

We have then defined five smart objects directly related to each motivation: a hamburger, a glass of water, a sofa, a desktop computer, and a toilet. The construction of these objects is described in the next section.

3. MODELING OF THE REQUIRED SMART OBJECTS

As already mentioned, each motivation of the actor is directly related to an object interaction. Even for the motivations of resting, eating and drinking, we have created smart objects, containing interactions to eat, drink and rest. The advantage to define such simple interactions with smart objects is that we can easily specify movements of reaching, grasping and taking objects to eat, or, for instance, to control sitting in a sofa. All motions are internally controlled in ACE with inverse kinematics.

Figure 3 shows a snapshot of the modeling phase of some of the used smart objects. It is possible to note the many geometric parameters used by the interaction plans, to initialize and control the actions inside ACE.

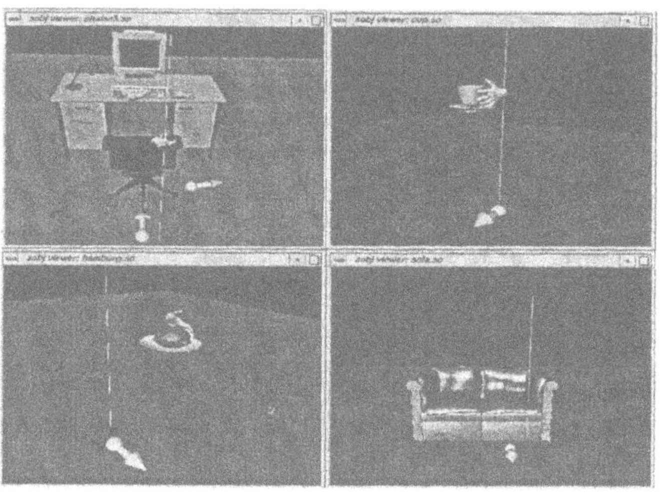

Figure 3. Modeling phase of some used smart objects.

The following table lists each used modeled smart object, with their main interaction capability:

Action	*Smart Object*	*Interaction*
Eat	hamburger	eat
drink	a cup of coffee	drink
resting	sofa	sit
work	computer and desk	sit and type
go to the toilet	toilet	use

Somod is used to create each smart object, in particular to define the behavioral and interaction information. For instance, figure 4 shows the programmed interaction plans used for the toilet model.

From ACE, only the given name of each interaction is seen and available for selection. When smart objects are loaded, the system only exposes the possible interactions of each object, hiding the internal interpretation of the interaction plans from the user, which is transparently executed by ACE.

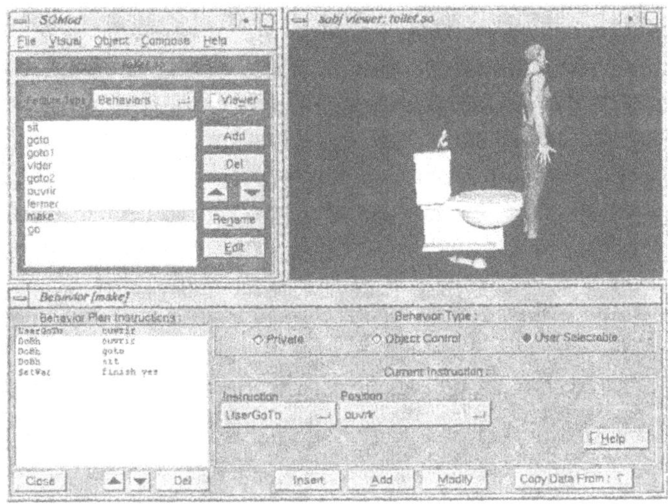

Figure 4. Modeling the interaction plan of a "simplified toilet".

Figure 5 shows the ACE system being used to test the interaction capabilities of the modeled desk. The user can easily select (from Python, or from an user interface) the interaction plans available in the object.

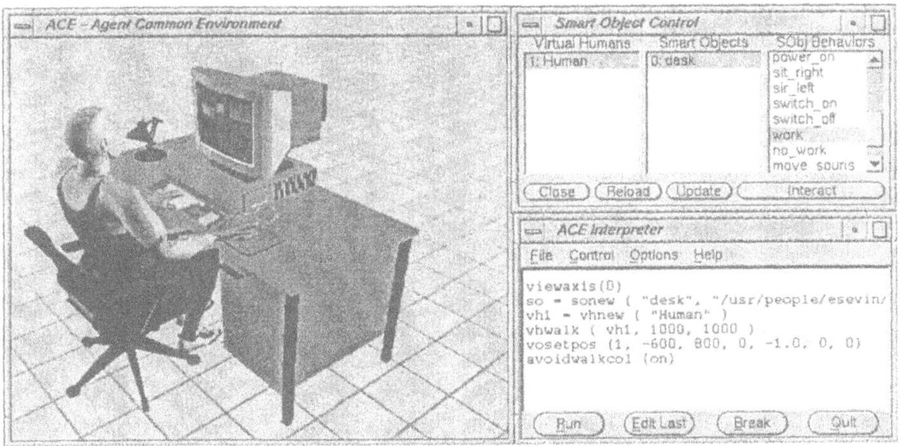

Figure 5. Testing the interaction capabilities of the desk model.

4. OBTAINED SIMULATION IN ACE

The action selection model was entirely developed in Python. The script makes use of two threads: one controlling the graphical refresh of the environment, and one controlling the continuously evaluation of parameters in the hierarchical action selection model.

The obtained simulation shows the virtual human actor living autonomously in the virtual environment, as exemplified in figure 6.

When the simulation starts, the actor has the initial behavior to explore the environment, collecting perceived information regarding the position of useful objects, like the hamburger and the coffee. After some time, the energy level drops, and the action to eat or drink is selected, according to the evaluation of the action suitability to perform. Other parameters regarding working, resting or the need to go to the toilet also change, controlling the actor accordingly.

Figure 6 also shows the variation of the motivational parameters at different levels in the hierarchical selection model.

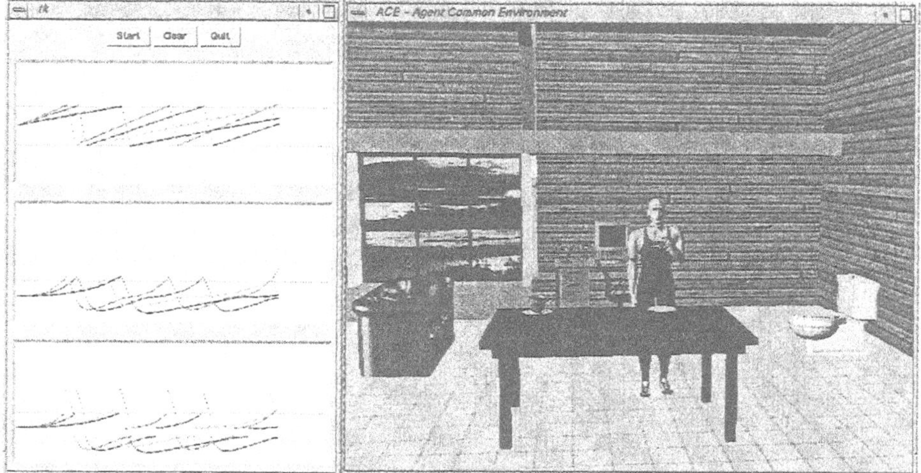

Figure 6. A snapshot of the achieved simulation. The curves on the left show the variation of the internal motivational parameters of the virtual human, at different levels in the hierarchy.

5. CONCLUDING REMARKS

We have shown in this article our approach to construct complex autonomous actors simulations, which is based on three main steps: definition of the required actor-object interactions, modeling of the interactive smart objects, and simulation inside ACE using Python scripts.

The advantages of our approach are mainly due to the modularity achieved, specially regarding the separation of the object interaction information from the behavioral action selection module, which is programmed in a high level scripted language as Python.

Many enhancements are being done to this system, as for instance, the integration of a complete navigation planning module that will enable us to perform tests with simulations in much larger environments, and also with many actors at a same time.

6. ACKNOWLEDGMENTS

This research was supported by the Swiss National Foundation for Scientific Research and by the Brazilian National Council for Scientific and Technologic Development (CNPq).

7. REFERENCES

1. W. L. Johnson, and J. Rickel, "Steve: An Animated Pedagogical Agent for Procedural Training in Virtual Environments", Sigart Bulletin, ACM Press, vol. 8, number 1-4, 16-12, 1997.
2. K. Perlin, and A. Goldberg, "Improv: A System for Scripting Interactive Actors in Virtual Worlds", Proceedings of SIGGRAPH'96, 1996, New Orleans, 115-126.
3. Motivate product information, Motion Factory web address: http://www.motion-factory.com.
4. M. Kallmann and D. Thalmann, "A Behavioral Interface to Simulate Agent-Object Interactions in Real-Time", Proceedings of Computer Animation 99, IEEE Computer Society Press, 1999, Geneva, 108-146.
5. M. Lutz, "Programming Python", Sebastapol, O'Reilly, 1996.
6. N. Badler. "Animation 2000", IEEE Computer Graphics and Applications, January/February 1100, 28-29.
7. R. Boulic, N. Magnenat-Thalmann, and D. Thalmann, "A Global Human Walking Model with Real Time Kinematic Personification", The Visual Computer, 6, 344-358, 1990.
8. R. Boulic, P. Becheiraz, L. Emering, and D. Thalmann, "Integration of Motion Control Techniques for Virtual Human and Avatar Real-Time Animation", In Proceedings of the VRST'97, 111-118, 1997.
9. C. Bordeux, R. Boulic, and D. Thalmann, "An Efficient and Flexible Perception Pipeline for Autonomous Agents", Proceedings of Eurographics '99, Milano, Italy, 23-30.
10. P. Baerlocher, and R. Boulic, "Task Priority Formulations for the Kinematic Control of Highly Redundant Articulated Structures", IEEE IROS'98, Victoria, Canada, 1998.
11. T. Tyrrel, "Defining the Action Selection Problem", Proceedings of the Fourteen Annual Conference on Cognitive Science Society", Lawrence Erlbaum Associates, 1993.
12. J. Y. Donnart, and J. A. Meyer, "Learning Reactive and Planning Rules in a Motivationally Autonomous Animat". IEEE Transactions on Systems, Man, and Cybernetics, part B: Cybernetics, 26(3), 381-395, June, 1996.
13. M. Kallmann, J. Monzani, A. Caicedo, and D. Thalmann, "ACE: A Platform for the Real Time Simulation of Virtual Human Agents", EGCAS'1100 - 11th Eurographics Workshop on Animation and Simulation, Interlaken, Switzerland, 1100.

GPSR Compliance
The European Union's (EU) General Product Safety Regulation (GPSR) is a set of rules that requires consumer products to be safe and our obligations to ensure this.

If you have any concerns about our products, you can contact us on

ProductSafety@springernature.com

In case Publisher is established outside the EU, the EU authorized representative is:

Springer Nature Customer Service Center GmbH
Europaplatz 3
69115 Heidelberg, Germany

ntent.com/pod-product-compliance
Group UK Ltd.
nes, MK11 3LW, UK

02B/543

. 7 5 7 4 9 2 9 8 *